Chronic Pain Management for the Hospitalized Patient

T0323384

Chronic Pain Management for the Hospitalized Patient

EDITED BY

RICHARD W. ROSENQUIST, MD
Chair, Department of Pain Management
Cleveland Clinic
Cleveland, Ohio

DMITRI SOUZDALNITSKI, MD, PHD
Clinical Professor of Anesthesiology
Ohio University, Heritage College of Osteopathic Medicine
Director of Clinical Research
Center for Pain Medicine
Western Reserve Hospital
Cuyahoga Falls, Ohio

RICHARD D. URMAN, MD, MBA
Associate Professor, Harvard Medical School
Department of Anesthesiology, Perioperative, and Pain Medicine
Director of Anesthesia, Center for Perioperative Research
Director of Anesthesia Services, BWH HealthCare Center, Chestnut Hill
Medical Director, Sedation Services for Interventional Procedures
Brigham & Women's Hospital
Boston, Massachusetts

OXFORD
UNIVERSITY PRESS

OXFORD
UNIVERSITY PRESS

Oxford University Press is a department of the University of Oxford. It furthers
the University's objective of excellence in research, scholarship, and education
by publishing worldwide.Oxford is a registered trade mark of Oxford University
Press in the UK and certain other countries.

Published in the United States of America by Oxford University Press
198 Madison Avenue, New York, NY 10016, United States of America.

Library of Congress Cataloging-in-Publication Data
Chronic pain management for the hospitalized patient / edited by Richard W. Rosenquist,
Dmitri Souzdalnitski, Richard D. Urman.
p. ; cm.
Includes bibliographical references.
ISBN 978-0-19-934930-2 (alk. paper)
I. Rosenquist, Richard W., editor.   II. Souzdalnitski, Dmitri, editor.
III. Urman, Richard D., editor.
[DNLM: 1. Chronic Pain.   2. Pain Management.   3. Analgesics—therapeutic use.
4. Inpatients.   5. Pain—drug therapy.   6. Pain Measurement—methods. WL 704.6]
RB127
616'.0472—dc23
2015023131

9 8 7 6 5 4 3 2 1

Printed by Sheridan, USA

Contents

Part II   MANAGEMENT OF CHRONIC PAIN IN SELECTED SETTINGS   83

Part III   ROLE OF NURSING, PHARMACY SPECIALIST, AND OTHER HOSPITAL SERVICES IN MANAGEMENT OF CHRONIC PAIN PATIENTS   189

Preface

A 2011 Institute of Medicine Report *Relieving Pain in America: A Blueprint for Transforming Prevention*, Care, Education and Research, described chronic pain as a significant public health problem. It is estimated to affect more 100 million Americans with an associated cost to society of at least $560–$635 billion annually, which includes healthcare costs ranging from $261–$300 billion annually. The sheer numbers of individuals with chronic pain means that significant numbers of patients with chronic pain will be admitted to the hospital on a daily basis. These patients pose a challenge to the medical system as they are often admitted by physicians with little training or experience in the care of chronic pain patients. Once admitted, physicians and allied health care providers are faced with addressing the primary medical condition requiring evaluation or treatment as well as the chronic pain condition.

Chronic Pain Management for the Hospitalized Patient is the first evidence-based book to address the long standing need for a resource to help physicians manage chronic pain in hospitalized patients. At the present time, almost one in ten patients admitted to the hospital is receiving chronic opioids and it has been estimated that as many as one in four may have a substance use issue. These factors increase the complexity of managing these patients and often lead to under treatment and/or patient dissatisfaction. In some settings, physicians with formal training in pain medicine are available to provide consultation and direct appropriate care. However, in most settings, these resources are not available to guide and improve patient care and reduce uncertainty for the provider regarding the most appropriate way to provide care. This concise, yet exceedingly informative reference book emphasizes the multidisciplinary approach to inpatient pain management.

The textbook addresses pain in six sections:

1. Chronic pain as a disease and the challenges of chronic pain management in the hospital setting
2. Management of chronic pain in selected settings

3. Role of Nursing, Pharmacy Specialist, and Other Hospital Services in Management of Chronic Pain Patients
4. Management of chronic pain in selected patient categories
5. Perioperative chronic pain management
6. Patient Satisfaction and Quality Management of Hospitalized Chronic Pain Patients

The book covers a wide variety of topics related to the inpatient management of acute-on-chronic pain including epidemiology, clinical assessment, pharmacological treatment, interventional therapies, physical therapy and rehabilitation, integrative medicine, acupuncture, and psychological evaluation and treatment. It addresses issues unique to specific hospital units such as the emergency department, intensive care unit, operating rooms, surgical and medical wards, as well as pediatric, labor and delivery, psychiatric, geriatric and palliative care settings. It provides recommendations for the management of acute pain of hospitalized patients with pre-existing chronic pain, opioid dependency, and substance abuse disorders. In addition, it outlines practical strategies and recommendations for the management of pre-existing chronic pain in nursing homes, rehabilitation facilities and prisons. The importance of nurses, pharmacists and other healthcare providers in the successful management of these complex patients is emphasized. Finally, discharge criteria related to pain management and practical tools to improve patient satisfaction are explored in detail.

This book is intended for practicing physicians, physician assistants, nurse practitioners, registered nurses, pharmacists, physical therapists, psychologists, residents, medical students and individuals at any stage of training who aim to provide the most up-do-date, evidence-based care to patients with pain. Hospital administrators will also find this book helpful as it addresses issues of relevance to patient safety and satisfaction.

We would like the thank all of our collaborators for their hard work and their brilliance, our colleagues and trainees for their interest and encouragement, and our families for their patience and indispensable support.

Richard W. Rosenquist, MD
Cleveland Clinic
Dmitri Souzdalnitski, MD, PhD
Western Reserve Hospital
Richard D. Urman, MD, MBA
Brigham and Women's Hospital

Contributors

Syed Ali, MD
Staff Physician
Center for Pain Medicine
Western Reserve Hospital
Cuyahoga Falls, Ohio

Orvil Luis Ayala, MD
Adult and Pediatric Pain Medicine
    Physician
Raritan Valley Pain Medicine
    Associates
New Brunswick, New Jersey

Vijay Babu, MD
Anesthesiology and Pain Medicine
Synovation Medical Group
San Diego, California

**Kimberly Berger, MSN, RN,
ACCNS-AG, CHPN**
Clinical Program Developer
University of Cincinnati
    Medical Center
Cincinnati, Ohio

Adam Canter, MD
Anesthesiology Resident
Department of Anesthesiology
Albert Einstein College of Medicine
Montefiore Medical Center
Bronx, New York

Jianguo Cheng, MD, PhD
Professor of Anesthesiology
Director of Multidisciplinary Pain
    Medicine Fellowship Program
Departments of Pain Management
    and Neurosciences
Cleveland Clinic
Cleveland, Ohio

Jill Mushkat Conomy, PhD
Pain Psychologist
Department of Pain Management
Cleveland Clinic Foundation
Cleveland, Ohio

**David E. Custodio, MD,
MBA, FACEP**
Vice President, Medical Affairs &
    Quality
Summa Akron City and St. Thomas
    Hospitals
Akron, Ohio

Jennifer Drost, DO, MPH
Research Director
Post Acute and Senior Services
Summa Health System
Akron, Ohio

Alexander Feoktistov, MD, PhD
Staff Physician
Director of Clinical Research
Diamond Headache Clinic
Chicago, Illinois

Edward Garay, MD, PhD
Clinical Fellow
Department of Anesthesiology
University of Pittsburgh
    Medical Center
Pittsburgh, Pennsylvania

Karina Gritsenko, MD
Assistant Professor of Anesthesiology
Assistant Professor of Family and
    Social Medicine
Albert Einstein College of Medicine
Montefiore Medical Center
Bronx, New York

Maged Guirguis, MD
Staff Physician
Department of Pain Management
Ochsner Health System
New Orleans, Louisiana

Salim Hayek, MD, PhD
Professor of Anesthesiology
Case Western Reserve University
Chief, Division of Pain Medicine
University Hospitals of Cleveland
Cleveland, Ohio

Richard W. Hohan, PT
Executive Director
Center for Pain Medicine
Western Reserve Hospital
Cuyahoga Falls, Ohio

Yili Huang, MD
Anesthesiology Resident
Yale-New Haven Hospital
New Haven, Connecticut

Danielle Ingram, MD
Palliative Medicine Fellow
Palliative Care and Hospice Services
Summa Health System
Akron, Ohio

Todd Ivan, MD
Director, Consultation Liaison
    Psychiatry Service
Summa Health System
Akron, Ohio
Clinical Associate Professor of
    Psychiatry
Northeast Ohio Medical University
Rootstown, Ohio
Clinical Associate Professor of
    Psychiatry
Ohio University Heritage College of
    Osteopathic Medicine
Athens, Ohio

Hari Kalagara, MD
Anesthesiology Institute
Cleveland Clinic
Cleveland, Ohio

Yury Khelemsky, MD
Assistant Professor of Anesthesiology
Mount Sinai Hospital
New York, New York

Nicole Labor, DO
Staff Physician
Addiction Medicine Program Director
Summa Health System
Akron, Ohio

Daniel J. Leizman, MD
Physical Medicine & Rehabilitation
    Specialist
Staff, Pain Management Department
    Cleveland Clinic
Assistant Professor of Anesthesiology
Cleveland Clinic Lerner College of
    Medicine
Cleveland, Ohio

Imanuel R. Lerman, MD, MS
Clinical Assistant Professor
University of California San Diego
La Jolla, California

Andree Maureen LeRoy, MD
Instructor in Physical Medicine and
    Rehabilitation
Spaulding Rehabilitation Hospital
Harvard Medical School
Boston, Massachusetts

Marisa Lomanto, MD
Assistant Clinical Professor of
    Anesthesiology
Yale School of Medicine
VA Connecticut Healthcare System
West Haven, Connecticut

Michael C. Lubrano, MD, MPH
Resident Physician, Department of
    Anesthesia & Perioperative Care
University of California San Francisco
    (UCSF) Medical Center
San Francisco, California

Susan M. Ludwig, FNP-C
Hospital Clinic
Lahey Clinic
Burlington, Massachusetts

Ankit Maheshwari, MD
Louis Stokes Cleveland VA
    Medical Center
Cleveland, Ohio

Beth H. Minzter, MD
Department of Pain Management
Medical Director, Main Campus
Cleveland Clinic Foundation,
Cleveland, Ohio

**Pamela S. Moore, PharmD,
BCPS, CPE**
Clinical Lead Pharmacist, Pain &
    Palliative Care
Pharmacy Residency Program
    Director, PGY2 Pain &
    Palliative Care
Summa Health System
Akron, Ohio

Stefan C. Muzin, MD
Attending Physician
Beth Israel Deaconess Medical Center
Harvard Medical School
Boston, Massachusetts

Rod Myerscough, PhD
Clinical Psychologist
Summa Health System
Akron, Ohio

Eman Nada, MD, PhD
Resident Physician
University of Arkansas for Medical
    Sciences
Little Rock, Arkansas

Khodadad Namiranian, MD, PhD
Clinical Fellow
Department of Pain Management
Cleveland Clinic
Cleveland, Ohio

Samer N. Narouze, MD, PhD
Clinical Professor of Anesthesiology
    and Pain Management, Ohio
    University
Clinical Professor of Neurological
    Surgery, Ohio State University
Chairman, Center for Pain Medicine
Western Reserve Hospital
Cuyahoga Falls, Ohio

Carmen V. Natale
System Director
Summa Health System
Akron, Ohio

Shahbaz Qavi, MD
Pain Medicine Fellow
Weill Cornell Tri-Institutional Pain
  Fellowship
New York Presbyterian Hospital
Weill Cornell Medical Center
New York, New York

Glenn R. Rech, RPh
Lead Pharmacist, Pain Management
Center for Pain Medicine
Western Reserve Hospital
Cuyahoga Falls, Ohio
Clinical Assistant Professor of
  Pharmacy Practice
Northeast Ohio Medical University
Rootstown, Ohio

Steven Rosenblatt, MD
Section Head, General Surgery
Digestive Disease Institute
Cleveland Clinic
Cleveland, Ohio

Ellen Rosenquist, MD
Assistant Clinical Professor of
  Anesthesiology
Department of Pain Management
Cleveland Clinic Anesthesiology
  Institute
Lerner College of Medicine
Cleveland, Ohio

**Richard Rynaski, LAc, BSEE, MS
Acupuncture, NCCAOM Diplomate**
Acupuncturist
Rockfall, Connecticut

Tim Sable, MD
Pain Management Specialist
Staff, Center for Pain Medicine
Western Reserve Hospital
Cuyahoga Falls, Ohio

Samuel W. Samuel, MD
Associate Fellowship Director
Pain medicine fellowship
Celevland Clinic Foundation
Cleveland, Ohio

Danielle Sarno, MD
Chief Resident, Department of
  Rehabilitation Medicine
New York-Presbyterian/Columbia
  University
Weill Cornell Medical Center
New York, New York

**Kristianne Schultz LAc,
DiplOM, MAcOM**
Integrative Health Practitioner
Allina Health Abbott Northwestern
Allina Health St. Francis Regional
  Medical Center
Penny George Institute for Health and
  Healing
Adjunct Faculty at Northwestern
  Health Sciences University
Minneapolis, Minnesota

**Kristianne Schultz L.Ac.,
MAc.O.M, Dipl.O.M.**
Integrative Health Practitioner, Allina
  Health, Penny George Institute
  for Health and Healing and Saint
  Francis Regional Medical Center
Shakopee, Minnesota

Waleed Shah, MD
Anesthesia and Interventional Pain
    Management
Anesthesia Associates of York
Wellspan York Hospital
York, Pennsylvania

**Harsha Shanthanna, MBBS, MD,
DNB, FIPP, EDRA**
Assistant Professor of Anesthesiology
Michael G. DeGroote School of
    Medicine
McMaster University
Hamilton, Ontario, Canada

Michael P. Smith, MD
Staff Anesthesiologist—Department
    of Anesthesia
Akron City Hospital
Summa Health System
Akron, Ohio

Loran Mounir Soliman, MD
Anesthesiology Institute
Cleveland Clinic
Cleveland, Ohio

Melissa Soltis, MD
Program Director
Palliative Care and Hospice Services
Summa Health System
Akron, Ohio

Denis Snegovskikh, MD
Assistant Professor of Anesthesiology
Associate Director, Obstetrics &
    Gynecology Anesthesiology
Director, Obstetrics & Gynecology
    Fellowship
Yale University School of Medicine
New Haven, Connecticut

Alexandra Szabova, MD
Assistant Professor of Anesthesia
Program Director, Pediatric Pain
    Medicine Fellowship
Cincinnati Children's Hospital
    Medical Center
Cincinnati, Ohio

Pavan Tankha, DO
Assistant Professor of Anesthesiology
Yale School of Medicine
Staff Anesthesiologist, Pain
    Management Clinic
VA Connecticut Healthcare System
West Haven, Connecticut

Kathy Travnicek, MD
Staff Physician
Advanced Pain Management
Madison, Wisconsin

Alparslan Turan, MD
Associate Professor of Anesthesiology
Outcomes Research
Cleveland Clinic
Cleveland, Ohio

Bruce Vrooman, MD
Pain Management
Cleveland Clinic
Cleveland, Ohio

Joseph Walker III, MD
Assistant Professor of Orthopedics
University of Connecticut
Farmington, Connecticut

Dajie Wang, MD
Staff Physician,
Anesthesiology—Pain Management
Jefferson University Hospitals
Philadelphia, Pennsylvania

Haibin Wang, MD, PhD
Assistant Professor
Center for Pain Research
University of Pittsburgh
  Medical Center
Pittsburgh, Pennsylvania

Christine Wierzbowski,
BSN, RN-BC
Unit Manager
Center for Pain Medicine
Western Reserve Hospital
Cuyahoga Falls, Ohio

Jiang Wu, MD
Assistant Professor of
  Anesthesiology and Pain Medicine
University of Washington
  Medical Center
Seattle, Washington

Sherif Zaky, MD, MSc, PhD
Director, Pain Management Service
Firelands Regional Medical Center
Assistant Professor of Anesthesiology
  and Preoperative Medicine
Case Western Reserve University
Cleveland, Ohio

Part I

CHRONIC PAIN AS A DISEASE AND CHALLENGES OF CHRONIC PAIN MANAGEMENT IN HOSPITAL SETTINGS

1

Epidemiology of Chronic Pain and Opioid Use and Challenges of Chronic Pain Management in Hospital Settings

JIANG WU AND JIANGUO CHENG

KEY POINTS

- Chronic pain is one of the most common reasons for seeking medical care in the United States and is a major health problem in both pediatric and adult patient populations.
- It is estimated that up to 35% of adults presenting for surgery, or about 80 million adults worldwide, suffer from chronic pain. A substantial number of these patients use analgesics on a chronic basis.
- Healthcare providers need current, state-of-the-art education to assist them in developing the necessary skills to manage patients with persistent pain in the hospital setting, including skills needed to use opioid medications safely and effectively.

Introduction

By definition, *pain* is "an unpleasant sensory and emotional experience associated actual or potential tissue damage, or describe in terms of such damage." Although there is no universally accepted standard definition for chronic pain, the simplest definition of *chronic pain* is when "pain persists beyond the normal tissue healing time (usually 3 months)."[1]

Until the 1960s, pain was considered an inevitable sensory response to tissue damage. In recent years, however, pain has been considered a highly unpleasant sensation that results from an extraordinarily complex and interactive series of mechanisms integrated at all levels of the neuraxis, from the periphery to higher cortical structures. Although most modulations of central and peripheral nervous systems by acute tissue damage are of short duration, some may persist and lead to chronic pain states.[2] The factors that determine the transition from acute to chronic pain remain to be identified. Because chronic pain often loses its protective role and causes functional impairment and physical and emotional suffering, it is often categorized as a disease state rather than as simply a constellation of symptoms. Chronic pain is often a result of inability of the body to restore its physiological functions to normal homeostatic levels,[2] as evidenced by functionally, anatomically, and neurochemically altered brains[3] and the dynamic and intricate interplay among the nervous, immune, and endocrine systems in patients with chronic pain.[4]

Epidemiology of Chronic Pain

Chronic pain is one of the most common reasons for seeking medical care in the United States and is a major health problem in both pediatric and adult patient populations.[5-7] Pain disorders and chronic pain are commonly reported in the literature from a static or cross-sectional view, with very limited longitudinal data. According to a 2011 Institute of Medicine report, *Relieving Pain in America*, approximately 116 million American adults are burdened with chronic pain.[8]

In children and adolescent patient populations, persistent and recurrent pain is also prevalent, constituting a serious developmental health concern that can interfere significantly with children's daily functioning. The physical, psychiatric, and social impacts of chronic pain can extend into adulthood. Generally, girls experience more pain than boys, and the prevalence rates increase with age. The exception is abdominal pain, which tends to be more prevalent in younger children. The median prevalence rate of headache—the most concerning type of pain among youth—is 23%, while incidence of other types of pain, such as abdominal pain, back pain, musculoskeletal pain, and pain combinations, varies, with median prevalence rates ranging from 11% to 38%.[9]

In adult patient populations the prevalence of chronic pain is more overwhelming. The published prevalence estimates of adult persistent and recurrent pain within the United States vary widely, from 14.6% to 64%, with a median prevalence rate of 30%.[5,10-12] Among those 65 years of age or older, 3 in 5 persons experienced pain that lasted a year or more, with more than 60% of U.S. nursing home residents reporting pain and 17% having substantial daily pain.[7,8] The prevalence of persistent pain only among adult primary care patients was estimated at 22%, ranging from 5 to 33%.[13] Primary chronic pain was most commonly attributed to lower back pain (8.1%), followed by primary osteoarthritis pain (3.9%) and migraine or severe headaches. Headache, common at younger ages (i.e., 18–34 years), rapidly declines in prevalence thereafter. In contrast, the other two pain conditions are either more common with increasing age (e.g., arthritis) or peak at a later age than that for headaches (e.g., back pain).[12]

Despite the wide variance in published prevalence estimates of chronic pain, the results of studies examining sociodemographic factors associated with chronic pain have been generally consistent. Factors correlated with increased prevalence of chronic pain include female sex, increasing age, marital status of divorced or separated, and indicators of lower socioeconomic status, such as education level, employment status, and residence in public housing. Other factors, such as higher body mass index, stress, depression, anxiety, and poor self-assessed health, have also been associated with chronic pain.

Impact of Chronic Pain on Health and Economy

For the millions of Americans who experience persistent pain, the impact on function and quality of life can be profound.[6,7,15] Particularly, chronic non-cancer pain is a very common and disabling condition in the U.S. workforce. It was reported that 13% of the total workforce experienced loss in productive time during a 2-week period, due to a common pain condition.[14] The economic, societal, and health impacts of chronic pain, especially among working-age populations, are enormous. Lost productive time from common pain conditions among workers costs an estimated $61.2 billion per year, which accounts for 27% of the total estimated work-related cost of pain conditions in the U.S. workforce. Most of the cost is related to reduced performance at work. Headache is the most common (5.4%) pain condition resulting in lost productive time, followed by back pain (3.2%), arthritis pain (2.0%), and other musculoskeletal pain (2.0%).[14]

It was estimated that the healthcare cost for patients with chronic pain might exceed the combined cost of treating patients with coronary artery disease, cancer, and AIDS.[16] For instance, estimates and patterns of direct healthcare expenditures among individuals with back pain in the United States reached $90.7 billion for the year 1998.[17] The financial cost to society is about $150 billion per year.[3] The annual average of healthcare cost incurred by individual patients with chronic pain, excluding cost for surgical procedures, ranges from $12,900 to $18,883.[18,19] The estimated annual economic cost associated with chronic pain exceeds $560 billion in the United States.[8] Thus, chronic pain represents a national challenge.

Barriers Responsible for Undertreatment of Pain

Chronic pain has historically been considered an undertreated condition in the United States.[1] The barriers responsible for the undertreatment of pain have been recognized as multifactorial.[20]

Clinician-related barriers are prominent concerns.[21] Physicians and other healthcare providers make therapeutic decisions that may be influenced by their belief that pain is an inevitable and accepted part of life; by their ethnic, racial, or gender biases;[22] or by their negative feelings toward patients with pain, including fear, suspicion (of diversion and substance abuse), anger, resentment, revulsion, and denial. Additionally, as a result of lacking the fundamental knowledge and basic skills in risk assessment and management, some clinicians may harbor excessive or inaccurate concerns about drug abuse, addiction, overdose, and diversion, and fears of investigation or sanction by federal, state, and local regulatory agencies. These concerns, in turn, may increase their reluctance to intervene, even when an astute assessment supports the likelihood of benefits being greater than the risks.

Patient-related factors are also major drivers of undertreatment.[21] Some patients ignore or underestimate the level of pain and think one can "see the pain through." Some are unwilling to take medications or injections due to confusion or concerns about side effects of analgesics (including opioids) or even fear that pain portends a serious illness or poor diagnosis, while others report satisfaction with pain management, despite persistent moderate or severe pain.

Barriers to pain assessment and management that are related to the healthcare system include a historical absence of clearly established practice standards and failure to make pain relief a priority. The growth of managed care, the greater emphasis on outpatient treatment, and new reimbursement policies all have introduced barriers to pain management. In addition, fragmented patient care increases the risk of poor coordination of care across treatment settings. Furthermore, the use of gatekeepers and formularies by some managed care programs may impede access to pain specialists, comprehensive pain management facilities, and more effective treatment modalities.

State laws and regulations, state medical board oversight, and federal drug enforcement regulations are intended to impede diversion and inappropriate use of potentially addictive drugs by taking punitive actions against inappropriate prescription of opioids, among other disciplinary or legal actions. This highly regulated environment may have contributed to the conservative prescription of controlled prescription drugs, including opioids. This belief has led to dramatic changes in pain management practice.

Epidemiology of Opioid Use for Chronic Pain

In 1998 and 2004, in order to alleviate physician uncertainty about opioid use and encourage better pain control, the Federation of State Medical Boards (FSMB) issued model guidelines or policies for the use of controlled substances for the treatment of pain.[23] Subsequently, over half of the state medical boards have either adopted or modified these guidelines and implemented them in their states. Over one-third of state legislatures, influenced by advocacy groups, have instituted Intractable Pain Treatment Acts (IPTA) that provide immunity from discipline for physicians who prescribe opioids within the requirements of the statute.

Opioid use has increased substantially over the past two decades since the publication of guidelines regarding long-term opioid therapy in patients with moderate to severe chronic pain that adversely affects their daily functioning or quality of life.[24] A study in 2003 demonstrated that about 90% of patients were on opioids and 42% were on benzodiazepines prior to presenting to a multidisciplinary pain management center.[25] The frequency of overall opioid use among patients with back pain was reported to be approximately 12%.[26] Many of the patients also received more than one type of opioids, most commonly one for sustained release and one for breakthrough pain. In 2009, there were 234 million prescriptions dispensed in the United States for immediate-release (IR) opioids and 22.9 million for long-acting (LA) opioid formulations (including controlled-release [CR], extended-release [ER], and sustained-release [SR] formulations). The IR opioid figure represents an increase of almost 50% in total prescriptions dispensed since 2000.[27] The United States, with 4.6% of the world's population, consumes 80% of the world's opioids.

Impact of Chronic Opioid Use on Society, Health, and Economy

Although the increase in prescribing opioid medications may signify a greater effort to improve the overall treatment of chronic pain, it has also contributed inadvertently to the growing public health problem of opioids abuse, addiction, overdose, and deaths.[28,29] Illicit drug use and dose escalations have been demonstrated in a similar proportion of patients on long-acting and short-acting opioids.[30,31] Studies indicate that 12% to 34% of patients receiving opioid therapy for chronic pain at some point will abuse their medications.[29,32-34] Diversion of prescribed opioids is also common. A recently published national survey reported that among persons aged ≥12 years in 2009–2010 who used pain relievers for nonmedical purposes, 55.0% obtained the most recently used pain relievers from a friend or relative for free. Another 11.4% bought them from a friend or relative (a significantly higher figure than the 8.9% reported by the same annual survey for 2007–2008), and 4.8% took them from a friend or relative without asking. More than 1 in 6 (17.3%) indicated that they obtained the most recently abused drugs through a prescription from a single health care provider, whereas almost 1 in 20 users (4.4%) obtained from a drug dealer or other stranger. About 0.4% bought the abused drugs on the Internet.[35] Other sources of diverted opioids include theft and fraud in the form of "doctor shopping."[36,37]

Drug overdose deaths in the United States exceed 38,000 annually, with prescription drugs involved in more than 55% of such deaths. Prescription opioid drugs were involved in nearly 75% of the 22,000-plus prescription drug overdose deaths in the United States reported in 2010,[38] accounting for more drug-related overdose deaths than those from heroin and cocaine combined.[39,40] Indeed, unintentional drug overdose ranks second only to motor vehicle accidents as the leading cause of annual accidental death in the United States, with individuals in the 35- to 54-year-old age group having the highest rates of unintentional drug overdose deaths.[41,42] Many of the overdose deaths from prescription opioids involve at least one other drug. The combination of opioids and benzodiazepines is particularly dangerous.[43] Deaths caused by opioid prescription drug abuse in the United States have risen more than threefold in one decade, from 1999 (4000 deaths) to 2008 (15,000 deaths), leading the Centers for Disease Control and Prevention (CDC) to declare the problem an ongoing "national epidemic."

More than 15 million people admit to abusing prescription drugs—more than the combined number of those who admit abusing cocaine (5.9 million), hallucinogens (4 million), inhalants (2.1 million), and heroin (0.3 million).[44] Consequently, federal actions such as Food and Drug Administration (FDA)-mandated risk mitigation strategies for long-acting opioids, federal support for requiring mandatory education for Drug Enforcement Administration (DEA) registration, and state-based initiatives designed to more tightly regulate opioid use have emerged.

Challenges of Managing Chronic Pain in a Hospital Setting and Future Direction of Chronic Pain Management

Approximately 230 million major surgical operations are performed worldwide each year.[45] It is estimated that up to 35% of adults presenting for surgery suffer from chronic pain and that a substantial number of such patients are on chronic use of analgesics. Optimal pain control for patients on chronic analgesics is particularly challenging, given the complexity of chronic pain; high tolerance to opioids and increased sensitivity to painful stimuli. Consequently, perioperative pain on top of chronic pain often remains undertreated even with easy access to multiple analgesic modalities in hospital settings, with 47% of patients experiencing moderate pain and 39% experiencing severe to extreme pain.[46]

Priority for pain management must be established, consistent with the view that persistent pain is a potentially serious illness in its own right. Acute and chronic pain must be given a level of attention comparable to that of management of any underlying disease or comorbidity. Arguably, opioid therapy plays an important role in pain management and should be available when needed for the treatment of all kinds of pain, including non-cancer pain. The DEA has also taken the position that clinicians should be knowledgeable about using opioids to treat pain and should not hesitate to prescribe them when opioids are the best clinical choice of treatment.[47] Failure to treat severe pain, including postoperative pain, has been described as a fundamental breach of human rights.[48] However, meeting the needs of adequate pain management in a seriously ill and hospitalized patient typically requires the use of opioid analgesics that carry with them significant risks of adverse events, as well as the potential for abuse and addiction. These issues are of particular concern for patients entering the hospital on opioid analgesics for chronic pain. The perioperative management of patients receiving chronic opioid therapy poses a great challenge to clinicians who must exercise judgment to provide the benefits of effective opioid analgesia but also consider issues related to the illicit or nonmedical use of these analgesics.

Summary

Organizations such as the Joint Commission now are requiring that inpatient pain assessment and relief be monitored as indicators of quality of care, and more standards for quality improvement in pain management are becoming widely available. Healthcare providers need current, state-of-the-art education to develop necessary skills to manage patients with persistent pain in the hospital setting, including skills needed to use opioid medications safely and effectively. They need to be aware of any personal biases that interfere with clinical judgment and to apply knowledge in a rational, scientific manner. With many treatment options now available, and with the recognition of increased costs associated with undertreated pain, clinicians must be encouraged to assess and treat pain, in the most effective ways possible, including multimodal analgesia (MMA). More emphasis should be placed on personnel training/staffing and more effective multimodal approaches should be utilized in hospital settings to ensure better pain management.

References

1. Harstall C, Ospina M. How prevalent is chronic pain? *Pain Clin Updates*. 2003;11(2). http://www.iasp-pain.org/PublicationsNews/NewsletterIssue.aspx?ItemNumber=2136. Accessed July 21, 2015.
2. Loeser JD, Melzack R. Pain: an overview. *Lancet*. 1999;353(9164):1607–1609.
3. Tracey I, Bushnell MC. How neuroimaging studies have challenged us to rethink: is chronic pain a disease? *J Pain*. 2009;10(11):1113–1120.
4. Chapman CR, Tuckett RP, Song CW. Pain and stress in a systems perspective: reciprocal neural, endocrine, and immune interactions. *J Pain*. 2008;9(2):122–145.
5. Watkins EA, Wollan PC, Melton LJ, 3rd, Yawn BP. A population in pain: report from the Olmsted County Health Study. *Pain Med*. 2008;9(2):166–174.
6. Blay SL, Andreoli SB, Gastal FL. Chronic painful physical conditions, disturbed sleep and psychiatric morbidity: results from an elderly survey. *Ann Clin Psychiatry*. 2007;19(3):169–174.
7. Health, United States, 2014. http://www.cdc.gov/nchs/hus.htm. Assessed September 10, 2014.
8. Institute of Medicine. *Relieving Pain in America: A Blueprint for Transforming Prevention, Care, Education, and Research*. Washington, DC: National Academies Press; 2011.
9. King SA, Snow BR. Factors for predicting premature termination from a multidisciplinary inpatient chronic pain program. *Pain*. 1989;39(3):281–287.
10. Hardt J, Jacobsen C, Goldberg J, Nickel R, Buchwald D. Prevalence of chronic pain in a representative sample in the united states. *Pain Med*. 2008;9(7):803–812.
11. Portenoy RK, Ugarte C, Fuller I, Haas G. Population-based survey of pain in the United States: Differences among white, African American, and Hispanic subjects. *J Pain*. 2004;5(6):317–328.
12. Johannes CB, Le TK, Zhou X, Johnston JA, Dworkin RH. The prevalence of chronic pain in United States adults: results of an Internet-based survey. *J Pain*. 2010;11(11):1230–1239.
13. Gureje O, Von Korff M, Simon GE, Gater R. Persistent pain and well-being: A World Health Organization study in primary care. *JAMA*. 1998;280(2):147–151.
14. Stewart WF, Ricci JA, Chee E, Morganstein D. Lost productive work time costs from health conditions in the United States: Results from the American Productivity Audit. *J Occup Environ Med*. 2003;45(12):1234–1246.
15. Sawyer P, Lillis JP, Bodner EV, Allman RM. Substantial daily pain among nursing home residents. *J Am Med Dir Assoc*. 2007;8(3):158–165.
16. Hough J. Estimating the health care utilization costs associated with people with disabilities: data from the 1996 Medical Expenditure Panel Survey (MEPS). Presented at the annual meeting of the Association for Health Services Research, Los Angeles, CA, 2000.
17. Luo X, Pietrobon R, Sun SX, Liu GG, Hey. Estimates and patterns of direct health care expenditures among individuals with back pain in the United States. *Spine*. 2004;29:79–86.
18. Bell G, Kidd D, North R. Cost-effectiveness analysis of spinal cord stimulation in treatment of failed back surgery syndrome. *J Pain Sympt Manage*. 1997;13:286–295.
19. de Lissovoy G, Brown RE, Halpern M, Hassenbusch SJ, Ross E. Cost-effectiveness of long-term intrathecal morphine therapy for pain associated with failed back surgery syndrome. *Clin Ther*. 1997;19:96–112.
20. Fishman SM, Papazian JS, Gonzalez S, Riches PS, Gilson A. Regulating opioid prescribing through prescription monitoring programs: balancing drug diversion and treatment of pain. *Pain Med*. 2004;5:309–324.
21. Jacox A, Carr DB, Payne R, et al. *Management of Cancer Pain*. Clinical Practice Guideline No. 9. AHCPR 94-0592. Rockville, MD: U.S. Department of Health and Human Services; 1994.
22. Burgess DJ, Crowley-Matoka M, Phelan S, et al. Patient race and physicians' decisions to prescribe opioids for chronic low back pain. *Soc Sci Med*. 2008;67(11):1852–1860.

23. Model Policy for the Use of Controlled Substances for the Treatment of Pain. The Federation of State Medical Boards of the United States. *J Pain Palliat Care Pharmacother.* 2005;19(2):73–78.
24. Chou R. 2009 Clinical Guidelines from the American Pain Society and the American Academy of Pain Medicine on the use of chronic opioid therapy in chronic non-cancer pain: what are the key messages for clinical practice? *Pol Arch Med Wewn.* 2009;119(7-8):469–477.
25. Manchikanti L, Damron KS, McManus CD, Barnhill RC. Patterns of illicit drug use and opioid abuse in patients with chronic pain at initial evaluation: a prospective, observational study. *Pain Physician.* 2004;7:431–437.
26. Luo X, Pietrobon R HL. Patterns and trends in opioid use among individuals with back pain in the United States. *Spine.* 2004;29:884–891.
27. Governale L. Outpatient prescription opioid utilization in the U.S., years 2000–2009. Washington, DC: U.S. Food and Drug Administration; 2010. http://www.fda.gov/downloads/AdvisoryCommittess/CommittessMeetingMaterials/drugs/DrugSafetyandRiskManagementAdvisoryCommittee/UCM220950.pdf. Accessed May 11, 2012.
28. Paulozzi LJ, Kilbourne EM, Shah NG, et al. A history of being prescribed controlled substances and risk of drug overdose death. *Pain Med.* 2012;13(1):87–95.
29. Katz NP, Sherburne S, Beach M, et al. Behavioral monitoring and urine toxicology testing in patients receiving long-term opioid therapy. *Anesth Analg.* 2003;97(4):1097–1102, table of contents.
30. Manchikanti L, Manchukonda R, Pampati V, Damron KS. Evaluation of abuse of prescription and illicit drugs in chronic pain patients receiving short-acting (hydrocodone) or long-acting (methadone) opioids. *Pain Physician.* 2005;8:257–261.
31. Manchikanti L, Damron KS, Pampati V, McManus CD. Prospective evaluation of patients with increasing opiate needs: prescription opiate abuse and illicit drug use. Pain Physician 2004;7:339–344.
32. Chabal C, Erjavec MK, Jacobson L, Mariano A, Chaney E. Prescription opiate abuse in chronic pain patients: clinical criteria, incidence, and predictors. *Clin J Pain.* 1997;13(2):150–155.
33. Manchikanti L, Pampati V, Damron KS, Fellows B, Barnhill RC, Beyer CD. Prevalence of opioid abuse in interventional pain medicine practice settings: a randomized clinical evaluation. *Pain Physician.* 2001;4(4):358–365.
34. Fishbain DA, Cole B, Lewis J, Rosomoff HL, Rosomoff RS. What percentage of chronic nonmalignant pain patients exposed to chronic opioid analgesic therapy develop abuse/addiction and/or aberrant drug-related behaviors? A structured evidence-based review. *Pain Med.* 2008;9(4):444–459.
35. Substance Abuse and Mental Health Services Administration. Results from the 2010 National Survey on Drug Use and Health: summary of national findings. NSDUH Series H-41, HHS Publication No. (SMA) 11-4658. Rockville, MD: Substance Abuse and Mental Health Services Administration; 2011.
36. Joranson DE, Gilson AM. Drug crime is a source of abused pain medications in the United States. *J Pain Symptom Manage.* 2005;30(4):299–301.
37. Fass JA, Hardigan PC. Attitudes of Florida pharmacists toward implementing a state prescription drug monitoring program for controlled substances. *J Manag Care Pharm.* 2011;17(6):430–438.
38. Jones CM, Mack KA, Paulozzi LJ. Pharmaceutical overdose deaths, United States, 2010. *JAMA.* 2013;309(7):657–659.
39. U.S. Department of Health and Human Services, Centers for Disease Control and Prevention. Policy impact: prescription painkiller overdoses. Updated December 19, 2011. http://www.cdc.gov/homeandrecreationalsafety/rxbrief. Accessed May 9, 2012.
40. U.S. Department of Health and Human Services, Centers for Disease Control and Prevention. Vital signs: overdoses of prescription opioid pain relievers—United States, 1999–2008. *MMWR Morb Mortal Wkly Rep.* 2011;60:1487–1492.

41. U.S. Department of Health and Human Services, Centers for Disease Control and Prevention. Unintentional drug poisoning in the United States. July 2010. http://www.cdc.gov/HomeandRecreationalSafety/pdf/poison-issuebrief.pdf. Accessed July 11, 2012.

42. Warner M, Chen LH, Makuc DM. Increase in fatal poisonings involving opioid analgesics in the Unites States, 1999–2006. NCHS Data Brief No. 22. Hyattsville, MD: National Center for Health Statistics; 2009. http://www.cdc.gov/nchs/data/databriefs/db22.htm. Accessed April 19, 2012.

43. Zacny JP, Paice JA, Coalson DW. Separate and combined psychopharmacological effects of alprazolam and oxycodone in healthy volunteers. *Drug Alcohol Depend.* 2012;124(3):274–282.

44. Bollinger LC, Bush C, Califano JA, et al. Under the counter. The diversion and abuse of controlled prescription drugs in the U.S. The National Center on Addiction and Substance Abuse at Columbia University (CASA), July 2005. http://www.casacolumbia.org/sites/default/files/Under-the-counter-the-diversion-and-abuse-of-controlled-prescription-drugs-in-the-us_0.pdf

45. World Health Organization (WHO). Report on emergency and surgical care. http://www.who.int/surgery/en/index.html. Accessed May 15, 2012.

46. Apfelbaum JL, Chen C, Mehta SS, Gan TJ. Postoperative pain experience: results from a national survey suggest postoperative pain continues to be undermanaged. *Anesth Analg.* 2003;97(2):534–540, table of contents.

47. Drug Enforcement Administration. Physician's Manual: An Informational Outline of the Controlled Substances Act of 1970. Washington, DC: U.S. Department of Justice; 1990.

48. Mitra S, Sinatra RS. Perioperative management of acute pain in the opioid-dependent patient. *Anesthesiology.* 2004;101(1):212–227.

2

Molecular and Physiological Markers and Mechanisms of Chronic Pain

HAIBIN WANG AND EDWARD GARAY

KEY POINTS

- Normal pain perception is protective, transient, and proportional to peripheral sensory input and resolves once the tissue injury heals or the putative harm is no longer present.
- Under certain pathophysiological conditions, the perception of pain becomes disabling, persistent, and disproportionate and outlasts the actual inciting event.
- There are many regulatory steps involved in converting a peripheral stimulus into the perception of pain, and that can shift the homeostatic process in a way that pain becomes a chronic disorder.
- Nociceptors are pseudounipolar peripheral neurons, typically with free nerve endings specialized for specific sensory modalities (i.e., mechanical, thermal, and chemical).
- Nociceptor activation threshold and modality specificity can be described by fiber neurophysiology, peripheral terminal arborization, and transducer expression profile.
- The constituents of the local microenvironment (e.g., mast cells, glial cells, extracellular matrix) are important regulators in the functional modification of the peripheral and central terminals of the nociceptor.
- Stimulus transmission and transduction are pivotal processes subjected to sensitization mechanisms that change functional anatomy, cellular/ intracellular function, and signal fidelity.

Introduction

As one of the most important innate defense mechanisms to avoid ongoing or potential harms, *nociception* is the process by which intense, noxious thermal, mechanical, or chemical stimuli are detected by a subpopulation of peripheral sensory nerve fibers, called *nociceptors*.[1] Nociceptive sensory flow is subsequently relayed to central structures and undergoes further refinement, which leads to a series of complex neurophysiological events that may involve both discriminative and affective processes. As a result, pain is generated. Normally, once the tissue injury heals or the putative harm is no longer present, pain resolves accordingly. However, under certain pathophysiological conditions, the perception of pain becomes persistent and outlasts the actual inciting event. Consequently, chronic pain no longer provides a protective role for the body; rather, it becomes a disease in itself. Over the past several decades, scientific advances have shed light on the many regulatory steps involved in converting a peripheral stimulus into the perception of pain and how pain becomes chronic. In this chapter, we highlight peripheral and central mechanisms that govern nociception and the development of chronic pain status.

Dissecting the Pain Pathway

Classically, the pain pathway has been depicted as a unidirectional multistep relay. The reality is far more complicated. From peripheral to central (Figure 2.1) structures, it can be divided into transduction (represented by the activation of transducers expressed on peripheral terminals of nociceptors and that respond to specific stimulation modalities); conduction (the propagation of action potential impulses along the primary sensory afferents toward the dorsal horn of the spinal cord); transmission (the relay of stimulus from first- to second-order sensory neurons in the spinal cord); projection (the sensory information that projects to the thalamus and then to the sensory cortex and limbic system); perception (how stimulus is converted into pain perception by the brain); and descending modulation (the mechanism by which the brain can either facilitate or inhibit sensory information at the level of the spinal cord). Conceivably, maladaptation at any of these steps may contribute to the development of chronic pain. Among these steps, transduction and transmission have received the most attention from scientists, as they are the main sites for the two most critical mechanisms in the development of chronic pain—peripheral and central sensitization, respectively.

NOCICEPTOR CHARACTERISTICS

Sensory neurons are the primary means of collecting stimuli originating from the peripheral environment of innervated tissues and relaying the information to the spinal cord and brainstem for processing and decoding. The structure of a sensory afferent includes a peripheral axonal branch, a cell body, and a central

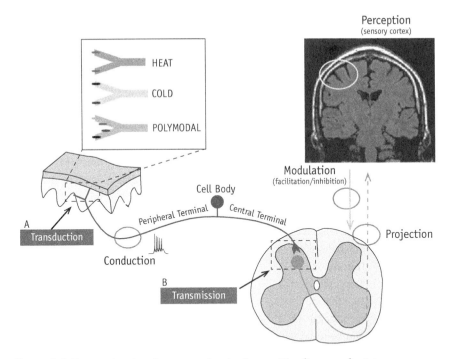

Figure 2.1 Two major sites for neuroplastic change. The diagram depicts a gross representation of the perception of pain signals that originate in peripheral structures. **A.** The transduction of noxious thermal, mechanical, or chemical signals is initiated by activation of specialized free nerve endings (boxed inset) characterized by distinct transducer expression profiles (described in Table 2.2) and neurophysiology (described in Table 2.1). Putative changes in pathological states modify these intrinsic mechanisms with a resulting magnification of signal transduction (i.e., peripheral sensitization). **B.** The transmission of nociceptive signals to central structures at the dorsal horn involves numerous mechanisms that are also susceptible to modification by pathological states (described in detail in Figure 2.2). Other mechanisms susceptible to modulation in pathological states, less represented in the literature, are highlighted by circles and include peripheral signal conduction, ascending/descending projections modulation, and central perception.

axonal branch (Figure 2.1). The cell bodies of these sensory neurons are located in the dorsal root (for the body), trigeminal (for the face), or nodose (visceral afferents) ganglia. From the cell body, a peripheral axon stalk extends to specific target tissues (e.g., skin, muscle, cartilage. or viscera) and a central axonal stalk extends toward the level-specific central nervous tissue (e.g., spinal cord). Sensory afferent fibers can be categorized according to their axon diameter, state of myelination, and conduction velocity (Table 2.1). In general, conduction

Table 2.1 **Nociceptor Fiber Neurophysiology**

Fiber Class*	Physical Features	Velocity Group**	Effective Stimuli
Aβ	Myelinated Large diameter Proprioception, light touch	Group II (>40–50 m/sec)	Low threshold Specialized nerve endings (e.g., pacinian corpuscles)
Aδ	Lightly myelinated Medium diameter Nociception	Group III (>10 and <40 m/sec)	Low threshold mechanical or thermal High threshold mechanical or thermal
C	Unmyelinated Small diameter Innocuous temperature, itch Nociception (peptidergic vs. non-peptidergic)	Group IV (<2 m/sec)	High threshold thermal, mechanical, or chemical Free nerve endings

velocity varies directly with axonal diameter and myelination. Thus, Aβ fibers are typically large diameter and myelinated and conduct fast; Aδ are smaller and less myelinated and conduct slower; C fibers are small and unmyelinated and conduct slowest. Different fibers respond most efficiently to a particular stimulus modality, which is determined by peripheral terminal properties. For example, the specialized terminal endings of Aβ fibers are optimized for detecting low-threshold mechanical perturbations and transducing innocuous tactile sensation. Regarding noxious stimuli, the terminal characteristics of some Aδ fibers and C fibers are optimized for detecting polymodal stimuli (Table 2.1) and, respectively, transducing acute, well-localized fast pain and poorly localized slow pain.[2]

Nociceptors, which are directly involved in transduction, conduction, and transmission steps in the pain pathway, have both a peripheral and central stalk that ends in a terminal arbor of "free unencapsulated" nerve endings. The branching pattern of the peripheral terminal arbor varies with the distinct effective stimuli and target of innervation. For example, in cutaneous tissue, higher spatial resolution for sensory discrimination is associated with a smaller terminal arbor. Some nociceptor subpopulations have been identified to maintain a specific terminal arbor structure that is dependent on its peptidergic function, for example, release of substance P or calcitonin gene–related peptide (CGRP).[3] Unlike the classic unipolar structure and unidirectional function of the prototypical neuron, the pseudounipolar structure of the nociceptor is optimized for bidirectional function. Proteins synthesized in the cell body are transported to peripheral and central terminals, reinforcing the functional equivalency of each terminal.[4] The nociceptor can receive and transmit messages from either end. A key example, similar to the release of neurotransmitters by the central terminal, is that the peripheral terminal can release various biochemically active molecules that influence the local microenvironment, a process termed *neurogenic inflammation*.[5,6] The central terminal also shares characteristic traits with the peripheral terminal in that it is designed to biochemically respond to endogenous molecules (e.g., H+, lipids, neurotransmitters) within its microenvironment.[7]

PERIPHERAL SENSITIZATION

Transduction and conduction are the two initial steps for sensing pain. Upon tissue injury, the inflammatory mediators may enhance the activity of a variety of transducers (Table 2.2) and conductors (e.g., voltage-gated sodium channels), which may lead to peripheral sensitization. The ability to become sensitized, that is, to increase its innate properties of excitability, is an important property of the nociceptor. Functionally, *peripheral sensitization* is defined as a reduction in the threshold needed for activation of nociceptors and an increase in the magnitude of response to previous noxious stimuli.[8] In addition, peripheral sensitization may also include the perception of pain from previously non-noxious stimuli and/or the development of ectopic activity.[7]

With significant scientific advances in recent years, now we have better understanding of the cellular and molecular basis for activation and sensitization of nociceptors. At the peripheral terminals, nociceptors express a variety of cell surface proteins that interact with the local microenvironment and serve as transducers in response to different noxious sensory modalities and ion channel conductors to generate and propagate action potentials. Concurrently, the peripheral terminals also express receptors for inflammatory mediators. These receptors have been shown to play a significant role in nociceptor response to acute tissue injury, associated with an activated inflammatory response, and upregulation of local inflammatory mediators. Receptor activation modulates intracellular signaling pathways that may either alter transducer or conductor's functional property via post translational modifications or directly influence the gene expression and upregulation of protein cellular content. This sensitization may only take a few minutes, through post translational modifications, or require a few hours or longer dependent on gene expression and protein translation mechanisms. Functionally modified and overexpressed transducers or conductors have been shown to contribute to the maintenance of pain.[8]

Among those transducers, the TRP (transient receptor potential) family of ion channels is of particular interest. The first member cloned in this family, TRPV1, has been extensively studied in its role in peripheral sensitization. TRPV1 is a major transducer for noxious heat (>43°C).[20] TRPV1 is important

Table 2.2 **Peripheral Transducers and Sensitization**

Transducer	Effective Stimulus	Role in Sensitization	Reference
Mechanical			
TRPV1	Role in response to hollow organ distension	Block central channel ↓ mechanical hyperalgesia	9
TRPV4	Direct activation by osmotic challenge	Visceral, cutaneous hypersensitivity in inflammation and nerve injury	10
ASIC3	Visceral afferents (↓ sensitivity in KO). Cutaneous afferents (↑, ↓, ↔ in KO)	Required for sensitization of colonic, muscle, and joint nociceptors	11
TREK1/2	Direct activation by mechanical stimuli	↑ Inflammatory hyperalgesia, potential role in neuropathic pain	12,13
P2X3	Indirect activation through ATP release from epithelial cells, hollow organ distension	Pronociceptive role in visceral and somatic pain associated with inflammation and nerve injury	14
Isoselectin B4	Role in response to direct mechanical activation in cultured DRGs. Interacts with extracellular chondroitin sulfate proteoglycan (veriscan)	Low pH-induced sensitization to mechanical activation regulated by varied concentraton of extracellular chondroitin sulfate	15
Thermal			
NaV1.8	Resistant to cold-induced inactivation. Indirectly essential for cold transduction	No published data	16
TRPM8	Direct activation by cold stimulus	Role in increased cold sensitivity after injury (KO studies)	17,18
TRPV1	Direct activation by heat stimulus	Multiple lines of evidence that TRPV1 is essential for thermal hyperalgesia associated with most types of tissue injury	19

Adapted from Gold and Gebhart.[8] KO, knockout.

for inflammatory thermal hyperalgesia.[21] Molecular analysis has demonstrated that TRPV1 contains multiple phosphorylation sites in its amino acid sequence. Phosphorylation of TRPV1 by protein kinase C (PKC)[22] or protein kinase A (PKA)[23] can modify TRPV1 function. Inflammatory mediators can upregulate TRPV1 function by employing PKC/PKA activity. For example, bradykinin secreted by mast cells has been shown to sensitize TRPV1 and lead to pain.[24]

Similar to TRPV1, the interaction between conductors and inflammatory mediators also play a significant role in developing and maintaining peripheral sensitization. Action potential generation is dependent on the summated activity of a variety of sodium channels. The functional states of sodium channels directly influence the conductivity of nociceptors, which may directly influence the propagation and intensity of action potentials that eventually reach the central synapses. A prototypical example is the sodium channel Nav1.7. Hyperactivity of Nav1.7 secondary to genetic aberrations has been linked to the development of erythromelalgia and paroxysmal extreme pain disorder, both diseases presenting with intense, burning pain.[25,26] Inflammatory mediators can upregulate Nav1.7 activity, leading to mechanical and thermal hypersensitivity.[27]

CENTRAL SENSITIZATION

Central sensitization is a process that generates hyperexcitability in the central nervous system and causes enhanced processing of pain information.[28] In contrast to wind-up, which is the phenomenon of a progressively increasing response during the course of sensory stimulation, central sensitization emphasizes the facilitation after the end of the conditioning.[29] Central sensitization is activity dependent, thus continuous peripheral inputs are essential. The sites for central sensitization can be at both the spinal and supraspinal levels. To date, the vast majority of studies have focused on the spinal cord dorsal horn, as it is the key juncture for relaying sensory flow (transmission). Among many of the mechanisms implicated in the development of central sensitization, there are three distinct mechanisms that appear to be essential: NMDA receptor-mediated hypersensitivity, loss of tonic inhibitory controls (disinhibition), and glial–neuronal interactions.[1]

In the dorsal horn of the spinal cord, peripheral sensory afferents transmit nociceptor electrical activity via releasing presynaptic neurotransmitters, for example, glutamate (Figure 2.2). Glutamate is a major excitatory amino acid and can directly excite postsynaptic neurons upon binding to its receptor (ligand-gated cation channels). Acute, transient pain perception is mainly characterized by glutamate binding to and activating AMPA receptors, which generally are not permeable to calcium ions. In contrast, when the nociceptive flow persists after tissue injury, glutamate may activate previously silent NMDA receptors. Unlike AMPA receptors, NMDA receptors are permeable to calcium. The calcium ions function as second messengers triggering a cascade of intracellular events,

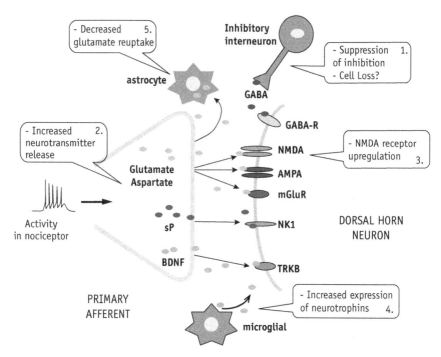

Figure 2.2 Central sensitization increases the gain of transmission. The diagram shows a few prominent mediators and cell–cell interactions in the spinal cord dorsal horn. Putative changes in pathological states include mechanisms involving 1. suppression of inhibition, 2. potentiation of presynaptic neurotransmitter release, 3. postsynaptic excitability, 4. release of neurotrophic factors from activated microglia, and 5. decreased glutamate reuptake by astrocytes. Overall, the result is a net increase in transmission of nociceptive input onto higher brain structures. BDNF, brain-derived neurotrophic factor; GABA, gamma-aminobutyric acid; mGluR, metabotropic glutamate receptor; NK1, neurokinin 1 receptor. sP, substance P.

which influence protein kinase (e.g., ERK1/2, cAMP, CAMKIV) activation and subsequent phosphorylation of target proteins (e.g., AMPA and NMDA receptors), ultimately changing their structure and function. Moreover, the intracellular signaling pathways increase the synapse-to-nucleus communication and modulate de novo gene expression of proteins pivotal to enhancing the transmission of peripheral signals to central structures.[30,31] As a result, NMDA receptor activation enhances the efficacy of transmission.

The excitatory activity at spinal cord dorsal horn is counterbalanced by a group of inhibitory interneurons. By releasing inhibitory neurotransmitters, such as GABA and glycine, these inhibitory interneurons can negatively control the net output of nociceptive sensory flow toward higher central structures. Tissue injury can decrease this tonic inhibitory effect from inhibitory interneurons—in other words, create disinhibition. Disinhibition facilitates spinal cord output in response to painful stimulation and contributes to central sensitization and chronic pain.[32] A growing body of evidence from preclinical studies has demonstrated that glial cells are involved in central sensitization. The interplay between glia and neurons is intricate. Different types of glial cells may employ different mechanisms to enhance neuronal activity and facilitate central sensitization (Figure 2.2). Upon activation, microglia can release brain-derived neurotrophic factor (BDNF) and other inflammatory mediators to sensitize the spinal neurons.[33] In response to enhanced neuronal and glial cell activity, astrocytes may decrease the reuptake of glutamate and essentially prolong the synaptic glutamate activity; increase the reuptake of GABA, and attenuate its inhibitory function.[34]

Summary

Peripheral and central sensitization are two pivotal processes in the development of pain hypersensitivity and chronic pain. Many cellular and molecular-level changes contribute to the development of peripheral and central sensitization. Our knowledge about this process is continuously expanding, fueled by the progress in basic and translational research. Additionally, perturbations in other components (e.g., signal conduction, descending modulation, and central perception) of the pain-processing pathway (Figure 2.1) may also play a significant role in various types of chronic pain. For example, cortical remapping (perception) is critical for phantom pain,[35] and altered descending modulation is involved in chronic migraine headaches.[36] Clarification of the underlying mechanisms that contribute to the development of chronic pain conditions could help direct investigational resources, assist in designing targeted interventions, and provide measures for ascertaining therapeutic outcomes. Ultimately, by decreasing the burden of disease, quality of life may be regained and work productivity restored.

References

1. Basbaum AI, Bautista DM, Scherrer G, Julius D. Cellular and molecular mechanisms of pain. *Cell*. 2009;139:267–284.
2. Meyer RA, Ringkamp M, Campbell JN, Raja SN. *Peripheral Mechanisms of Cutaneous Nocioception*. St. Louis, MO: Elsevier; 2008.
3. Zylka MJ, Rice FL, Anderson DJ. Topographically distinct epidermal nociceptive circuits revealed by axonal tracers targeted to Mrgprd. *Neuron*. 2005;45:17–25.
4. Fishman S, Ballantyne J, Rathmell JP, Bonica JJ. *Bonica's Management of Pain*. Baltimore, MD: Lippincott, Williams & Wilkins; 2010.
5. Kilo S, Harding-Rose C, Hargreaves KM Flores CM. Peripheral CGRP release as a marker for neurogenic inflammation: a model system for the study of neuropeptide secretion in rat paw skin. *Pain*. 1997;73:201–207.

6. White DM, Helme RD. Release of substance P from peripheral nerve terminals following electrical stimulation of the sciatic nerve. *Brain Res.* 1985;336:27–31.

7. Kuner R. Central mechanisms of pathological pain. *Nat Med.* 2010;16:1258–1266.

8. Gold MS, Gebhart GF. Nociceptor sensitization in pain pathogenesis. *Nat Med.* 2010;16:1248–1257.

9. Honore P, Wismer CT, Mikusa J, et al. A-425619 [1-isoquinolin-5-yl-3-(4-trifluoromethyl-benzyl)-urea], a novel transient receptor potential type V1 receptor antagonist, relieves pathophysiological pain associated with inflammation and tissue injury in rats. *J Pharmacol Exp Ther.* 2005;314:410–421.

10. Alessandri-Haber N, Dina OA, Chen X, Levine JD. TRPC1 and TRPC6 channels cooperate with TRPV4 to mediate mechanical hyperalgesia and nociceptor sensitization. *J Neurosci* 2009;29:6217–6228.

11. Page AJ, Brierley SM, Martin CM, et al. Different contributions of ASIC channels 1a, 2, and 3 in gastrointestinal mechanosensory function. *Gut.* 2005;54:1408–1415.

12. Maingret F, Patel AJ, Lesage F, Lazdunski M, Honore E. Mechano- or acid stimulation, two interactive modes of activation of the TREK-1 potassium channel. *J Biol Chem.* 1999;274:26691–26696.

13. Alloui A, Zimmermann K, Mamet J, et al. TREK-1, a K+ channel involved in polymodal pain perception. *EMBO J.* 2006;25:2368–2376.

14. Burnstock G. Purinergic mechanosensory transduction and visceral pain. *Mol Pain.* 2009;5:69.

15. Kubo A, Katanosaka K, Mizumura K. Extracellular matrix proteoglycan plays a pivotal role in sensitization by low pH of mechanosensitive currents in nociceptive sensory neurones. *J Physiol.* 2012;590:2995–3007.

16. Zimmermann K, Leffler A, Babes A, et al. Sensory neuron sodium channel Nav1.8 is essential for pain at low temperatures. *Nature.* 2007;447:855–858.

17. Bautista DM, Jordt SE, Nikai T, et al. TRPA1 mediates the inflammatory actions of environmental irritants and proalgesic agents. *Cell.* 2006;124:1269–1282.

18. McKemy DD, Neuhausser WM, Julius D. Identification of a cold receptor reveals a general role for TRP channels in thermosensation. *Nature.* 2002;416:52–58.

19. Gold MS, Caterina MJ. *Molecular Biology of Nociceptor Transduction.* San Diego, CA: Academic Press; 2008.

20. Tominaga M, Caterina MJ, Malmberg AB, et al. The cloned capsaicin receptor integrates multiple pain-producing stimuli. *Neuron.* 1998;21:531–543.

21. Caterina MJ, Leffler A, Malmberg AB, et al. Impaired nociception and pain sensation in mice lacking the capsaicin receptor. *Science.* 2000;288:306–313.

22. Bhave G, Hu HJ, Glauner KS, et al. Protein kinase C phosphorylation sensitizes but does not activate the capsaicin receptor transient receptor potential vanilloid 1 (TRPV1). *Proc Natl Acad Sci U S A.* 2003;100:12480–12485.

23. Bhave G, Zhu W, Wang H, et al. cAMP-dependent protein kinase regulates desensitization of the capsaicin receptor (VR1) by direct phosphorylation. *Neuron.* 2002;35:721–731.

24. Mizumura K, Sugiura T, Katanosaka K, Banik RK, Kozaki Y. Excitation and sensitization of nociceptors by bradykinin: what do we know? *Exp Brain Res.* 2009;196:53–65.

25. Estacion M, Dib-Hajj SD, Benke PJ, et al. NaV1.7 gain-of-function mutations as a continuum: A1632E displays physiological changes associated with erythromelalgia and paroxysmal extreme pain disorder mutations and produces symptoms of both disorders. *J Neurosci.* 2008;28:11079–11088.

26. Fertleman CR, Baker MD, Parker KA, et al. *SCN9A* mutations in paroxysmal extreme pain disorder: allelic variants underlie distinct channel defects and phenotypes. *Neuron.* 2006;52:767–774.

27. Nassar MA, Stirling LC, Forlani G, et al. Nociceptor-specific gene deletion reveals a major role for Nav1.7 (PN1) in acute and inflammatory pain. *Proc Natl Acad Sci U S A* 2004;101:12706–12711.

28. Woolf CJ. Evidence for a central component of post-injury pain hypersensitivity. *Nature*. 1983;306:686–688.

29. Woolf CJ. Central sensitization: implications for the diagnosis and treatment of pain. *Pain*. 2011;152:S2–S15.

30. Cheng HY, Pitcher GM, Laviolette SR, et al. DREAM is a critical transcriptional repressor for pain modulation. *Cell*. 2002;108:31–43.

31. Latremoliere A, Woolf CJ. Central sensitization: a generator of pain hypersensitivity by central neural plasticity. *J Pain*. 2009;10:895–926.

32. Moore KA, Kohno T, Karchewski LA, et al. Partial peripheral nerve injury promotes a selective loss of GABAergic inhibition in the superficial dorsal horn of the spinal cord. *J. Neurosci*. 2002;22:6724–6731.

33. Gosselin RD, Suter MR, Ji RR, Decosterd I. Glial cells and chronic pain. *Neuroscientist*. 2010;16:519–531.

34. Ji RR, Berta T, Nedergaard M. Glia and pain: is chronic pain a gliopathy? *Pain*. 2013;154(Suppl 1):S10–S28.

35. Knecht S, Henningsen H, Elbert T, et al. Reorganizational and perceptional changes after amputation. *Brain*. 1996;119(Pt 4):1213–1219.

36. Noseda R, Burstein R. Migraine pathophysiology: anatomy of the trigeminovascular pathway and associated neurological symptoms, cortical spreading depression, sensitization, and modulation of pain. *Pain*. 2013;154(Suppl 1): S44–S53.

3

Psychological and Social Markers
of Chronic Pain

JILL MUSHKAT CONOMY

KEY POINTS

- There are distinct psychological and social markers of chronic pain, reflecting the impact of chronic pain on all aspects of an individual's life.
- The psychological factors incorporate the emotional and cognitive aspects of chronic pain.
- Social factors extend to issues related to family, friends, work, recreation, and financial and legal components. It is virtually impossible to extricate the individual components from their relationship to one another.
- It is important to assist the individual to understand chronic pain exacerbation during hospital admission, develop realistic expectations for treatment, and encourage the patient to take an active role in his/her own improvement.
- It is important to assure the patient you believe the chronic pain to be genuine; consider a referral to the hospital psychologist to help with acquisition of skills for managing pain.

Introduction

John Bonica and Wilbert Fordyce were pioneers in developing the field of pain management as a specific discipline, recognizing that it is an interdisciplinary endeavor focusing on treating the individual and all aspects of his/her life as affected by the distress of chronic pain.[1] It is interesting to watch as other areas of medicine are earning accolades for "newly" discovering this treatment model which Dr. Fordyce described in his renowned 1976 book.[2] One of the most important aspects of this paradigm is that chronic pain has an impact on all aspects of an individual's life.

Impact of Chronic Pain: The BioPsychoSocial Model

The BioPsychoSocial model of pain management functions on a model of chronicity.[3] Acute pain incorporates the expectation that, as damage heals, so pain will heal as well. Unfortunately, as conditions of chronic pain and/or chronic illness demonstrate, pain does not necessarily heal to the premorbid state. It becomes imperative to recognize the impact of chronic pain on all aspects of an individual's life.[4] This includes biological factors, psychological factors, and social factors—thus the biopsychosocial model. The biological factors include physiological and chemical components of chronic pain. This begins with the initial trauma or illness and continues with the sequelae of the various factors that interact with the illness, including substances which overlap with the psychological, behavioral and social factors. The psychological factors incorporate the emotional and cognitive aspects of chronic pain.[5] Social factors extend to issues related to family, friends, work, recreation, financial and legal components. It is virtually impossible to extricate the individual components from their relationship to one another. This design acknowledges that we must recognize and treat the impact of chronic pain on the entire life of an individual, while also appreciating the impact it has on the other people in that person's life as well as extending to society in general. As we ascertain the many factors identified in this model, it is readily evident that no one healthcare professional is able to address all of these concerns. Chronic pain management mandates a multidisciplinary approach to provide input from many specialties to attain optimal results.[6]

The biopsychosocial model reflects concerns for the impact of chemical factors on chronic pain, be they prescribed medications; drugs obtained from family, friends, or off the street; alcohol; caffeine; or nicotine. Basic physics tells us that for every action there is a reaction. The reaction to opioid medications may include depression. The reaction to antidepressant medications may include sexual dysfunction and loss of libido, which may already be impaired because of the pain itself. Treating one problem may incur another. Steroid injections may provide some relief; they may also contribute to weight gain, a concern of many patients who may have eliminated exercise and an active lifestyle because of pain. Pain may interfere with sleep, yet the person who consumed quantities of caffeinated beverages and/or nicotine in the past, may be unable or unwilling to recognize such consumption may contribute to sleep disturbance. One factor cannot be extricated from all the others (Figure 3.1).[7]

As the individual begins to address these tumultuous biological and chemical changes, s/he may be asked to see a psychologist. Not infrequently, by the time a patient arrives at a chronic pain management program, that person may have encountered someone who said, inferred, orwas perceived to imply "the

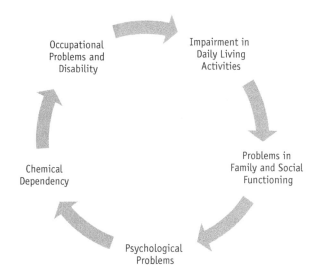

Figure 3.1 Biological and social features of chronic pain. Reprinted with permission from Souzdalnitski D, Walker J, Rosenquist RW. Chronic pain patient and other co-existing conditions (substance abuse, psychiatric). In: Urman R, Vadivelu N, eds. *Perioperative Pain Management*, 1st ed. Oxford University Press; 2013:83–93.

pain is all in your head." This is an all too commonly heard phrase from patients. Imagine how disconcerted a person become when the pain management specialist, whether physician, nurse, physician's assistant, or other healthcare professional, says, "I'd like you to see our psychologist." That person may view the pain management center as the last stop on a frustrating road to recovery. Now the worst fear is validated: no one believes the pain is real. Allaying that fear is critical in making that initial referral to the pain management psychologist, who can further reassure the patient that this is not the case. It may be beneficial for the healthcare professional to provide a handout explaining what a pain management psychologist does, the role that is an integral a part of the treatment team, and, most particularly, why this in no way reflects concerns that the pain is not real.

The pain psychologist validates the impact of chronic pain on all aspects of an individual's life, recognizing among the psychological factors that it is normal to have depression, anxiety, trepidation, anger, and a vast array of emotions as a reaction to the pain, reflective of concerns for normal people caught up in an abnormal situation. It is incumbent upon the psychologist to evaluate the individual patient and then engender an understanding of the impact of the biological factors on the psychological and social well-being of the person and provide reassurance that chronic pain management recognizes the need to treat the entire person and the impact the illness and/or injury has imposed on all aspects of the individual's life. People often lose self-esteem, are readily frustrated when unable to do simple activities that had previously been done by rote, and may generally feel overwhelmed by what they no longer feel capable of accomplishing. Some feel helpless, some hopeless, some even suicidal. Feelings of guilt may be pervasive and may have an impact on or be reinforced by family and friends. People may become desperate and ready to try anything that may offer the least modicum of hope that the pain may be relieved or even cured. For some there is a propensity for denial; for others, perhaps self-pity. There may be loss of a sense of humor, or an easy loss of temper, with anger directed particularly toward those closest—family, friends, coworkers—who then may become alienated. For many, pain is a great distractor; it becomes difficult to concentrate, causing people to question if there really is something wrong with their head. Pain may create a loss of physical, social, vocational, and avocational activities; this can lead to boredom, which is every bit as stressful as having too much to contend with. Of all the psychological factors affecting a patient with pain, perhaps the greatest and most distressing is the perception of a loss of control. The pain is in control of what one does, how much one does, how often one does it, and whether or not one enjoys what used to be pleasurable endeavors. The greatest contribution of the pain management psychologist may be in assisting the person in the acquisition of skills directed toward regaining that internal locus of control.

The psychologist, psychiatrist, or social worker who specializes in pain management also recognizes the impact that chronic pain has on the social aspects of an individual's life, the final component of the biopsychosocial model. There may be a loss of job, loss of income, financial constraints, loss of social activities, including involvement with family and friends, and loss of physical activities, including sports. There may be a loss of sexual activity, which is incorporated across all three components of this paradigm. People may not be able to engage with their children in physical activities and play. Walking the dog may appear to be a Herculean task. Household chores and repairs remain unaccomplished. There may be a power struggle with a spouse, a role reversal in the family. The only muscles receiving a regular workout may be the thumbs from operating remote control devices for the television and video games. There may be inattention to physical appearance, extending to lack of care and even lack of bathing. Isolation may be prevalent. These factors and more are pervasive across biological, psychological, and social domains when dealing with the impact of chronic pain.

Evaluation

First and foremost in the treatment process is to obtain an initial evaluation that explores the history of the illness or injury and the impact it has had on the

Table 3.1 **Evaluation of a Patient with Chronic Pain—Key Points**

Presenting Problem	Current, Past Medications/ Allergies	Emotional and Cognitive Status
Circumstances of onset	Substance use/abuse	Goals and expectations
Interview and observations	Family history and issues	Test data
History of illness/injury	Education/employment	Impressions
Other physical conditions	Interview and observations	Recommendations
Relevant treatment history	Current and past activities	

individual and his or her family, friends, and colleagues, and how the person is dealing with the pain and its repercussions. It is critical that this evaluation be performed specifically by a pain management psychologist and not just by a general practitioner. Patients must trust that the psychologist has an understanding of what their pain problem is from a medical vantage point, how it affects them, and options for treatment. Table 3.1 reflects what might be included in a basic pain management psychology evaluation.

Factors addressed in this evaluation are specifically past and current treatment, including what has and has not worked, substance issues involving alcohol, prescription medications, and illicit drugs. Family history looks at the impact of pain on the family, and may address issues of behavior and reinforcement, as well as abuse, which includes physical, psychological, and/ or sexual. The interview process to assesses the emotional status and cognitive functioning while also observing behavior, appearance, and interactions with others, including family or other support. Concerns regarding depression, anxiety, anger, frustration, memory, concentration, stressors, mood changes, and irritability are evaluated. Suicidal ideation is addressed. The impact of sleep disturbance is also considered. Activities should be reviewed, including activities of daily living, household chores, social and leisure activities relinquished those maintained. Coping strategies and adaptability are also reviewed. Motivation, goals, and expectations, realistic or otherwise, need to be considered. Standardized tests are often used as aids in the assessment process, as well as providing baseline data for follow-up assessment of treatment outcomes.

The evaluator needs to be trained in the fields of pain management and psychology/psychiatry or a related field, be able to assess the pain problem and the impact it has on various aspects of a person's life, and have an understanding of the implications for treatment inherent in these factors. This includes a basic understanding of relevant medical conditions and of related issues the physician may consider regarding treatment options. The evaluator also needs an understanding of the role of other disciplines, such as physical therapy, occupational therapy, pharmacotherapy, vocational rehabilitation, and acupuncture, in treating individuals with a pain problem. The psychological evaluation, often referred to as a behavioral medicine evaluation, should take into account the contributions available from other members of the treatment team as impressions are formed, recommendations made, and communication maintained among members of the team.

While the psychological treatment of chronic pain patients in the hospital setting is discussed in detail elsewhere in this book. It is important to note at the outset that, as the bio-psycho-social model suggests, a multitude of issues need to be addressed in the management of chronic pain. A sample of pain psychology questions and answers is presented in this chapter's Appendix.

Summary

There are distinct psychological and social markers of chronic pain, reflecting the impact of chronic pain on all aspects of an individual's life. The psychological factors incorporate the emotional and cognitive aspects of chronic pain. Social factors extend to issues related to family, friends, work, recreation, and financial and legal components. It is virtually impossible to extricate the individual components from their relationship to one another. Therefore, is it critical to recognize and treat the impact of chronic pain on the entire life of an individual, while also appreciating the impact it has on the other people in that person's life, an impact that extends even to society in general. Chronic pain management mandates a multidisciplinary approach that provides input from many specialties to obtain optimal results.

References

1. Turk DC, Robinson JP. Multidisciplinary assessment of patients. In: Ballantyne J, Rathmell J, Fishman S, eds. *Bonica's Management of Pain*, 4th ed. Philadelphia: Lippincott Williams & Wilkins; 2010:288–301.
2. Fordyce WE. Pain and suffering. A reappraisal. *Am Psychol*. 1988;43:276–283.
3. Turk DC, Monarch ES. Biopsychosocial perspective on chronic pain. In: DC Turk, RJ Gatchel, eds. *Psychological Approaches to Pain Management: A Practitioner's Handbook*, 2nd ed. New York: Guilford Press; 2002:3–29.
4. Apkarian AV, Baliki MN, Geha PY. Towards a theory of chronic pain. *Prog Neurobiol*. 2009;87(2):81–97.
5. Arntz A, Lousberg R. The effects of underestimated pain and their relationship to habituation. *Behav Res Ther*. 1990;28:15–28.
6. Vowles KE, McCracken LM, Eccleston C. Processes of change in treatment for chronic pain: the contributions of pain, acceptance, and catastrophizing. *Eur J Pain*. 2007; 2007;11(7):779–787.
7. Oslund S, Robinson RC, Clark TC, et al. Long-term effectiveness of a comprehensive pain management program: strengthening the case for interdisciplinary care. *Proc (Bayl Univ Med Cent)*. 2009;22(3):211–214.

Appendix: Common Questions and Answers

If I am referred to a psychologist, does it mean my doctor thinks my pain is just in my head and not real?

No. We recognize that your pain is real. Our goal is to help you acquire skills to manage it more effectively, to teach you HOW to live with it, rather than simply expecting you to live with it. We want you to increase function and return to a full and active lifestyle.

What will the psychologist do?

The Psychologist will perform an initial evaluation to learn about your pain, how it affect you specifically, how it may affect others, including your family, and to assess the skills you currently have that work for you, and the skills you have tried that do not work effectively. Testing may be used to better understand the impact of your pain.

What happens in treatment?

After the initial assessment, a treatment plan is formulated with you. It generally focuses strongly on skill acquisition, including relaxation skills, sleep management, pain and stress management, and general coping strategies. Issues of the impact of pain on families and loved ones will also be addressed. Sexual concerns related to chronic pain may be addressed. The overall goal is to increase coping skills and functional activities. Cognitive Behavioral therapy is used to help you adjust your perspective regarding your pain and the impact it has on your life.

Will the psychologist prescribe medicine?

No. A psychologist has a doctoral degree, but is not a doctor of medicine; that person is not licensed to prescribe medication. However, he or she can discuss medication concerns with you and your physician.

4

Pain Assessment Scales, Clinical Tools and Techniques

ANKIT MAHESHWARI AND RICHARD D. URMAN

KEY POINTS

- The accurate assessment of hospitalized chronic pain patients is essential for effective acute pain control.
- Simple measures of pain assessment such as the numerical rating scale (NRS) are applicable in most chronic pain patients. However, in select patient populations such as older adults with severe dementia and patients with complex chronic pain conditions, specialized multidimensional tools are required for assessment and treatment.
- Common freely available tools can be incorporated in routine clinical practice or help must be sought from the pain specialist to assess patients with complex pain in to prevent undertreatment of patients who cannot express their pain and overtreatment of patients who report high pain intensity scores.
- The baseline pain score should be highlighted. Generally, it is not realistic to expect mild pain scores—less than 4/10—during hospital admission for someone whose baseline pain score has been severe for a long time prior to admission.

Introduction

Pain is considered the sixth vital sign; it is a performance measure for hospitals and an important patient satisfaction parameter.[1] Most importantly, it is a cause of distress for patients and must be treated appropriately. Therefore, accurate assessment and reporting of pain is very important. Pain assessment may be difficult for patients with chronic pain conditions and for children and cognitively impaired adults. This chapter presents pain assessment scales and clinical tools which are commonly used for pain assessment in hospitalized patients.

Pain Assessment in Patients with Chronic Pain

SIMPLE PAIN SCALES

Single-item measures of pain intensity are the most commonly used measures in clinical practice. The three used most are the visual analog scale, numerical rating scale, and verbal rating scale (Figure 4.1).

Visual Analog Scale (VAS)
A VAS consists of a line, usually 100 mm long, with the ends of the line labeled with descriptors of the intensity of pain ("no pain" to "extreme pain"). Respondents place a mark along the line, which represents their intensity of pain. The mark is then measured using a scale and the value recorded in millimeters. The VAS is well validated and shows sensitivity to changes in the intensity of pain with treatment.[2,3] The VAS has the advantage of having a higher number of response categories (0–100 mm), thus making it more sensitive to assess response to treatment. It can be easily administered to even sick elderly patients who are cognitively intact.

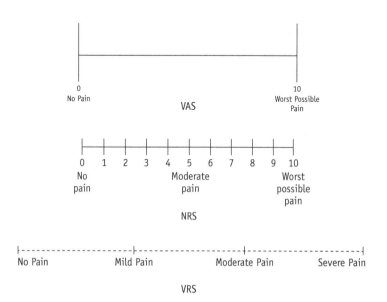

Figure 4.1 Visual analog pain scale (VAS), numerical rating scale (NRS), and verbal rating scale (VRS).

Numerical Rating Scale (NRS)

An NRS consists of a range of numbers (usually 0–10). Respondents are told that the lowest number represents no pain and the highest number represents the worst pain you can imagine. Like the VRS, the NRS has also been demonstrated to be sensitive to treatment of pain.[4] It is easy to administer and is one of the most common tools used with hospitalized patients for the assessment of pain. It shows strong associations with other pain rating scales.[5]

Visual Rating Scale (VRS)

The VRS consists of a list of descriptors such as none, mild, moderate, and severe. Each of the descriptors is associated with a number, which helps in objectively recording the response—for example, none is 0 and severe is 4. Studies have described VRS use with anywhere from 4 to 15 descriptors of pain intensity. Like the VAS and NRS, the VRS demonstrates sensitivity to changes in pain with treatment.[6] Of the three, this is the least common method used with hospitalized patients, although the term *VRS* is sometimes used loosely to refer to either the NRS or VAS. This scale assumes that patients comprehend the meaning of the descriptors in the same way. This assumption may not be reasonable when patients have diverse cultural and educational backgrounds.

It is important to define the meaning of the numbers on the VRS as well as the line on the VAS each time one is administered to the patient. Merely asking patients to assign their pain a number from 0 to 10 may result in overtreatment. In addition to the scale, it is important to use other descriptors of pain to truly assess the nature of pain and to differentiate the patient's acute pain from a chronic pain condition. A Dutch study showed that a majority of patients did not want to be treated with opiate medications despite reporting a pain score >4, which is conventionally used as a guide to treatment.[7]

MULTIDIMENSIONAL PAIN SCALES

Multidimensional pain scales measure the sensory, affective, and cognitive components of pain. Pain has sensory and affective qualities in addition to intensity. While cumbersome, these scales can provide more objective information regarding these components of pain. Use of standardized pain questionnaires when managing patients' chronic pain can reduce patient reporting biases. Selected questionnaires are specific for specific pain problems such as neuropathic pain, arthritic pain, cancer pain, and headache. A pain specialist may be involved in the care of patients who appear to have complex pain problems. A detailed discussion regarding the specialized pain scales and their validity with specific pain conditions is beyond the scope of this chapter; however, some of the commonly used pain questionnaires in the hospital setting are discussed next.

McGill Pain Questionnaire (MPQ)

The McGill Pain questionnaire is a common tool and may be especially helpful in assessing patients with chronic pain conditions. It has 78 descriptors classified in 20 categories.[8]

Brief Pain Inventory (BPI)

The BPI was designed for assessment of cancer pain but it is also widely used to assess other types of pain. It is easier to administer than several other questionnaires and has been well validated for a variety of chronic pain conditions.[9]

PAIN ASSESSMENT IN SELECTED PATIENT POPULATIONS

Pediatric Patients

Assessment of pain in this patient population may have to rely on surrogate measures of pain, such as vital signs and behaviors.

Behavioral changes include crying, grimacing, consolability, sleep state, and movements of the limbs and body. Cry can be described in terms of pitch and duration. Facial expressions may include brow bulge, eye squeeze, nasolabial furrowing, open lips, and taut tongue.[10] The reliability and validity of these measures are highest for acute and post-procedural pain. Overlap may occur with other states such as sleep deprivation and hunger.

The Face, Legs, Activity, Cry, Consolability (FLACC) scale[11] and Children's Hospital of Eastern Ontario Pain Scale (CHEOPS)[12] have been well validated for assessment of acute post-procedural pain. Another good composite scoring system is the COMFORT scale, which can be used across a wide variety of ages.[13] The key characteristics of these scales are summarized in Table 4.1. Actual scales can be obtained for clinical use after proprietary approval.

Changes in physiological parameters which have been associated with post-procedural pain include changes in heart rate, respiratory rate, blood pressure, palmar sweating, tissue oxygenation, and intracranial pressure, where applicable. The specificity of these measures is not high and the context of changes in these parameters has to be considered. During a procedure, these measures may be good markers of pain.

Several pain scales have been designed for the neonate and premature infant. Similarly, there are specific pain scales to assess pain in children with cognitive impairment, such as the Non-Communicating Children Pain Scale (NCCPC).[14] These scales are important to use because it has been shown that pain in non-communicating children may be undertreated. Pain assessment by clinicians and even by parents using surrogate markers such as crying does not correlate well with the actual pain in this patient population.

The older child may be provided a VAS-type scale with facial expressions (e.g., Wong Baker Faces Pain Rating Scale, depending on their comprehension level.

Table 4.1 **Pain Assessment Scales**

Pain Scale	Nonverbal Signs	Age Group
CHEOPS	Cry Facial Expression Verbal expression Torso position Touch Leg position	1–7 years
FLACC	Face Legs Activity Cry Consolability	Children
COMFORT Scale	Alertness Calmness Respiratory response Physical movement Muscle tone Facial expression Mean arterial pressure Heart rate	Newborn to adolescent

CHEOPS: Children's Hospital of Eastern Ontario Pain Scale; FLACC: Face, Legs, Activity, Cry, Consolability.

Elderly Patients

The elderly patient population is complex given the presence of more than one complaint and comorbidities affecting pain while the person is hospitalized.

In elderly patients with severe dementia, nonverbal cues may have to be used for pain assessment (Table 4.2), although, it has been shown that self-report of pain may still be reliable and valid for most of these patients.[15,16] Therefore, obtaining self-report of pain is advocated whenever possible.

Tools like the VAS, NRS, and VAS can be effectively used in this patient population to evaluate pain intensity. In addition, the Wong-Baker Faces scale and color-coded scales that range from blue (no pain) to bright red (severe pain) may be helpful. A problem with simply assessing intensity of pain is that clinicians may discount self-reports of pain from patients with cognitive impairment because of inconsistencies in self-report.[17]

ICU Patients

Inconsistent or ambiguous documentation of pain scores has been reported for intensive care unit (ICU) patients.[18] Simple pain scales may not be easily

Table 4.2 **Nonverbal Indicators of Pain in Cognitively Impaired Older Adults**

Behaviors	Agitation
	Anger
	Uneasiness
	Wincing
	Grimacing
	Sad/depressed
	Withdrawn
Vocalizations	Crying
	Grunting
	Groaning
	Moaning
	Shouting
Physical features	Guarding
	Limping
	Abnormal posture or weight bearing
	Decreased level of activity
	Decreased appetite
	Poor sleep
	Rubbing
	Restlessness: arm, leg and body
	repositioning
	Clenched fists
	Heavy breathing

administered in this patient population. Intubated but coherent patients can be asked about pain intensity using the NRS, VAS, or VRS and asked to mark the most appropriate response. Being intubated and mildly sedated does not preclude directly assessing pain intensity by self-report.

The intubated and sedated patient should be assessed using other surrogate markers, including limb movements and body movements, and physiological markers such as heart rate and blood pressure should be used in the context of a painful intervention such as endotracheal tube suctioning or a bedside procedure. The Richmond Agitation and Sedation Score (RASS), though not designed for pain, is a good scale to use when attempting to achieve comfort for these patients.[19]

Cancer Patients

Cancer-related pain is complex and clearly multidimensional because of the sensory and affective components involved. It may also be diffuse and involve several anatomical areas. A body chart (figure of the human body) to mark areas of pain may be helpful in treating pain appropriately. Cancer pain affects several domains of life; most validated assessment tools include other parameters that measure not only measure pain but its impact on life. Commonly used specialized pain scales available for assessing these patients include the MD Anderson Symptom Assessment Scale[20] and the BPI.[9]

Anxiety and depression may be closely associated with pain in these patients, thus comprehensive evaluation using validated scales is recommended. Several other validated scales are available to assess the impact of anxiety and depression on pain and the impact of the disease condition on function and activities of daily living. While it is hard to routinely implement these complex scales in clinical practice, they should be used when the intensity of pain alone is not adequate for pain treatment.

Summary

Accurate assessment of pain in hospitalized patients is necessary for effective treatment. Simple measures of pain assessment, such as the NRS, are applicable in most uncomplicated scenarios. However, in select patient populations, such as elderly persons with severe dementia and patients with complex chronic pain conditions, specialized multidimensional tools are required for assessment and treatment. Common freely available tools can be incorporated in routine clinical practice, or help must be sought from a pain specialist to assess patients with complex pain. This prevents undertreatment of patients who cannot express their pain and overtreatment of patients who report high pain intensity scores.

References

1. The Joint Commission. Pain management standards. Vol. 2000. http://www.jointcommission.org/topics/pain_management.aspx, Accessed July 24 2015.
2. Joyce CRB, Zutshi DW, Hrubes V, et al. Comparison of fixed interval and visual analog scales for rating chronic pain. *Eur J Clin Pharmacol*. 1975;8:415–420.
3. Joshi GP, Viscusi ER, Gan TJ, et al. Effective treatment of laparscopic cholecystectomy with intravenous followed by oral COX-2 specific inhibitor. *Anesth Analg*. 2004;98:336–342.
4. Chesney MA, Shelton JL. A comparison of muscle relaxation and electromyography biofeedback treatments for muscle contraction headache. *J Behav Ther Exp Psychiatry*. 1976;7:221–225.
5. Kremer EF, Atkinson JH Jr, Ignelzi RJ. Measurement of pain: patient preference does not confound measurement. *Pain*. 1981;10:241–248.
6. Fox EJ, Melzack R. Transcutaneous electrical stimulation and acupuncture: comparison of treatment for low back pain. *Pain*. 1976;2:141–148.

7. van Dijk JFM, Kappen TH, Schurmaans MJ, et al. The relationship between patients' NRS pain scoresand their desire for additional opioids after surgery. *Pain Practice*. 2014. doi:10.1111/papr.12217.

8. Melzack R. The McGill Pain Questionnaire: major properties and scoring methods. *Pain*. 1975;1:277–299.

9. Cleland CS, Ryan KM. Pain assessment: global use of the brief pain inventory. *Ann Acad Med*. 1994;23:129–138.

10. Craig KD. The facial display of pain. In: Finley GA, McGrath PJ, eds. *Measurement of Pain in Infants and Children. Progress in Pain Research and Management*, Vol. 10;IASP Press. Seattle, WA: 1998:103–122.

11. Merkel SI, Voepel-Lewis T, Shayevitz JR, et al. The FLACC: a behavioral scale for scoring post operative pain in young children. *Pediatr Nurs*. 1997;23:293–297.

12. McGrath PJ, Johnson G, Goodman JT. CHEOPS: a behavioral scale for rating post operative pain in children. In: Fields HL, Dubner R, Cervero F, eds. *Advances in Pain Research and Therapy*, Vol. 9. New York: Raven Press; 1985:395–402.

13. Ambuel B, Hamlett KW, Marx CM, et al. Assessing distress in pediatric intensive care environments: the COMFORT scale. *J Pediatr Psychol*. 1992;17:95–109.

14. McGrath PJ, Rosmus C, Camfield C, et al. Behaviors caregivers use to determine pain in non-verbal cognitively impaired individuals. *Dev Med Child Neurol*. 1998;40:340–343.

15. Feldt KS, Ryden MB, Miles S. Treatment of pain in cognitively impaired compared with cognitively intact older adult patients with hip fratures. *J Am Geriatr Soc*. 1998;46(9):1079–1085.

16. Ferrell BA, Ferrell BR. Pain assessment among cognitively impaired nursing home residetns. *J Am Geriatr Soc*. 1993;41:24.

17. Sengstaken EA, King SA. The problems of pain and it's detection among geriatric nursing home residents. *J Am Geriatr Soc*. 1993;41:541.

18. Haslam L, Dale C, Knechtel L, et al. Pain descriptors for critically ill patients unable to self report. *J Adv Nurs*. 2012;68:1082–1089.

19. Ely EW, Truman B, Shintani A, et al. Monitoring sedation status over time in ICU patients: the reliability and validity of the Richmond Agitation Sedation Scale (RASS). *JAMA*. 2003;289:2983–2991.

20. Cleland CS, Mendoza TR, Wang XS, et al. Assessing symptom distress in cancer: the MD Anderson Symptom Inventory. *Cancer*. 2000;89:1634–1646.

5

Opioids: An Overview

DANIEL J. LEIZMAN, ALPARSLAN TURAN, AND SHAHBAZ QAVI

KEY POINTS

- The U.S. Food and Drug Administration (FDA) defines opioid tolerance as use of 60 mg morphine equivalence for 7 days or longer. A significant number of hospital admissions would meet this definition of opioid tolerance.
- Management of opioid-dependent patients' pain in the hospital setting can be challenging for the physician as well as for nursing staff and other healthcare providers.
- It is advisable that the same maintenance dosage of opioids be continued for chronic pain patients in the hospital unless contraindicated; one can consider increasing the dose for acute pain or surgery.
- Conversion and rotation of opioids should be carried out effectively and safely in hospitalized patients.
- Patients who state a better effect of one opioid than that of another should not be categorized as "drug seekers" because genetic and other individual variations may influence individual sensitivity to opioid pharmacotherapy.
- Inpatient pain management care of hospitalized patients serves as the foundation of their treatment plan and as a conduit for what is done subsequently for them as outpatients.

Introduction

Opioids are often used as a component of treatment for moderate to severe chronic, nonmalignant pain. The past 15 years have seen an increase in prescriptions of opioids for treating chronic pain, as well as increases in opiate diversion and abuse, in overdose-related deaths, and in the number of individuals being treated for opiate addiction.[1,2] The guiding therapeutic goal of opioid therapy for chronic pain management should be achieving satisfactory patient analgesia and maximizing functional ability. Use of the lowest possible dose is recommended, to decrease the likelihood of side effects and physical and behavioral complications. Behavioral and psychosocial complications of opioid therapy include concomitant substance abuse (including concomitant illicit opioid use), addiction, multisourcing opioids from various providers, diversion, use of prescription opiates to achieve an opiate high, and self-medicating mood disturbances. The success of opioid therapy for chronic pain management should be assessed subjectively in terms of self-reported patient pain levels but also, more importantly, objectively in terms of functional outcome measurement. Inpatient pain management care of hospitalized patients serves as the foundation of their treatment plan and as a conduit for what is done subsequently for them as outpatients.

In terms of the history of opioid use, it is not known where and when the first opium poppy was first cultivated. The first written records of historical use of opioids for therapeutic benefit dates back to the third century b.c.e. Their introduction into Western medicine for the relief of pain has earned these drugs a unique place in medical and public perception.[3] While the term *opiate* is commonly used as a synonym for opioid, the appropriate use of this term is restricted to the natural alkaloids found in the opium poppy (*Papaver somniferum*). Conversely, the term *opioid* refers to both synthetic substances and opiates, as well as to opioid peptides.

Opioids exert their main analgesic activity on opioid receptors. Opioids are known to be the most potent analgesics available. Thus with the imperative to treat patients' moderate to severe pain, opioids have been established as the most important tool in the treatment of pain usually associated with cancer and pain associated with terminal illness.[4] Patients with moderate to severe chronic nonmalignant pain are also commonly prescribed opiate medications.[5,6]

Epidemiological studies indicate that use of opioids for chronic non-cancer pain has increased substantially over the last two decades. In one large U.S. survey, the proportion of office visits for chronic musculoskeletal pain in which any opioids were prescribed doubled from 8% in 1980 to 16% in 2001.[2] Use of more potent opioids (such as morphine, hydromorphone, oxycodone, and fentanyl) has also increased.[7] Over the same two decades, the proportion of office visits in which prescriptions for potent opioids were given increased from 2% to 9%.[2]

The etiologies of these non-cancer chronic pain conditions are often musculoskeletal and neurological in origin.[8,9] Examples include cervical spinal stenosis, cervical spondylosis, cervical radicular pain, lumbar spinal stenosis, lumbar degenerative disc disease, lumbar radicular pain, degenerative joint disease, traumatic orthopedic injuries, postherpetic neuralgia, and various types of neuropathic pain of peripheral and central origin.[8-11]

Although the term *chronic non-cancer pain* encompasses pain associated with a wide diversity of conditions, common treatment goals, regardless of the underlying cause, are pain relief and/or improvement in physical and psychological functioning. Physicians should limit long-term opioid prescribing to patients with well-defined pain conditions who have not responded to non-opioid treatments and for whom opioids have been shown to be effective. The prescribing physician is often challenged with the need to treat chronic pain by relieving pain and improving function yet minimizing unwanted side effects and the risk of complications.

With this framework in mind, this chapter discusses the concepts and use of opioid therapy for managing chronic non-cancer pain. It includes descriptions of various chemical groups of opioids and delivery routes of opioid therapy. Common side effects and concerns of using opioid therapy area also presented, as is evidence of the efficacy of opioid therapy for chronic pain management. Opioid conversion and opioid rotation are defined, and examples of application in patient care are given. Finally, recommended principles for guiding chronic pain management are summarized.

Opioid Compounds and Treatment Options

Opioid compounds have been classified as short- or long-acting on the basis of their duration of action. The short-acting compounds have a more rapid increase and decrease in serum levels compared to long-acting compounds. Long-acting opioids have less fluctuation in plasma concentration, which is associated with higher patient satisfaction because of fewer inadequate pain control periods. Studies comparing short-acting to long-acting opioids in regard to analgesia have shown inconsistent results, with no superiority of one over the other. When dosed on a fixed schedule, they have very similar total systemic opioid concentrations and pain control. Decisions regarding which type to use to treat chronic pain should be individualized to patient needs and response to treatment regimens.

Opioids are also classified as full agonists, partial agonists, or mixed agonist-antagonists, depending on their effect on opioid receptors. Most commonly used drugs, such as morphine, hydromorphone, codeine, oxycodone, oxymorphone, hydrocodone, methadone, levorphanol, and fentanyl, are classified as full agonists. Partial agonists (e.g., buprenorphine) have a ceiling effect and are less effective at opioid receptors. Mixed agonist-antagonists (e.g., pentazocine, butorphanol, and nalbuphine) either block or don't affect one opioid receptor while activating a different opioid receptor (Table 5.1).

IMMEDIATE-RELEASE MEDICATIONS

Immediate-release medications are designed for occasional and temporary pain relief because they work fast, but this pain relief is usually short-lived. Thus these

Table 5.1 **Opioid Classifications Based on Source and Related Structural Group**

Opioid Analgesic	Source of Chemical	Morphine-Related Structure with 6-Hydroxyl Group	Related Structural Group
Alfentanil	Synthetic		Meperidine
Alphaprofine	Synthetic		Meperidine
Buprenorphine	Semi-synthetic	No	Morphine
Butophanol	Synthetic	No	Morphine
Codeine	Natural	Yes	Morphine
Dezocine	Synthetic		Morphine
Dihydrocodeine	Semi-synthetic	Yes	Morphine
Fentanyl	Synthetic		Meperidine
Hydrocodone	Semi-synthetic	No	Morphine
Hydromorphone	Semi-synthetic	No	Morphine
Levorphanol	Semi-synthetic	No	Morphine
Meperidine	Synthetic		Meperidine
Methadone	Synthetic		Unique
Morphine	Natural	Yes	Morphine
Nalbuphine	Semi-synthetic	Yes	Morphine
Oxycodone	Semi-synthetic	No	Morphine
Oxymorphone	Semi-synthetic	No	Morphine
Pentazocine	Synthetic		Morphine
Propoxyphene	Synthetic		Methadone
Sufentanil	Synthetic		Meperidine
Tramadol	Synthetic		Unique

short-acting medications are used "as needed for pain," but they can also be used as scheduled drugs. Commonly used medications include morphine, hydromorphone, oxymorphone, codeine, fentanyl, hydrocodone, and oxycodone. Codeine, hydrocodone, and oxycodone are also available in combination with acetaminophen or a nonsteroidal anti-inflammatory drug (NSAID).

INTRAVENOUS MEDICATIONS

Intravenous pain medications are most commonly employed during the immediate postoperative period. Intravenous opioids are usually given alone, and most commonly include morphine sulfate, fentanyl, hydromorphone, and, rarely, meperidine and tramadol (Table 5.2). The intravenous route has several advantages, including absorption and bioavailability, ability to bypass the

Table 5.2 **Commonly Used Intravenous Drugs**

Opiod	PRN Dosing	PCA On-demand Dosing
Morphine	1–4 mg	0.5–1.0 mg
Hydromorphone	0.5–2 mg	0.1–0.3 mg
Fentanyl	25–100 µg	5–25 µg

oral route when oral administration is not available or not indicated, and ease of administration on a scheduled or as-needed basis. There are also a number of disadvantages of intravenous application: the need to maintain an indwelling intravenous catheter, potency of drugs, increased risk of incorrect dosage or drug misidentification, possibility of infection, and requirement of having a healthcare professional to administer medications.

PATIENT-CONTROLLED ANALGESIA

Patient-controlled analgesia (PCA) is an effective and unique method for administering opioids to patients for pain relief, and it gives patients a sense of control over their pain. The drugs are given via the help of a pump and require an indwelling intravenous, transdermal, intrathecal, or incisional articular catheter. PCA provides significant benefit to nurse-administered medications because response time is minimal and patient satisfaction is higher with PCA. The pumps are usually easy to operate, and limited dosing is accepted as safe. Even pediatric patients have been able to use PCA successfully. A very important safety feature of PCA is that patients who are oversedated will not be able to press the button to obtain dangerous doses of the drug. This safety feature is only overridden if someone else pushes the button for them. Patients must be cognitively and physically capable of understanding the use of PCA, which limits use in many pediatric patients and in confused, elderly patients. Another critical factor in decreasing errors with use of PCA is patient and family education.

Common indications for PCA are postoperative pain, severe acute pain, cancer pain, or the patient being unable to tolerate oral medications. Most common medications used are opioids—morphine, fentanyl, and hydromorphone; local anesthetics—bupivacaine and ropivacaine; or clonidine or baclofen. Sometimes a combination of these drugs is used—specifically, local anesthetics are combined in epidural or intrathecal use to achieve synergistic effect at lower doses without increasing the side effects that would result if used alone at higher doses. The PCA is employed until transition to oral medications is possible, the pain is well controlled, and the patient can tolerate oral medications.

The PCA device can be used with or without a background infusion. If a background is used, then a continuous rate needs to be included in the settings. Settings include a bolus dose (patient demand dose); a period when the patient cannot obtain the medication, called a lockout period; and number of doses per hour, defining the maximum amount of medication that can be delivered. The number of unsuccessful demands a patient makes is often used as a guide to adjusting the settings of PCA. However, there may be other reasons for increased demand rate other than pain, including anxiety, patient confusion, or inappropriate patient use.

Most cancer and chronic pain patients will need PCA demand and continuous dosing. Studies have shown conflicting results as to whether opioid use with PCA is more effective than using conventional methods of opioid analgesia. There also seems to be no consensus on difference in incidence of side effects; however, respiratory depression due to oversedation seems to be less common with PCA.

Non-opioid analgesic drugs, such as ketamine, and/or antiemetics like ondansetron have been added to the opioids in PCA to improve analgesia and possibly decrease side effects. Currently, there is no clear evidence to suggest any benefit from the combination over independent administration of the same drug.

ORAL MEDICATIONS

Morphine

Morphine is one of the most commonly used and oldest known prototype of pure μ-agonist. Only about 40% of the administered dose reaches the central compartment because of presystemic elimination (i.e., metabolism in the liver). Morphine has two active metabolites, morphine-6-glucuronide and morphine-3-glucuronide. Morphine-6-glucuronide binds to the opioid receptor and is responsible for long duration of action in patients with renal failure. Morphine-3-glucuronide contributes to some adverse effects, such as myoclonus and confusion. These side effects are much more apparent in patients with renal failure. Morphine is available in immediate-release and extended-release formulations. Immediate-release and extended-release formulations seem to vary little in their degree of pain relief, side effects, or adverse events.

Immediate-release oral morphine drugs achieve steady state in 24 hours when given in a fixed dosing regimen. Although there is no relationship between blood levels and analgesic effect, efficient analgesia will not occur below certain minimum blood levels. The elimination of morphine occurs primarily as renal excretion of active metabolites. A small portion of the glucuronide conjugate is excreted in the bile. The elimination half-life of morphine is between 2 and 4 hours.

Morphine immediate-release tablets are available; dosing is 5–30 mg PO every 4 hours in opioid-naïve patients. Oral solution dosing is 10–20 mg PO every 4 hours in opioid-naïve patients. In addition, 5 mg oral immediate-release morphine is usually given for rescue.

Hydromorphone (Dilaudid)

Hydromorphone is a semi-synthetic opioid (hydrogenated ketone of morphine) agonist that was introduced into clinical practice in the 1920s. Hydromorphone has a short half-life (2 to 3 hours), which facilitates dose titration but complicates efforts to use it for chronic pain. Compared to morphine, hydromorphone is more potent. The equianalgesic ratio in the literature ranges from 2 to 12; however, the most commonly accepted ratio is about 7:1 (morphine to hydromorphone). Side effects with hydromorphone are similar to those of opioids in general and most often include constipation, nausea, and sedation. Hydromorphone is metabolized in the liver, with approximately 62% of the oral dose being eliminated by the liver on the first pass. For orally administered immediate-release preparations, the onset of action is approximately 30–40 minutes and duration is 3–4 hours. Hydromorphone is preferred over morphine for patients with decreased renal clearance, to decrease the risk the toxicity from accumulation of morphine metabolites. Patients with hepatic and renal impairment should be started on a lower starting dose. Hydromorphone is metabolized to 3-glucoronide metabolite, which has been associated with dose-dependent excited behaviors, including allodynia, myoclonus, and seizures in animal models.

Hydromorphone is available not only in tablets but also in an oral liquid form, which makes it more suitable for patients who have swallowing and gastrointestinal problems. The usual starting dose for hydromorphone tablets is 2 mg to 4 mg, orally, every 4 to 6 hours, and for oral liquid is 2.5 mL to 10 mL (2.5–10 mg), every 3 to 6 hours. Furthermore, a breakthrough dose should be given. It is important that dosage is individualized because adverse events can occur at doses that may not provide complete relief from pain.

Oxycodone

Oxycodone is a phenanthrene class opioid provided in pure form, or in combination with acetaminophen or aspirin. Bioavailability of oxycodone is high and the half-life is 3 hours. It is metabolized in the liver by glucuronidation to noroxycodone, and by 2D6 to oxymorphone, which is excreted in urine. Since oxycodone is dependent on the cytochrome P450 (CYP) 2D6 pathway for clearance, it is possible that drug–drug interactions can occur with CYP 2D6 inhibitors. Furthermore, there is considerable variation in the efficiency and amount of CYP 2D6 enzyme produced between individuals. Unpredictable individual responses to treatment are sometimes related to these properties of the drug.

Oxycodone tablets contain different amounts of acetaminophen—325, 500, and 650—and 2.5 mg, 5 mg, 7.5 mg, and 10 mg active drug. When these drugs are used, care must be taken to not exceed the recommended maximal dose of the coanalgesic (for example, 4 g or less of acetaminophen per day). The modified-release formulation of oxycodone is now widely used for management of chronic pain.

Methadone

Methadone is a synthetic medication used to treat opioid addiction and is prescribed as an opioid of choice for patients with chronic pain and comorbid substance use disorders. Methadone occurs in R- and S-enantomeric forms. The R-form binds to opioid receptor and S-form blocks the N-methyl-D-aspartate (NMDA) receptor. Methadone is rapidly absorbed from the stomach, with 60%–70% bioavailability, and analgesic effect starts in 30 to 60 minutes. Analgesia from methadone lasts for 4-6 hours, thus a dosing of up to 3–4 times per day is suggested for analgesia. Methadone is metabolized to inactive forms by liver and intestinal CYP 3A4 and CYP 2D6. Metabolites of methadone are then excreted in feces and urine. Mild and moderate liver and renal disease do not seem to affect pharmacokinetics. Age doesn't seem to affect clearance. Patients with end-stage renal disease require a 50% decrease in dosing.

The most frequent side effects seen with methadone are respiratory depression and sedation. Methadone has been associated with prolongation of the QT interval, which can cause life-threatening cardiac arrhythmia. Methadone dosing requires close monitoring, use of low starting doses, an adequate interval between dose changes, and caution when treating patients who have heart disease or use medications that have effects on the QT interval. Weight gain, sexual dysfunction, decrease in testosterone levels, constipation, and cognitive slowing are some of the common side effects related to chronic methadone use.

Equianalgesic doses for methadone and other opioids are not well defined. Usually, chronic pain treatment with methadone should begin with a low dose (5 mg 2–3 times a day) and then gradually increase, depending on the response. Low cost and long half-life make it affordable for patients who cannot otherwise obtain sustained-release opioids. The opioid equianalgesic table is located on the cover of this book.

Levorphanol

Levorphanol is a synthetic morphine analogue and the optical isomer of dextromethorphan. It has μ, κ, and δ agonist, as well as NMDA antagonist effects. The NMDA antagonist effect makes it more suitable for treating neuropathic pain. Levorphanol is well absorbed after oral administration and reaches peak plasma concentrations in approximately 1 hour. It is metabolized in the liver and is eliminated as the glucuronide metabolite through the kidneys. It has a similar degree of respiratory depression properties to those of other opioids.

Like methadone, there is a variable dosing equivalent: for morphine doses less than 100 mg, the conversion factor is 12:1, while doses over 600 mg may need a conversion factor of 25:1. There is cross-tolerance among opioids when converting a patient from morphine to levorphanol. The total daily dose of oral levorphanol should begin at approximately 1/15 to 1/12 the total daily dose of oral morphine that the patient previously required. It should then be adjusted in accord with the patient's clinical response.

BUCCAL MEDICATIONS

Fentanyl

Fentanyl is a highly lipophilic opioid that can be absorbed through membranes, including transmucosal membranes. Transmucosal fentanyl absorption, through oral mucosa, is more rapid than oral absorption. It is better tolerated in patients with dysphagia, nausea, or vomiting and minimizes first-pass metabolism.

The very first fentanyl intended for oral transmucosal use was introduced in 1999. *Oral transmucosal fentanyl citrate* (OTFC) is a buccal formulation of a fentanyl lozenge on a lollipop. Fentanyl is available in six strengths: 200 μg, 400 μg, 600 μg, 800 μg, 1200 μg, and 1600 μg. The patient places and then rubs the fentanyl against the mucosa, which dissolves over 15 minutes. One-quarter of the OTFC`s total dose is absorbed by the buccal mucosa, and 75% of the dose is swallowed and then absorbed from the gastrointestinal tract, where two-thirds is eliminated via first-pass metabolism. The bioavailability of OTFC is therefore ~50% of the total dose. The main use of these drugs is for breakthrough pain (BTP) in chronic pain or acute postoperative pain. When compared with an intravenous route, pain relief is lower, but ease of use brings advantages. Second generations of delivery systems, like buccal tablets and buccal soluble film, provide a refinement enabling better drug absorption.

Fentanyl buccal soluble film is approved for treatment of BTP. Fentanyl is included in a film that adheres to the buccal mucosa inside of the cheek, dissolving within 15–30 minutes, releasing fentanyl, which passively diffuses into the bloodstream. It requires a minimal quantity of saliva. The proportion of the fentanyl that undergoes transmucosal absorption is approximately 50%, and the absolute bioavailability is approximately 71%. The usual starting dose is 200 μg per episode and can be increased by 200 μg increments. For persisting pain, an 800 or 1200 μg dose can be given as well. Each dose must be separated by 2 hours.

Fentanyl buccal tablets have been designed to treat episodes of BTP. Fentanyl buccal tablets involve an effervescent drug-delivery system to penetrate across the buccal mucosa. Dosing is 100, 200, 400, 600, and 800 μg and can be repeated after 30 minutes if pain control is insufficient. The median time to peak plasma concentration is about 50 minutes, possibly due to a large dose absorbed transmucosally. In studies, patients stated that the 30-minute post-dose medication performance was "good" to "excellent" in 41% of BTP episodes, compared with

26% of episodes treated with oxycodone ($p < 0.0001$), and more patients preferred fentanyl buccal tablets over oxycodone.

All of the transmucosal versions of the fentanyl start to be effective after
30 minutes, with similar analgesic efficacy; treatment selection should be
based on side-effect profiles, ease of use, and suitability for the individual
patient.

EXTENDED-RELEASE MEDICATIONS

Extended-release medication by definition means that these drugs slowly
release in the body over an extended period of time. Extended-release and long-
acting opioids are available in several forms—tablets, liquids, and skin patches.

Efficacy of Long-Term Opioid Therapy for Treatment of Chronic Nonmalignant Pain

Opioid medication therapy is typically very efficacious in relieving acute pain;
however, there is limited information in the literature regarding long-term use.
Available data have demonstrated modest benefit in relation to pain intensity.[12]
Recent reviews evaluating long-term use of opioids found only modest evidence
of efficacy,[13] and there are few trials comparing opioids with other drugs.[14]
Currently, there is no high-quality evidence to suggest superior efficacy of any
specific opioid preparation or formulation in long-term use.[15]

EFFICACY OF OPIOID THERAPY FOR CHRONIC PAIN MANAGEMENT WITH FUNCTIONAL OUTCOME MEASUREMENT

Data demonstrating improvements in quality of life and/or functional
improvement with opioid therapy are lacking in the literature. Additionally,
general physical activity monitoring in chronic pain rehabilitation is usually
limited to functional indices like range of motion, endurance exercises, or
self-reporting.[16,17]

Side Effects of Opioid Therapy and Related Concerns

Treating chronic pain with long-term opioid usage comes with particular concerns. These include opioid tolerance, opioid-induced hyperalgesia, drug/dose
escalation, overdose-associated death, abuse, and diversion.[18-20] Prescription
opioid abuse is currently an epidemic in the United States, causing addiction,

greater healthcare utilization, and 70% drugs going to abusers.[21,22] The common side effects and complications of opioid therapy are as follows:

- Constipation
- Decreased testosterone
- Opioid-induced hyperalgesia
- Overdose
- Opioid dependence
- Opioid-dependent neonates
- Opioid tolerance, efficacy issues, drug/dose escalation issues
- Misuse and/or addiction (19%–26% of hospitalized patients have substance use disorders)
- Respiratory depression (though not common in chronic usage if being used regularly according to instructions)

Use of the newer opioid antagonists with only peripheral action may help avoid some of the side effects without losing the central opioid analgesic effects. This is possible because of either limited systemic bioavailability of these medications or a peripherally restricted site of action, as they don't cross the blood-brain barrier. One of the available medications, alvimopan, may help with ileus associated with opioid use. It is important to note, however, that alvimopan is contraindicated in patients taking therapeutic doses of opioids for more than 7 days. Another peripherally acting μ-receptor antagonist, methylnaltrexone, can be used as well. It is a quaternary naltrexone derivative, which is restricted from crossing the blood-brain barrier. It blocks peripheral opioids' side effects on the gastrointestinal tract, mainly constipation. It is administered subcutaneously. Because of limited systemic availability of the extended-release naloxone formulation, a combination of extended-release naloxone with extended-release oxycodone can be used during the rehabilitation phase to lessen the degree of opioid-induced motor stasis of the bowels without decreasing its analgesic effects. Naloxegol is an oral agent which has been recently approved for opioid-induced constipation.

Another common side effect of opioids is itching. The precise control of opioid-induced itching through peripherally acting opioid receptor antagonists has not yet been successful, however, possibly because of a central component in the mechanism of opioid-induced itching.

Opioid-dependent patients typically experience less nausea and itching than their opioid-naïve counterparts. Respiratory compromise, however, and unwarranted sedation are quite common. One of the reasons for these effects is concomitant use of benzodiazepine anxiolytics and other sedative agents, which invariably are requested by many opioid-dependent patients. Consumption of high doses of opioids can bring about circumstances in which an intensive care team needs be involved to save the patient's life. Patients with impaired kidney function or other significant comorbidities, morbidly obese patients, children, and older adults are particularly at high risk. Telemetry and other tools for monitoring these patients are important to set up when significant doses of opioids are used in managing acute or chronic pain in opioid-dependent patients. However, even with thorough monitoring, untoward events are common. The opioid-sparing approaches discussed elsewhere in this book are thus recommended for management of acute or chronic pain in opioid-dependent patients.

Efficacy Related to Formulation and Route of Delivery

Recently developed long-acting opioids provide convenient dosing and uniform blood levels, resulting in uninterrupted analgesia.[23] Properties of long-acting opioids are reported to contribute to better pain control, improvement in functional outcomes, and a decrease in the tendency of escalation in dosing, resulting in a better safety profile.[24,25] Furthermore, lower peak serum levels of long-acting opioids, compared to those with short-acting opioids, are expected to induce less psychoactive effects (abuse potential).[24] Still, available studies do not adequately address the possible beneficial effects of long-acting opioids or compare them with most commonly prescribed short-acting opioids. Therefore, more extensive studies with long-term follow-up are warranted.

Tamper-resistant drugs have formulations modifying the tablet, capsule, or patch in order to neutralize the active component and make it undesirable for abuse or unintended use.[26,27] These formulations aim to address concerns regarding abuse of opioids, however, they cannot address situations where individuals take more drugs in order to experience euphoria.[26] Benefits of these products need to be evaluated in expansive long-term clinical trials looking at different aspects of abuse.

Opioid Conversion and Rotation

It is advisable that the same maintenance dose of opioids be continued for chronic pain patients in the hospital, unless contraindicated, and that one consider increasing the dose for acute pain or surgery. Therefore, conversion and rotation of opioids in hospitalized patients are predictable. The distinction between conversions and rotation is as follows.

Opioid conversion involves using the same opioid compound but through different route of delivery. Examples of conversion include intravenous fentanyl to transdermal fentanyl, intravenous morphine to oral morphine, and intravenous methadone to oral methadone (see Appendix A).

Opinions vary regarding the conversion of oral opioids to intravenous and back, and regarding opioid rotation. Most parenteral doses of opioids can be decreased from oral doses because intravenous or intramuscular administration bypasses bowel absorption and first-pass hepatic metabolism. This is unambiguously the case with intravenous hydromorphone and morphine, which have about three times greater bioavailability and systemic potency than equianalgesic oral preparations. The exception is oxycodone and its extended-release formulations, which have substantial oral bioavailability but low intravenous bioavailability. Individual patient differences should be taken into consideration when conversion options are considered. Related factors include individual pain perception, age, gender, medical conditions, and genetic variations that may alter the metabolism and excretion of medications.

Opioid rotation is changing one opioid to another. The drug is typically administered via the same route, but a different chemical compound is used. The switch from one opioid to another is made usually because the parenteral form of medication is unavailable (for example, the patient has been taking oxycodone at home but is now in the hospital and NPO). Another reason for using opioid rotation is to improve treatment response or to reduce side effects. The definitive mechanisms by which opioid rotation improves overall response to treatment are not yet known. Positive therapeutic effect may be related to incomplete cross-tolerance to dissimilar opioids that act differently on diverse types and subtypes of opioid receptors. As a result, opioid rotation may decrease tolerance, help lower the opioid dose, and thus decrease unfavorable effects. For example, methadone is an opioid receptor agonist and also an NMDA receptor antagonist. Rotation to methadone has been shown to be effective for decreasing the equivalent opioid requirement and reducing acute or chronic pain in the hospital setting.

The disadvantage of using rotation and conversion of opioids during hospitalization is that they raise the risk of medical errors. Active involvement of pharmacy services in management of acute or chronic pain in the hospital setting may increase the safety of opioid use dramatically (discussed in detail elsewhere in this book). In addition, new research may make opioid rotation more effective and safer, by exploring additional factors in its use, such as the role of genetic variations in opioid rotation and conversion.

Summary

The U.S. Food and Drug Administration (FDA) defines opioid tolerance as use of 60 mg morphine equivalence for 7 days or longer.[28] A significant number of hospital admissions meet the definition of opioid tolerance.[29] Management of opioid-tolerant and opioid-dependent patients in the hospital setting can be challenging for the physician, as well as for nursing staff and other care providers. Most important to the success of inpatient chronic pain management is attentive management of a patient's pain, with judicious use of opioids. This must be followed with quality care in the outpatient setting. Patients who are

---

Box 5.1 **Objectives of Inpatient Opioid Therapy**

1. Promote adequate analgesia.
2. Prevent drug abstinence and withdrawal.
3. Identify and address related social, mental health, and behavioral issues.
4. Set up patient pain management plan for hospitalization proactively, before elective hospitalization, whenever possible.

---

engaged in their own care and are motivated to improve and maximize their well-being physically and mentally, despite having a chronically painful condition, will likely fare best. In order to achieve successful chronic pain management, a partnership between patient and physician is required, with a strong commitment to maximizing the total well-being of the patient. If this has not been achieved for the patient as an outpatient, the physician and patient can each be faced with an array of issues during a hospitalization, which may already be a stressful situation. Providing high-quality outpatient chronic pain management will allow for the most ease and least stress of managing chronic pain when the patient is hospitalized, electively or emergently.

The objectives listed in Box 5.1 should be kept in mind with regard to opioid therapy in the management of chronic pain for inpatients.

The practice tools listed in Box 5.2 may help to avoid use of opioids for treatment of acute or chronic pain in patients during hospitalization.

Box 5.2 **Opioid-Sparing Techniques**

1. Consider weaning patients off chronic opioids or at least reducing dosage prior to elective surgery.
2. A multidisciplinary team approach is often needed and is beneficial for the inpatient; the team may include a psychiatrist, addiction specialist, and/or social worker.
3. Consider initial intravenous patient-controlled analgesia (PCA) to achieve adequate analgesia with opioids and to establish 24-hour total dosage of opioid required for satisfactory pain control prior to conversion/rotation to the at-home prescription.
4. Use adjunct medications for treatment of acute or chronic pain, including ketamine, muscle relaxants, membrane stabilizers, beta-blockers (perioperatively), and other agents.
5. Prescribe physical modalities, including heat/cold, orthotics, and assistive devices.
6. Integrate peripheral nerve block and anesthetic infiltration techniques.

Further medical research is needed to elucidate the role of opioids in the treatment of acute or chronic non-cancer pain in the hospital setting. This research needs to focus on the safety of high-dose opioid therapy required for treating acute pain and objective measurable functional outcomes for chronic pain following discharge from the hospital. The physician must do what is best medically for the patient's well-being, not necessarily what best pleases the patient or is least taxing or least confrontational for the physician. This can be a difficult task when dealing with patients with chronic pain. Providing this type of care takes extra time and effort, and it requires physician knowledge, empathy, and good judgment, and strong ethical conviction.

References

1. Huxtable, CA, Roberts, LJ, Somogyi, AA, Macintyre, PE. Acute pain management in opioid tolerant patients: a growing challenge. *Anaesth Intensive Care*. 2011;39:804–823.
2. Savage SR, Kirsh KL, Passik SD. Challenges in using opiods to treat pain in persons with substance use disorders. *Addict Sci Clin Pract*. 2008;4(2):4–25.
3. Brownstein MJ. A brief history of opiates, opioid peptides, and opioid receptors. *Proc Natl Acad Sci USA*. 1993;15(90):5391–5393.
4. Stannard CF. Opioids for chronic pain: promise and pitfalls. *Curr Opin Support Palliat Care*. 2011;5:150–157.
5. Gilson AM, Ryan KM, Joranson DE, et al. A reassessment of trends in the medical use and abuse of opioid analgesics and implications for diversion control. 1997-2002. *J Pain Symptom Manage*. 2004;28:176–188.
6. Caudill-Slosberg MA, Schwartz LM, Woloshin S. Office visits and analgesic prescriptions for musculoskeletal pain in US: 1980 vs. 2000. *Pain*. 2004;109:514–519.
7. Portenoy RK. Appropriate use of opioids for persistent non-cancer pain. *Lancet*. 2004;364:739–740.
8. Kalso E, Edwards JE, Moore RA, et al. Opioids in chronic non-cancer pain: systematic review of efficacy and safety. *Pain*. 2004;112:372–380.
9. Stein C, Reinecke H, Sorgatz H. Opioid use in chronic non-cancer pain: guidelines revisited. *Curr Opin Anaesthesiol*. 2010;23:598–601.
10. Eisenberg E, McNicol E, Carr DB. Opioids for neuropathic pain. *Cochrane Database Syst Rev*. 2006;(3):CD006146.
11. Ballantyne JC, Shin NS: efficacy of opioids for chronic pain. *Clin J Pain*. 2008;24:469–478.
12. Noble M, Treadwell JR, Tregear SJ, et al. Long-term opioid management for chronic non-cancer pain. *Cochrane Database Syst Rev*. 2010;CD006605.
13. Furlan A, Sandoval JA, et al. Opioids for chronic non-cancer pain: a meta-analysis of effectiveness and side effects. *CMAJ*. 2006;174:1589–1594.
14. Finnerup NB, Otto M, McQuay HJ, et al. Algorithm for neuropathic pain treatment: an evidence based proposal. *Pain*. 2005;118:289–305.
15. Chou R, Carson S. Drug class review on long-acting opioid analgesics: final report update 5. Portland, OR: Oregon Health & Science University; 2008. http://www.ncbi.nlm.nih.gov/books/NBK10648/pdf/TOC.pdf
16. Soin A, Cheng J, Brown L, Moufawad S, Mekhail N. Functional outcomes in patients with chronic nonmalignant pain on long-term opioid therapy. *Pain Pract*. 2008;8(5):379–384.
17. Schofferman J. Restoration of function: the missing link in pain medicine? *Pain Med*. 2006;7(Suppl 1):S159–S165.
18. Gironda RJ, Lloyd J, Clark ME, Walker RL. Preliminary evaluation of reliability and criterion validity of Actiwatch-Score. *J Rehabil Res Dev*. 2007;44(2):223–230.

19. Franklin GM, Mai J, Wickizer T, Turner JA, Fulton-Kehoe D, Grant L. Opioid dosing trends and mortality in Washington State workers' compensation, 1996-2002. *Am J Ind Med*. 2005;48(2):91–99.

20. Chou R, Fanciullo GJ, Fine PG, et al. American Pain Society–American Academy of Pain Medicine Opioids Guidelines Panel. Clinical guidelines for the use of chronic opioid therapy in chronic non-cancer pain. *J Pain*. 2009;10(2):113–130.

21. Office of National Drug Control Policy. Epidemic: responding to America's prescription drug abuse crisis, 2011. http://www.whitehouse.gov/sites/default/files/ondcp/issues-content/prescription-drugs/rx_abuse_plan_0.pdf. Accessed April 26, 2012.

22. Substance Abuse and Mental Health Services Administration. Results from the 2009 National Survey on Drug Use and Health: Vol. I. Summary of National Findings. Washington, DC: Dept. of Health and Human Services, SAMHSA, Office of Applied Studies; 2010.

23. Zorba Paster R. Chronic pain management issues in the primary care setting and the utility of long-acting opioids. *Expert Opin Pharmacother*. 2010;11(11):1823–1833.

24. Wilsey BL, Fishman S, Li CS, Storment J, Albanese A. Markers of abuse liability of short- vs long-acting opioids in chronic pain patients: a randomized cross-over trial. *Pharmacol Biochem Behav*. 2009;94(1):98–107.

25. Fine PG, Mahajan G, McPherson ML. Long-acting opioids and short-acting opioids: appropriate use in chronic pain management. *Pain Med*. 2009;10(Suppl 2):S79–S88.

26. Schneider JP, Matthews M, Jamison RN. Abuse-deterrent and tamper-resistant opioid formulations: what is their role in addressing prescription opioid abuse? *CNS Drugs*. 2010;24(10):805–810.

27. Brems C, Johnson ME, Wells RS, Burns R, Kletti N. Rates and sequelae of the coexistence of substance use and other psychiatric disorders. *Int J Circumpolar Health*. 2002;61(3):224–244.

28. FDA blueprint for prescriber education for extended-release and long-acting opioid analgesics. http://www.fda.gov/downloads/Drugs/DrugSafety/InformationbyDrugClass/UCM277916.pdf Accessed November 30, 2014.

29. Committee News: patients and their pain experience in the hospital: the HCAHPS imperative with payments at risk in value-based purchasing environment. https://www.asahq.org/For-Members/Publications-and-Research/Newsletter-Articles/2014/March-2014/committee-news-on-pain-medicine.aspx Accessed November 30, 2014.

6

Non-Opioid Medications

ADAM CANTER, VIJAY BABU, AND KARINA GRITSENKO

KEY POINTS

- Non-opioid medications may have a significant opioid-sparing effect in the hospital setting.
- Weighing the risks and benefits with regard to the mechanism of action as well as the side-effect profile of each non-opioid agent applied is important.
- A delicate balance is necessary for each individual patient, based on history, physical exam, comorbidities, medication profile, and specific acute or chronic pain needs.

Introduction

More than 100 million adult Americans suffer from chronic pain—disease states that are so pervasive they require medical attention and often pharmacological management.[1] As stated by the American Chronic Pain Association (ACPA) Resource Guide, "an essential concept in pain management is that each patient is different and will respond differently to situations, interventions, surgeries, and medications."[2] Thus, targeting nociceptive, neuropathic, and psychogenic pain with appropriate treatment is an integral part of a multimodal treatment approach.

In determining a treatment regimen for the chronic pain patient, pain scales, diagrams, questionnaires, and other modalities of evaluation are employed, along with a history and physical examination, imaging studies, electromyography, and nerve studies to find a possible physiological etiology of one's chronic pain. The fact that various modes of evaluation are necessary to properly assess the chronic pain patient only reinforces the complexity of chronic pain.[3]

As an example, cancer-related pain represents a paradigm of chronic pain where the source of the pain may come from the malignant lesion itself, associated sequelae, or therapy. Often these patients require opiates in addition to adjuvant medications.[3] Other conditions such as fibromyalgia, myofascial pain, and neuropathy/neuralgia may require antidepressants, topical local anesthetics, muscle relaxant options, and NSAIDs, as well as membrane stabilizers, respectively. As the etiology of pain may be multifactorial, the respective pathologies and treatment options capture the parallel between their understood etiology and the applied pharmacology.[3]

In this chapter, we focus on the discussion of *non-opioid medications* as an essential component of the armamentarium in the treatment of chronic pain.

Advantages and Disadvantages of Analgesic Agents

When choosing an analgesic agent, there are risks and benefits to various categories of medications used. In terms of opioid medication options, the pharmacodynamics of fentanyl provides a good example for both the benefits and risks of opioid use. Fentanyl remains a potent analgesic that is 100-fold the strength of morphine[4] and very useful as an acute pain analgesic perioperatively or for chronic pain in the select chronically ill patient. At increasing doses, fentanyl can cause sedation, euphoria, bradycardia, cough suppression, vasodilation, ventilatory depression, increased biliary pressure, muscle rigidity, depressed cellular immunity, ileus, delayed gastric emptying, nausea, and miosis.[5] All of these side effects can be equally as detrimental to the patient as the pain the patient is experiencing. In addition, assessment of side effects and sequelae becomes even more important if an escalating dose of opioids is being provided, as this may lead to hyperalgesia.

In contrast, non-opioid medications are essential in targeting the neuropathic, psychogenic, and nociceptive aspects of chronic pain. While non-opioid agents, such as non-steroidal anti-inflammatory drugs (NSAIDs), have less potent analgesic properties than those of opioids, they carry fewer (and different) systemic side effects and do not exhibit a potential for dependence. That being said, these benefits must be weighed against potential side effects for each class of medication. NSAIDs are associated with platelet dysfunction, renal damage, and gastric ulcers. Other non-opioid agents, such as tricyclic antidepressants (TCAs), monoamine oxidase inhibitors (MAOIs), selective serotonin reuptake inhibitors (SSRIs), and neuroleptic drugs, may have significant side effects ranging from urinary retention and heart block to somnolence and peripheral edema. These latter medications may have significant interactions with other medications but also remain the cornerstone of therapy for neuropathic pain.[5] Some non-opioid medications such as botulinum toxin, topical lidocaine, and ziconotide have dose-dependent toxicities which must be considered.[6] In the next sections we describe many of the options of non-opioid medications for analgesic options, including risks and benefits (Table 6.1).

Table 6.1 **Advantages and Disadvantages of Non-Opioid Medications in Treatment of Acute or Chronic Pain**

Advantages	Disadvantages
Targeted therapy	Extensive side effects (TCA, steroids, NSAIDs, neuroleptics, anticonvulsants, etc.)
Less addictive properties (apart from ketamine and benzodiazepines)	Less potent than opiates (for certain types of chronic pain)
Less tolerance	Drug interactions (MAOI and SSRI)
Synergistic when combined with opiates (acetaminophen combo-drugs)	Variable efficacy as monotherapy
Anti-inflammatory/antipyretic (acetaminophen, NSAIDs, steroids)	Potential lethal withdrawal states (benzodiazepines)
Improved prevention of breakthrough pain	Limited antagonists (flumazenil)
OTC access and inexpensive	OTC access

MAOI, monoamine oxidase inhibitor; NSAID, nonsteroidal anti-inflammatory drug; OTC, over the counter; SSRI, selective serotonin reuptake inhibitor; TCA, tricyclic antidepressant.

Nonsteroidal Anti-Inflammatory Drugs

Nonsteroidal anti-inflammatory drugs are some of the most commonly used medications for pain control. This family of medications can be administered orally, intramuscularly, and intravenously for treatment of a wide variety of ailments, such as headaches, osteoarthritis, radicular pain, and as an early step in the World Health Organization (WHO) ladder in the treatment algorithms for cancer pain.[7] NSAIDs are weak organic acids, containing one or more aromatic rings that are attached to an acidic functional group. The pKa values for these medications range from 3 to 3.5 and thus are readily absorbed through the gastrointestinal (GI) tract. They are metabolized by the liver and are predominantly protein bound.[8]

The mechanism of action is through inhibition of prostaglandin synthesis. When phospholipids are metabolized, they produce arachidonic acid, which in turn is broken down into a leukotriene pathway and a prostaglandin/thromboxane pathway. NSAIDs inhibit cyclooxygenase I and II with variable selectivity. By inhibiting this pathway, production of prostacyclins, prostaglandin E and F, thromboxane A, and leukotriene B, C, and D is blunted (Figure 6.1).

The prostacyclins generate significant potentiation of inflammatory molecules such as serotonin, histamine, and bradykinin, which are released in response to tissue damage.[8] Table 6.2 highlights the sites of action of this heterogeneous group of medications and the potential adverse effects.[3]

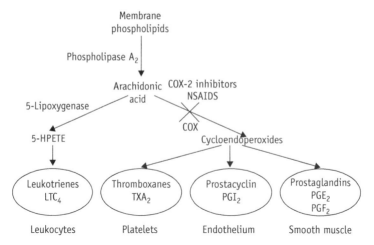

Figure 6.1 NSAID action on the arachidonic acid pathway. Reprinted with permission from Subongkot S, Frame D, Leslie W, Drajer D. Selective cyclooxygenase-2 inhibition: a target in cancer prevention and treatment. *Pharmacotherapy.* 2003;23(1):9–28.

NSAID CATEGORIES

NSAIDs are grouped into salicylates, proprionic acids, indols, COX-2 inhibitors, and p-aminophenols.

Salicylates
Aspirin is the quintessential salicylate; however, its use in the management of chronic pain is limited due to its effects on the GI tract and platelets. Aspirin is used commonly for cardiac disease and vascular disease. It remains the most commonly used medication for headaches.[9]

Proprionic Acids
The proprionic acids consist of ibuprofen and naproxen. These medications have efficacy in the treatment of joint pain, myalgias, migraines, tension headaches, and mild to moderate cancer pain.[8] Specifically, osteoarthritis (OA) and rheumatoid arthritis (RA) are responsive to the proprionic acids in both topical and oral forms. They provide an anti-inflammatory property that is targeted at the degenerative disease process of OA and in modulation of the inflammatory products released in type 3 hypersensitivity diseases such as RA. The therapeutic regimens for these diseases usually incorporate diet change, exercise, weight loss, corticosteroids, and disease-modifying antirheumatic drugs (DMARDs). Nevertheless, the American College of Rheumatology emphasizes that NSAIDs do not alter disease-modifying outcomes but serve to reduce pain, inflammation, and preserve joint function.[9]

Table 6.2 **Arachidonic Acid Metabolite Actions**

PGI1	Fever, vascular smooth muscle relaxation and contraction, increased GI motility, inhibition of gastric acid secretion, production of gastric mucosal lining, renal blood flow and Na/K exchange, potentiation of other pain mediators, sensitization of nociceptors, inhibition of platelet aggregation
PGI2	Contraction of uterine smooth muscle, bronchial constriction, inhibition of platelet aggregation
PGE	Fever, vascular smooth muscle relaxation, contraction of uterine smooth muscle, bronchial smooth muscle relaxation
TXA	Vascular smooth muscle contraction, bronchial constriction, increased platelet aggregation
LTB	Capillary permeability
LTC	Bronchial constriction
LTD	Bronchial constriction

From Ballantyne (2006)[8], p. 93.

Low back and radicular pain benefits more from NSAIDs when it is acute rather than chronic.[9] It has been shown that tissue removed during surgeries for ruptured discs showed synovial fluid that contained between 20- and 100-fold the PLA2 levels known to liberate arachidonic acid from the cells and thus inflammatory byproducts.[10] NSAIDs are a targeted therapy toward this inflammatory process; specifically, naproxen, diclofenac, and ibuprofen have been found to be successful in the management of back and radicular pain.

Indol
Ketorolac is one of the most commonly used indols. It was released in 1990 in the United States and has been used widely for postoperative analgesia because of its potency. It is often given parenterally but can be administered orally and intramuscularly. Due to possible development of renal and GI side effects, the use of ketorolac is primarily in the acute pain setting or in chronic pain limited to breakthrough or periodic adjuvant therapy.[8]

COX-2 Inhibitor
In the United States, the only approved COX-2 inhibitor is celecoxib. Compared to nonselective NSAIDs, COX-2 selectivity reduces the risk of GI ulcers as well as platelet inhibition. Other previously available COX-2 inhibitors were removed from the market, secondary to an increased risk of thromboembolic events and cardiac valvular issues when these agents were used chronically.[5,11] In combination with pregabalin, celecoxib has been shown to be more effective in the treatment of chronic lower back pain than therapy with celecoxib or pregabalin alone (monotherapy).[12]

P-aminophenol

Acetaminophen is synthesized from p-aminophenol, and its mechanism of action is thought to be largely through central action on the spinal cord and cerebral cortex. It also causes a minor central inhibition of prostaglandin synthetase.[13] In cancer pain therapy, acetaminophen with or without opiates is used effectively for management of mild to moderate pain.[1] In fact, the WHO three-step analgesic ladder for treatment of cancer pain includes acetaminophen as a primary treatment for mild pain and an adjuvant treatment for management of moderate and severe pain.[14] Acetaminophen doses should not exceed 4 g per day because of the risk of hepatoxicity.[11] Kaufman et al. conducted a study looking at the prevalence of individuals exceeding the 4 g daily maximum dose. They found that almost 5% of the sample group exceeded the dose, and of the population of people who exceeded the dose, 1 in 5 took more than double the maximum daily dose.[15] Recently, the 4 g dose has been suggested by some medical societies to be scaled down to 3 g per day, due to the substantial risk of hepatotoxicity.

The cytochrome P450 enzymes in the liver metabolize acetaminophen. N-acetyl-p-benzoquinone imine, one of the highly reactive intermediate byproducts, is eliminated by conjugation with glutathione. At high doses of acetaminophen, glutathione is depleted and N-acetyl-p-benzoquinone imine cannot be adequately cleared. This accumulation of N-acetyl-p-benzoquinone imine in the liver results in necrosis and can lead to liver failure. N-acetylcysteine is the primary treatment for acetaminophen toxicity, replenishing glutathione levels.[16]

Depression and Analgesia, Use of Antidepressant Agents

Regarding the relation between depression and chronic pain, 75%–80% of patients with depression exhibit some somatic pain symptoms and, conversely, patients who initially present with chronic pain present with depression in 40% of cases.[17] When treating patients with both chronic pain and depression, it is important to understand the chronology of their symptoms and to address all components of the clinical presentation. Patients with both depression and chronic pain have an increased risk of suicide and can undergo a more difficult treatment course.[17] Specific agents can be considered which can address two pathologies simultaneously.

TRICYCLIC ANTIDEPRESSANTS (TCAs)

Tricyclic antidepressant medications are used in the treatment of neuropathic pain such as diabetic neuropathy and postherpetic neuralgia. The first usage of such medications for chronic pain dates back to 1960 and has since become an effect tool in targeted treatment of chronic pain. TCAs work primarily by reducing the uptake of norepinephrine (NE) and serotonin; in doing so, the elevated levels of neurotransmitters serve to augment activation of descending inhibitory neurons.[17–19] Treatment effectiveness with TCAs is independent of the patient's psychiatric comorbidities. TCAs are effective against burning-type pain and lancinating pain. They are considered first line for the treatment of neuropathic pain by the International Association for the Study of Pain (IASP), as this category of medications requires the lowest number of patients needed to treat for a positive analgesic result.[20] However, TCAs have not been shown to be effective for spinal cord injury pain, HIV neuropathy, and pain related to chemotherapy.[17] Extensive meta-analysis has shown that TCAs are effective in fibromyalgia and are likely effective against irritable bowel syndrome (IBS).[17] IASP guidelines place TCAs as a first-line agent in chronic central pain management.[20]

MONOAMINE OXIDASE INHIBITORS (MAOIs)

Due to substantial side effects and interactions with many drugs (Table 6.3), the use of MAOIs has fallen out of favor. MAOIs irreversibly inhibit monoamine oxidase, resulting in an impaired metabolism of NE, dopamine (DA), and serotonin. There are two subgroups of MAO enzymes, A and B—A selectively metabolizes serotonin (5-HT) and NE and is used mostly for depression and anxiety treatment; B metabolizes DA, tyramine, and phenethalymine and is primarily used in the treatment of Parkinson's disease.[21] Another mechanism of anti-nociception is through monoamine modulation and through interaction with opioid receptors. These medications may stimulate the release of endogenous opioids.[13] Phenelzine has been used to treat chronic fatigue syndrome, migraines, and atypical facial pain.[8]

Table 6.3 **Polypharmacological Interaction**

Drug Associations	Effect
TCA + amphetamine or methylphenidate	Hypertensive crises
TCA + SSRI	Serotoninergic syndrome
TCA + sedatives	Oversedation
Chlomipramin E + modafinil (inhibition of P450)	TCA intoxication
MAOI + methylphenidate/TCA/SSRI/IRNS	Hypertensive crises
MAOI + selegiline	Hypertensive crises
SSRI + selegiline	Serotoninergic syndrome
TCA + selegiline	TCA intoxication

For abbreviations see Table 6.1.
From the Brazilian Guidelines for the Treatment of Narcolepsy,[47] p. 311.

SELECTIVE SEROTONIN REUPTAKE INHIBITORS/ SEROTONIN-NOREPINEPRHINE REUPTAKE INHIBITORS (SSRIs/SNRIs)

SSRIs are used alone or in combination with other agents for the treatment of fibromyalgia, neuropathic pain, and depression.[3] These medications act on the presynaptic serotonin reuptake pump by selective inhibition.[8] The side-effect profile produced by SSRI/SNRIs is much more limited than that with TCAs and MAOIs.[21] Although SSRI appear safer, there are fewer data to show the effectiveness of SSRI when treating neuropathic pain.[22] Meta-analysis pooled from the Cochrane study did not show efficacy in the treatment of migraines when compared with placebo.[23] On the other hand, it has been shown that SNRIs are effective for fibromyalgia and neuropathic pain.[17,22,24] Clinically, these medications exhibit variable efficacy, indicative of the complex nature of chronic pain and the patient-specific presentation. SNRIs are considered first line by IASP, even though they are less efficacious than TCAs[20]

Anticonvulsants (Membrane Stabilizers)

Useful in the treatment of posttraumatic neuralgia, painful diabetic neuropathy, postherpetic neuralgia, trigeminal neuralgia, and radiculopathy, anticonvulsants act as neuromodulators.[8,13] They are most effective for treatment of "lancinating or burning pain," such as neuropathic-type pain associated with trigeminal neuralgia.[8] This group of drugs acts on sodium, potassium, and calcium channels in the neuronal membrane. The commonly used agents in the treatment of chronic pain include carbamazepine, oxcarbazepine, topiramate, levetiracetam, pregabalin, zonisamide, gabapentin, and lamotrigine.[8,10]

Carbamazepine is thought to block sodium channels and inhibit norepinephrine uptake and decrease nerve impulse firing.[8] Agranulocytosis and critical hyponatremia are feared side effects with carbamazepine. Therefore, routine hematological and electrolyte monitoring is required.[13] In a meta-analysis of 15 studies pooled from the Cochrane Database, it was shown that carbamazepine is effective in the treatment of chronic neuropathic pain; however, because the study durations did not span longer than 4 weeks, there should be some reluctance in extrapolating such results to projected effectiveness in chronic treatment.[25]

Oxcarbazepine is structurally related to carbamezepine and acts on sodium channels in addition to increasing conductance of potassium and modulation of neural calcium channels. Like carbamazepine, hyponatremia is also a documented side effect, so routine chemistries must be reviewed. Since oxcarbazepine has less dramatic side effects than those of carbamazepine, it has taken over as a first-line treatment for trigeminal neuralgia.[8]

Topiramate has been shown to be effective in the treatment of chronic lumbar and radicular pain via inhibition of voltage-gated sodium channels and calcium channels, as well as inhibition of GABA, AMPA, and kainite glutamate receptors.[1,26]

Levetiracetam acts by reducing conductance through high-voltage calcium channels, impacting potassium channel conductance, and preventing inhibition of GABA and glycine channels.[8] There is a paucity of studies showing the efficacy of levetiracetam in chronic pain management.

Gabapentin is a structural analog of GABA that modulates the alpha2-delta subunit of N-type calcium channels. The medication has few side effects and is usually well tolerated.[13,27] Used successfully in the treatment of painful diabetic neuropathy and other peripheral neuropathies, gabapentin also improves sleep. With long-term use, gabapentin can cause weight gain, which can be problematic in the diabetic patient.[27]

Pregabalin is an enantiomer of GABA; its mechanism of action is currently unknown; however, it has been found to act as a GABA analog, increasing neuronal GABA levels and glutamic acid decarboxylase activity.[8] Pregabalin binds to (alpha2-delta) calcium channels and modulates pain transmission much like the anticonvulsant medications. However, pregabalin has a much more preferable side-effect profile.[28] Another advantage of pregabalin is that it can be titrated more quickly than gabapentin and some other anticonvulsant medications. Case reports have shown effectiveness in patients with ankylosing spondylitis with pain refractory to opioids.[28] Multiple randomized control studies have shown improved quality of life and improved sleep in patients with chronic painful diabetic neuropathy, thus pregabalin, along with alpha2 agonists, is a first-line agent. Using quantitative sensory test evaluation, Olesen et al. found that pregabalin is successful in treating chronic pancreatitis pain.[29] Pregabalin has indications for both fibromyalgia and diabetic nerve pain. Unlike TCAs, there is level A evidence, according to the American Academy of Neurology recommendations, that pregabalin is successful in treating specifically diabetic neuropathic pain.[27,30]

Zonisamide is a sulfonamide anticonvulsant used primarily for treatment of seizures in adults. Its mechanism of action is not known; however, like the other drugs discussed in this section, it acts on sodium channels, calcium channels, and GABA receptors through modulation. In various small studies, zonisamide has been shown to be effective in the treatment of neuropathic pain and migraines. There is a lack of randomized control data to show efficacy of zonisamide's use in pain management.[31]

Lamotrigine acts by inhibiting voltage-gated sodium channels and glutamate release. At therapeutic doses, lamotrigine has been effective in the treatment of trigeminal neuralgia, HIV neuropathy, spinal cord injury pain, and post-stroke pain.[13] One of the limitations of lamotrigine is the fact that it must be titrated slowly to therapeutic levels in order to reduce the risk of Steven-Johnson syndrome.[32]

Benzodiazepines

Benzodiazepines act on GABA-A receptors to increase chloride conductance, resulting in hyperpolarization of the postsynaptic neuron. These medications are typically prescribed for anxiety, insomnia, or spasticity and are administered orally.[6] Most of the literature studying benzodiazepine use in chronic pain has been conducted using an animal model, so application in the clinical setting is not well established. Another limitation of benzodiazepine use for chronic pain is the ability of patients to develop tolerance or addiction. Withdrawal from benzodiazepines may be fatal secondary to intractable seizure activity; therefore, they should not be abruptly withdrawn. Sedation during daytime activity is not well tolerated. There are 19 subunits of the GABA receptor; novel uses have arisen from different allosteric stimulation of the various subunits such that agents with less sedative properties have been produced. Many patients with generalized anxiety disorders, posttraumatic stress disorder (PTSD), or obsessive-compulsive disorder (OCD) have somatic symptoms along with their psychological pathology. While benzodiazepines serve to treat the anxiety and may improve secondary symptoms, they should be used extremely carefully when used simultaneously with opioids because they may mutually potentiate sedation and respiratory depression.[8]

Muscle Relaxants

Antispasmodic agents or muscle relaxants consist of baclofen, cyclobenzaprine, and tizanidine. Baclofen is useful in the treatment of trigeminal neuralgia spastic conditions that may arise from multiple sclerosis or spinal cord lesions.[8] Intrathecally administered baclofen has been shown to be effective in the management of pain generated from spastic muscle contractions but not from neuropathic pain directly.[14] By acting on the GABA-B receptors, baclofen inhibits monosynaptic and polysynaptic reflexes at the spinal level.[33] It is thought that through modulation and reduction of excitatory neurotransmitter, baclofen is able to decrease the spinal and cerebral spasticity in upper motor neuron lesions.[33]

Cyclobenzaprine is structurally similar to TCAs and has a similar side-effect profile; it is contraindicated in concomitant use with MAOIs.[8,34] The medication is effective in the treatment of purely muscular pain. When used for spastic pain of neurogenic etiology, cyclobenzaprine is ineffective.[8] Tizanidine is an alpha-2 agonist that acts on spinal and cerebral receptors and has been shown to be effective in the treatment of spastic muscle pain in multiple sclerosis, spinal cord injury, and post-stroke. Unlike baclofen and cyclobenzaprine, it does not cause muscle weakness or have soporific properties.[15] Compared with benzodiazepines and dantrolene, medications used to treat spasticity that affects the activities of daily life, tizanidine does not exhibit the respective sedative properties and muscle weakness of these drugs.[35]

Corticosteroids

Typically not used as a primary or first-line agent, corticosteroids are nonetheless effective in the treatment of rheumatic, radicular, and cancer chronic pain. The mechanism of action of steroids in the treatment of chronic pain is not completely understood.[8] In a study conducted by Vachon-Presseau et al., an examination of the analgesic effect of acute pain and the cortisol response was performed. The study focused on the spinothalamic tract and used MRI to observe the downregulation in neural activity in the dorsal horn due to increased levels of endogenous cortisol. In animal models, steroids have been shown to decrease neural activity at the dorsal horn. The study concluded that steroids decrease acute responses to noxious stimuli; however, extrapolation to chronic pain populations was not examined.[23] When examining sciatic pain, steroids provide relief in the short term but not immediately, likely secondary to a decreased nerve root inflammation rather than downregulation of neural activity.[36]

Steroids are an essential component of basal homeostasis and the stress response. They uphold functionality of immune and inflammatory response and act centrally on the brain and pituitary axis. By negative feedback mechanisms, steroids regulate nearly all facets of the body and, as such, can have significant systemic side effects when exogenous steroids are given in either high-dose or long treatment course. Thus, steroid use in chronic pain treatment is limited by the iatrogenic systemic side effects and time course (Table 6.4).[37]

Local Anesthetics

By acting on neuronal sodium channels and inhibiting the expression of nitric oxide and thus preventing the release of proinflammatory cytokines, local

Table 6.4 **Side Effects of Steroids**

Increased infection/thrush	Impaired wound healing	Adrenal suppression
Dermatitis	Acne	Cushinoid habitus
Increased Appetite	Mood swings/depression	Hyperglycemis
Edema	Glaucoma	Hoarseness
Weight gain	Osteoporosis	Hypertension

Modified from mayoclinic.com.

anesthetics provide analgesia for postherpetic neuralgia, peripheral neuropathic pain, painful diabetic neuropathy, HIV-induced neuropathy, radicular pain, myofascial pain, and osteoarthritic pain. This group of medications also provides prolonged relief thought to be secondary to reduced activation of microglia and astrocytes.[38] Lidocaine and prilocaine are approved in the United States for use topically. Eutectic mixture of local anesthetic (EMLA) cream is a combination of prilocaine 2.5% and lidocaine 2.5% and is effective in the treatment of postherpetic neuralgia. Topical lidocaine in high concentrations (5%) appears to be effective in the treatment of neuropathic pain in patients refractory to other treatments. Most of the patients studied who experienced relief exhibited burning or shock-type pain.[39] All of these formulations, when administered transdermally, have the benefit of local rather than systemic effects; nevertheless, local anesthetic toxicity can occur and is dose dependent. Toxicity is characterized by central nervous system (CNS) disturbances, seizure activity, and cardiac arrhythmias and arrest. The most common side effects consist of burning, dermatitis, pruritis, rash, and erythema.[13]

In addition to transdermal administration, local anesthetics can be given via the epidural space for radicular pain ("sciatica") and systemically for nerve injury pain, diabetic neuropathy, cancer pain, and herpetic neuralgia.[13] Lidocaine has been shown to be more effective systemically when given intravenously; procaine has the advantage of less toxicity but the disadvantage of a very short half-life.[13] The benefits of intrathecal administration of local anesthetics are avoidance of the blood-brain barrier, the ability to achieve continuously titratable doses of medication, the avoidance of systemic metabolism, and direct access to receptors in the CNS.[40] Limitations of intrathecal administration are invasiveness in the application, potential transient sympathectomy, expense, and risks associated with any neuraxial techniques, including bleeding, infection, and trauma to the neuraxial space.

Miscellaneous and Newer Non-Opioid Agents

Capsaicin is primarily used for arthritic and neuropathic pain; it is derived from chili peppers and is commonly used in a topical preparation. Capsaicin is thought to deplete the levels of substance P in afferent neurons. Disadvantages of the medication are that it must be applied repeatedly throughout the day and it causes burning initially. The efficacy is relatively high and toxicity is not an issue.[27,41]

Ketamine is a noncompetitive antagonist of NMDA receptors. It acts both peripherally and centrally and blocks calcium channel activity in addition to reducing sodium channel depolarization and cholinergic discharge. Ketamine has been used effectively to treat peripheral neuropathy, postherpetic neuralgia, cancer pain, fibromyalgia, and complex regional pain syndromes. Addictiveness and extensive psychomotor effects limit its use outside a controlled environment.[13]

Botulinum toxin is one of the most potent toxins that exist. It causes a temporary halt in the presynaptic release of acetylcholine from nerve endings, resulting in paralysis. It is thought that botulinum toxin blocks both the motor neuron and nociceptive transmission. The medical preparation is of use in disease states that may be caused by spastic muscular tension, such as myofascial syndrome, arthritis, and neuropathic pain, as well as chronic back and pelvic pain. When injected in temporal, glabellar, occipital, and supraorbital sites, it has use in migraine treatment and is FDA approved for this purpose. Systemic toxicity and limitation of mobility are setbacks.[42]

Cannabinoids act on CB1R and CB2R, which are G-protein-coupled cannabinoid receptors, to generate a variety of effects. The majority of studies performed have been on animal models or on patients suffering from multiple sclerosis or cancer. The efficacy of cannabis as a monotherapy for severe pain is poor. Meta-analysis suggests that cannabis may provide analgesia for mild to moderate pain and is more effective as an adjuvant or in combination with other medications.[43]

Clonidine is an alpha-2 adrenergic agonist that has been shown to generate relief from neuropathic cancer pain when administered intrathecally. Clonidine can cause cardiovascular depression and is soporific. Tests on animal models with neuropathic pain regularly showed downregulation of opioid receptors and thus a lesser response to opioids. However, alpha-2 agonists are found to be more potent under these conditions. Clonidine, in combination with opioids, intrathecally delivered, is an effective treatment for severe neuropathic pain.[24]

Ziconitide is approved for intrathecal use only. It is derived from the venom of the sea snail *Conus magus*. A synthetic peptide, ziconitide, antagonizes voltage-gated N-type calcium channels primarily in the presynaptic nerve terminals of the dorsal horn.[44] Ziconitide binds to the substantia gelatinosa of the dorsal spinal lamina. This is an important site for nociceptive processing. The medication does carry a risk of nonspecific CNS side effects when given in high doses.[45]

New therapeutic targets include the A3 adenosine receptor (A3AR). It was shown that that increasing endogenous adenosine levels through selective adenosine kinase inhibition produces powerful analgesic effects in an experimental setting with a novel and highly selective A3AR agonist.[46] It was also demonstrated that these effects were prevented by blockade of spinal and supraspinal A3AR. In addition, these powerful analgesic effects were lost in A3AR knockout mice. The analgesia produced by A3AR activation is independent of opioid and endocannabinoid pathways. Importantly, the A3AR activation decreases the excitability of spinal wide dynamic-range neurons and produces supraspinal inhibition of spinal nociception through activation of serotonergic and noradrenergic bulbospinal circuits, which may have a critical role in non-opioid treatment and selective alleviation of persistent neuropathic pain.

Summary

There are many subtypes of pain that require treatment in patients with chronic pain. Thus, not only must one distinguish between neuropathic and somatic pain, but one also must individualize care by weighing the risks and benefits with regard to the mechanism of action as well as the side-effect profile of each agent applied. In this chapter, specific non-opioid agents have been addressed, with an emphasis on mechanism of action, side-effect recognition, and efficacy, especially with regard to neuropathic pain needs. Also, we must realize that many analgesic agents can be used in a multimodal fashion. There must be a delicate balance in treatment for each individual patient, based on history, physical exam, comorbidities, medication profile, and specific pain needs.

References

1. Muehlbacher M, Nickel MK, Kettler C, et al. Topiramate in treatment of patients with chronic low back pain: a randomized, double-blind, placebo-controlled study. *Clin J Pain.* 2006;22(6):526–531.

2. Feinberg S, et al. *ACPA Resource Guide to Chronic Pain Medication and Treatment, 2013 Edition.* Rocklin, CA: American Chronic Pain Association; 2013.

3. Butterworth J, IV, Mackey DC, Wasnick JD. *Morgan & Mikhail's Clinical Anesthesiology,* 5th ed. New York: McGraw-Hill; 2013.

4. Duke J. *Anesthesia Secrets,* 4th ed. Philadelphia: Mosby Elsevier; 2011.

5. Miller RD, Pardo MC, Jr. *Basics of Anesthesia,* 6th ed. Philadelphia: Elsevier Saunders; 2011.

6. Rudolph U, Knoflach F. Beyond classical benzodiazepines: novel therapeutic potential of GABAa receptor subtypes. *Nat Rev Drug Discov.* 2011;10(9):685–697.

7. Schug SA, Zech D, Dorr U. Cancer pain management according to WHO Analgesic Guidelines. *J Pain Sympt Manage.* 1990;5(1):27–32.

8. Ballantyne JC. *The Massachusetts General Hospital Handbook of Pain Management,* 3rd ed. Philadelphia: Lippincott Williams & Wilkins; 2006.

9. Herndon CM, Hutchison RW, Berdine HJ, et al. Management of chronic nonmalignant pain with nonsteroidal anti-inflammatory drugs. *Pharmacotherapy.* 2008;28(6):788–805.

10. Barash PG, Cullen BF, Stoelting RK. *Clinical Anesthesia,* 5th ed. Philadelphia: Lippincott Williams & Wilkins; 2006.

11. Wagner T, Poole C, Roth-Daniek A. The capsaicin 8% patch for neuropathic pain in clinical practice: a retrospective analysis. *Pain Med.* 2013;14:1202–1211.

12. Romano CL, Romano D, Bonora C, Mineo G. Pregabalin, celecoxib and their combination for treatment of chronic low-back pain. *J Orthopaed Traumatol.* 2009;10(4):185–191.

13. Wallace MS, Staats PS. *Pain Medicine and Management: Just the Facts.* New York: McGraw-Hill; 2005.

14. Long MD. *Contemporary Diagnosis and Management of Pain,* 2nd ed. Newton, PA: Handbooks in Health Care; 2001.

15. Kaufman DW, Kelly JP, Rohay JM, Malone MK, Weinstein RB, Shiffman S. Prevalence and correlates of exceeding the labeled maximum dose of acetaminophen among adults in a U.S.-based Internet survey. *Pharmacoepidemiol Drug Saf.* 2012;21(12):1280–1288.

16. Ben-Shachar R, Chen Y, Luo S, Hartman C, Reed M, Nijhout HF. The biochemistry of acetaminophen hepatotoxicity and rescue: a mathematical model. *Theor Biol Med Model.* 2012;9:55.

17. Verdu B, Decosterd I, Buclin T, Stiefel F, Berney A. Antidepressants for the treatment of chronic pain. *Drugs.* 2008;68(18):2611–2632.

18. Arnold LM, Lu Y, Crofford LJ, et al. A double-blind, multicenter trial comparing duloxetine with placebo in the treatment of fibromyalgia patients with or without major depressive disorder. *Arthritis Rheum.* 2004;50:2974–2984.

19. Max MB. Endogenous monoamine analgesic systems: amitriptyline in painful diabetc neuropathy. *Anesth Prog.* 1987;34:123–127.

20. Ballantyne J, ed. Pharmacological management of neuropathic pain. International Association For the Study of Pain. Pain: Clinical Updates. November 2010; Vol. XVIII, Issue 9. http://iasp.files.cms-plus.com/Content/ContentFolders/Publications2/PainClinicalUpdates/Archives/PCU_18-9_final_1390260608342_7.pdf. Accessed July 24, 2105.

21. Stahl MS, Felker A. Trends in psychopharmacology: monoamine oxidase inhibitors: a modern guide to an unrequited class of antidepressants. *CNS Spectr.* 2008;13:10.

22. Lee YC, Chen PP. A review of SSRIs and SNRIs in neuropathic pain. *Expert Opin Pharmacother.* 2010;11(17):2813–2825.

23. Vachon-Presseau E, et al. Acute stress contributes to individual differences in pain and pain-related brain activity in healthy and chronic pain patients. *J Neurosci.* 2013;33(16):6826–6833.

24. Martin TJ, Eisenach JC. Pharmacology of opioid and nonopioid analgesics in chronic pain states. *J Pharmacol Exp Ther.* 2001;299(3):811–817.

25. Wiffen PJ, Derry S, Moore RA, McQuay HJ. Carbamazepine for acute and chronic pain in adults. *Cochrane Database Syst Rev.* 2011;1:CD005451.

26. Khoromi S, Patsalides A, Parada S, et al. Topiramate in chronic lumbar radicular pain. *J Pain.* 2005;6(12):829–836.

27. Kontoangelos KA, Kouzoupis AV, Ferentinos PP, Xynos ID, Sipsas NV, Papadimitriou GN. Pregabalin for opioid-refractory pain in a patient with ankylosing spondylitis. *Case Rep Psychiatry.* 2013;2013:912409.

28. Vinik AI, Casellini CM. Guidelines in the management of diabetic nerve pain: clinical utility of pregabalin. *Diabetes Metab Syndr Obes.* 2013:6:57–78.

29. Olesen SS, Graversen C, Bouwense SA, van Goor H, Wilder-Smith OH, Drewes AM. Quantitative sensory testing predicts pregabalin efficacy in painful chronic pancreatitis. *PLoS ONE.* 8(3):e57963.

30. Ohta H, Oka H, Usui C, et al. A randomized, double-blind, multicenter, placebo-controlled phase III trial to evaluate the efficacy and safety of pregabalin in Japanese patients with fibromyalgia. *Arthritis Res Ther.* 2012;14:R217. http://arthritis-research.com/content/14/5/R217

31. Krusz JC. Treatment of chronic pain with zonisamide. *Pain Pract.* 2003;3(4):317–320.

32. Moulin DE, Clark AJ, Gilron I, et al. Pharmacological management of chronic neuropathic pain—consensus statement and guidelines from the Canadian Pain Society. *Pain Res Manage.* 2007;12(1):13–21.

33. Ucar T, Kazan S, Turgut U, Smanci NK. Outcomes of intrathecal baclofen (ITB) therapy in spacticity. Turk Neurosurg. 2011;21(1):59–65.

34. Argoff CE. Pharmacologic management of chronic pain. *J Am Osteopath Assoc* 2002;102(9 Suppl 3):S21–S27.

35. Gelber DA, Good DC, Dromerick A, Sergay S, Richardson M. Open-label dose-titration safety and efficacy study of tizanidine hydrochloride in the treatment of spasticity associated with chronic stroke. *Stroke.* 2001;32(8):1841–1846.

36. Pinto RZ, Maher CG, Ferreira ML, et al. Drugs for relief of pain in patients with sciatica: systematic review and meta-analysis. *BMJ.* 2012;344:e497.

37. Chrousos GP, Kino T. Glucocorticoid signaling in the cell: expanding clinical implications to complex human behavioral and somatic disorders. *Ann N Y Acad Sci.* 2009;1179:153–166.

38. Toda S, Sakai A, Ikeda Y, Sakamoto A, Suzuki H. A local anesthetic, ropivicaine, suppresses activated microglia via a nerve growth factor–dependent mechanism and astrocytes via a nerve growth factor–independent mechanism in neuropathic pain. *Mol Pain.* 2011:7:2.

39. Delorme C, Navez ML, Legout V, Deleens R, Moyse D. Treatment of neuropathic pain with 5% lidocaine-medicated plaster: five years of clinical experience. *Pain Res Manage.* 16(4):259–263.

40. Belverud SA, Mogilner AY, Schulder M. Intrathecal bupivicaine for head and neck pain. *Local Reg Anesth*, 2010;3:125–128.

41. Park HJ, Moon DE. Pharmacologic management of chronic pain. *Korean J Pain.* 2010;23(2):99–108.

42. Sim WS. Application of botulinum toxin in pain management. *Korean J Pain.* 2011;24(1):24(1):1–6.

43. Kraft B. Is there any clinically relevant cannabinoid-induced analgesia? *Pharmacology.* 2012;89:237–246.

44. Buga S, Sarria JE. The management of pain in metastatic bone disease. *Cancer Control.* 2012;19(2):154–166.

45. Yaksh TL, de Kater A, Dean R, Best BM, Miljanich GP. Pharmacokinetic analysis of ziconotide (SNX-111), an intrathecal N-type calcium channel blocking analgesic, delivered by bolus and infusion in the dog. *Neuromodulation.* 2012;15(6):508–519.

46. Little JW, Ford A, Symons-Liguori AM, et al. Endogenous adenosine A3 receptor activation selectively alleviates persistent pain states. *Brain.* 2015;138(Pt 1):28–35.

47. Aloe F, et al. Brazilian guidelines for the treatment of narcolepsy. *Rev. Bras. Psiquiatr.* 2010;32(3):294–305.

7

How and When You Should Get a Pain Medicine Consult and What You Should Ask—Establishing Treatment Goals

ABDUL KANU AND ELLEN ROSENQUIST

KEY POINTS

- The pain management specialist serves as a consultant to hospitalists and other specialists for treating the patient with acute or chronic pain and managing it in the hospital setting.
- It is important to understand the scope of training and expertise of your consulting pain provider so that you can match your patient's needs with the provider's expertise.
- If the initial upward titration of pain medications failed to control acute pain in a patient with chronic pain, then a chronic pain service should be consulted.
- It is essential that primary physicians are familiar with the general principles of operation of implantable devices and with initial management of common complications.

Introduction

An increasing percentage of hospitalized patients carry the diagnosis of chronic pain. Chronic pain is a complex clinical entity that is often associated with other comorbidities.[1] This chapter provides a general framework for how to approach treatment of a patient's chronic pain and how to consult a chronic pain service. An important concept to understand is the fundamental difference between acute pain and chronic pain, which is a common source of confusion. *Acute pain* is typically correlated with the severity of physical injury and is responsive to opioids.[2] *Chronic pain*, by contrast, may not be responsive to opioids. Some common types of medications for chronic pain, such as membrane stabilizers, serotonin-norepinephrine reuptake inhibitors (SNRIs), or tricyclic antidepressants (TCAs), usually take several weeks before clinical pain relief is appreciated. Chronic pain and acute pain can also present at the same time, which can be tremendously confusing for any clinician. Understanding the breadth of treatment options can help one to direct patients to the right specialist for the most tailored treatment plan. Generally, any physician who has completed an accredited pain fellowship by the American Council for Graduate Medical Education (ACGME) will have the expertise necessary to handle or triage most acute pain or chronic pain issues. Some of the most common clinical scenarios are reviewed in this chapter to illustrate how to approach treatment for a typical chronic pain patient.

When calling on a consultant, it is important to know the unique training that goes into producing a pain physician. Most practitioners are trained in a primary medical specialty, such as anesthesiology, neurology, physiatry, or psychiatry, and then elect to pursue subspecialty training in pain management. In general, their expertise is in medical (opioid and non-opioid) management and interventional pain procedures. Physiatrists can elect to pursue elective training in pain management by completing interventional spine fellowships. These fellowships enable physiatrists to be comfortable with medical management as well as some interventional procedures.[3,4] Pain fellowships in the United States are typically accredited by the ACGME, however, non-ACGME accredited fellowships do exist. ACGME-accredited fellowships undergo a continuous rigorous evaluation and vetting process, whereas non-ACGME-accredited fellowships are not as highly regulated for quality. Despite this discrepancy, non-ACGME-accredited fellowships can still provide excellent training in the management of chronic pain. Although pain specialists vary greatly in their expertise, any physician who has elected to pursue a pain fellowship will have the knowledge to medically treat patients with chronic pain and direct such patients to any avenues of treatment that may lie outside their specific area of expertise.

One must take the consultant provider's training into consideration when referring an inpatient or outpatient for consultation. For instance, if one wants to refer a patient for a celiac plexus for abdominal pain secondary to pancreatic cancer, one may elect to choose a pain physician trained in anesthesia. If one wants to refer a patient for psychogenic pain, one may consider a practitioner who has training in psychiatry. Pain patients are quite complex; therefore, it is best to a find a practitioner that best matches the likely etiology of a patient's pain. This expedites the healing process and decreases the potential frustration of pain patients seeing multiple physicians without significant relief.

General Principles of Use of Chronic Pain Consultants

With the increasing medical complexity and aging of patients, primary care providers have increased their use of medical consultants. Unfortunately, education in chronic pain has not been a standard part of the medical school curriculum. This has led to a knowledge gap in treating an extremely common medical issue. An important aspect of using a consultant is providing a concisely defined clinical question for the pain practitioner. This clarity will be most helpful to a consultant in providing recommendations for addressing a specific medical issue. Communicating the role of the consultant provider to the patient is essential to establishing a trusting relationship between all parties.[5] The consultant and primary care provider must constitute a unified front when dealing with pain issues.

A pain history should include not only clinical symptoms but also previous treatment(s) and physicians consulted. The physical exam and history for chronic pain is similar to that for any medical condition; however, in this case it is important to focus on certain aspects in order to provide a consultant with a clear clinical picture. Knowledge of the training and abilities of the consultant provider can help direct patients to the correct specialist. It is important to realize that pain physicians are usually trained in neurology, physiatry, psychiatry, or anesthesiology, but they can also come from primary care. For instance, implantation of devices is typically performed by anesthesiology pain physicians, whereas biofeedback and relaxation therapy may be given by psychiatry pain physicians.

Chronic pain consultants need to illicit an appropriate pain history and independent physical exam. Based on the history and exam, the consultant will make recommendations that encompass a treatment plan to address the clinical question at hand. Recommendations should be brief, concise, and explicit about the course of action, including drug dosage and duration. In addition, follow-up with primary providers increases the likelihood that the recommendations will be implemented.[6]

What to Tell Your Chronic Pain Consultant

CLINICAL HISTORY OF ACUTE OR CHRONIC PAIN

When consulting a pain specialist, it is important to illicit a relevant pain history.[7] It is very common for patients to mention pain in multiple anatomic locations during their history. By focusing questions and redirecting patients to the relevant portions of their pain history, one can get clarity on the most urgent symptoms (Table 7.1).

Table 7.1 **History of Present Illness with Focus on Pain**

Factors	Questions
Onset	When did the pain start? Was there an inciting event or trauma? Was the pain gradual in onset with increasing severity?
Provocative/alleviating factors	Is there any specific position or activity that reproduces the pain? Is there any specific position or medication that completely relieves the pain?
Quality	What one word best describes the pain? It may be useful to have the patient choose from specific words, such as *burning, aching, sharp, numbness, tingling, throbbing, pounding.*
Radiation/region of pain	Can you point with one finger where the pain is most intense? Does the pain radiate from this point? If so, where does this pain radiate?
Severity	On a scale of 1 to 10 (10 being the worst pain you have ever experienced), what would you rate your pain?
Time/temporal factors	Is there a consistent time during the day when the pain is most intense?

Questions need to be specific and focused in such a way as to minimize circuitous answers. As with any medical history, it is important to obtain a chief complaint, current medications (both dosage and frequency of administration), history of illicit drug use, review of systems, vocational history (disabled, worker's compensation, retired, etc.), and psychiatric conditions. It is important to illicit the information a pain physician will need to most effectively provide recommendations.

There are several specific clinical descriptors used by pain physicians to describe types of pain (Table 7.2). Although none of these descriptors[8] are

Table 7.2 **Common Descriptors Used to Describe Chronic Pain**

Descriptor	Definition
Allodynia	A painful response to a stimulus that is normally not painful—for instance, lightly touching an extremity, causing a painful response
Hyperalgesia	A painful stimulus causing a response that is out of proportion to the painful stimulus—for instance, testing a pinprick sensation in a patient to see if it causes a significant amount of pain
Paresthesia	An abnormal sensation that is elicited after any type of stimulus
Dysesthesia	An unpleasant sensation that is elicited after any type of stimulus

Table 7.3 **Common Terms Related to Chronic Opioid Use**

Term	Definition
Tolerance	An increasing dose of medication is needed for the same clinical effect.
(Pseudo)addiction	Increasing dosage is requested by a patient for pain, but the pursuit of medication ceases after pain relief is obtained.
Addiction	Maladaptive behaviors exhibited by a patient to obtain medications
Withdrawal	Clinical symptoms that present with cessation of a medication

specific to chronic pain, each type of descriptor may hint at the mechanism of pain. For instance, paresthesia and dysesthesia may hint at a diseased or malfunctioning peripheral nerve. In addition, the adjectives given in the table will help you elucidate the etiology of a patient's pain, move your thought process toward using a consultant, and communicate relevant information to the consultant.

The common descriptors of chronic opioid use are listed in Table 7.3 and are discussed in detail elsewhere in this book (e.g., see Chapter 5).

CHRONIC PAIN, ANXIETY, AND DEPRESSION

Historically, pain has been viewed as a noxious sensation in reaction to a stimulus, such as trauma, surgery, or bodily injury. Physicians often use pain as a marker for the intensity and severity of physical injury. For instance, a severed limb should invoke a greater pain response than a sprained ankle. Most diagnostic tools, especially imaging modalities, are intended to seek evidence of physical pathology. The development of chronic pain involves neuroplastic changes that occur in the dorsal root laminae and other central nervous system structures.[9,10] Therefore, nerves that normally sense light touch may activate a pathway intended for severe pain or depression. These changes can vary greatly from individual to individual. Hence, the same mechanism of chronic pain may cause significant depression, anger, suffering, and restriction of activities in one individual while another individual may continue to engage in daily activities of living without restriction.

Chronic pain is known to be linked in some patients to depression and an inability to cope with other aspects of life. These individuals have a great deal of frustration toward physicians, employers, family members, and insurance providers, who all can at times provide obstacles to obtaining relief. When evaluating a patient for chronic pain, always consider the benefit of psychological counseling as a strategy to overcome pain.[11]

PHYSICAL EXAMINATION

Although covered earlier, it is important to review parts of the clinical exam that will be valuable to a consulting physician.[12] First, it is important to assess mental status, by asking the patient to provide the patient's name, date, year, and the current president. Deficits in mental status could point to side effects of pain medications, such as difficulty with concentration or sedation. Some patients may express discontent with answering "erroneous" questions, which could point to emotional issues.

Cranial nerve examination should be thorough. In addition to positive findings, certain aspects of the examination may aid in the diagnosis of common facial pain syndromes. Test sensation by light touch and pinprick along the three major branches (V1, V2, V3) of the trigeminal nerve. In hospitalized patients, trigeminal neuralgia and atypical facial pain are common causes of facial pain that could be confused with other types of headaches.[13] The rotation of the neck and palpation of the bilateral occiput may point to cervicalgia and occipital neuralgia, respectively.

For the motor exam, it is important to document the strength of the muscle being tested. Briefly, 5/5 is full range of motion with full resistance, 4/5 is full range of motion with some resistance, 3/5 is range of motion with gravity, and 2/5 is range of motion with gravity eliminated. In addition, documenting the tone of the muscle can point to the chronicity of the disease process. The sensation exam should test both light touch and pinprick sensation. It is important to compare each side of the body and test along symptomatic dermatomes and/or peripheral nerves. If necessary, it may be helpful to consult a dermatome chart.

Deep tendon reflex testing can point to an upper or lower motor neuron deficit. The most commonly tested reflexes are biceps (C5), triceps (C7), patellar (L4), and Achilles (S1). It is important to document the response. Briefly, (2+) is a normal response, (1+) sluggish, (3+) slightly hyperactive, and (4+) hyperactive with clonus.

An often simple but overlooked portion of the exam is analyzing the patient's gait. It is important to look for issues with balance, such as wide gait and ataxia. One should examine the level of the hips because a product as simple as new orthotic shoes can help with back pain. Assist devices such as canes, crutches, and walker should be examined and optimized for the patient's mobility.

A pain consultant will, of course, independently examine the patient thoroughly; however, it is important to include this information in the referral. A concise and focused physical examination can help the referring provider in developing will provide clarity toward focused clinical questions to ask the consulting pain providers.

CHRONIC VERSUS ACUTE PAIN

Chronic pain is defined as pain of at least 3 to 6 months' duration,[14] whereas acute pain is defined as pain less than 30 days' duration. It is extremely important to distinguish between these two clinical entities. Acute pain is typically handled in a hospital setting by consulting operating room anesthesiologists, although other specialists may handle acute pain consults. These patients have pain that is usually responsive to opioids and anti-inflammatory medications. Most hospitals will have protocols for acute pain management; however, some patients may have pain that exceeds these parameters. At this point in time, patient-controlled analgesia can prove helpful.[21] When management of intravenous opioid pain medications required is beyond the comfort level of a provider, it may be helpful to ask for assistance from an acute pain specialist.

Chronic pain, by contrast, is a completely different classification of pain and is managed completely differently in most situations. This is a great source of confusion for referring providers. Chronic pain is usually not responsive to escalating doses of opioids in the acute setting. Medications used to treat chronic pain have slow onset and can take several weeks of titration before a significant clinical effect is appreciated.[15] Interventional procedures are especially helpful; however, these elective procedures are not typically performed on hospitalized patients. Many of these patients have had chronic pain long before ever being hospitalized. The likelihood of "curing" the chronic pain during a brief hospitalization is extremely small. The referring provider must think about the value of a chronic pain consult in the hospital setting in terms of significantly reducing a patient's chronic pain. It may be useful to discuss realistic goals of chronic pain control in the hospital. Chronic pain consultants should set up an outpatient chronic pain services follow-up upon patient discharge to provide continuity of care or start a chronic pain patient's journey to pain relief.

When to Call a Chronic Pain Consultant

ACUTE PAIN ON CHRONIC PAIN: ESTABLISHING TREATMENT GOALS

The management of acute pain in the patient with chronic pain presents a common clinical scenario when hospitalized patients are referred to pain specialists. First, one must look at how pain is typically assessed in the hospital setting. A healthcare provider, typically a nurse, asks the patient to rate the current pain on a scale from 1 to 10.[16] Pain below a rating of 3 may not be treated pharmacologically. Pain that is moderate (4 to 7) may be treated with oral medications. Severe pain (7–10) may require intravenous medications. For an opioid-naïve patient, after the first several doses of intravenous opioids, side effects such as sedation and respiratory depression may be evident. The opioid-tolerant patient may continue to receive pain medications without side effects until the comfort level of the healthcare provider has been exceeded. Even after this point, the patient will continue to report a high intensity of pain. Therefore, the goals of pain control should be realistic: it is not reasonable to expose chronic pain patient to the risk of overdose of pain medications to bring his or her pain to the level of 4/10, acceptable for most inpatient population, when the baseline pain level is high, for example, 8/10.

In this scenario, it is important to differentiate the acute pain from the coexisting chronic pain. Interestingly, most patients will be able to distinguish between their background chronic pain and the acute pain. Setting a goal of treating the acute pain in the hospital while discussing management of chronic pain is typically useful. Upward titration of opioids and adjunct pain medications may work for acute pain in patients with chronic pain. If the chronic pain patient has a nil per os (NPO) order, the daily dose of chronic oral opioid is converted to intravenous opioids and then titrated upward as necessary when there is acute on chronic pain. Patient-controlled analgesia can be started for the chronic pain patient during hospital admission in an attempt to improve patient satisfaction. Some patients, especially those with neuropathic pain, can benefit from the addition of membrane-stabilizing medication such as gabapentin. As previously discussed, it is important to let the patient know that chronic pain will likely not be cured during this hospitalization. A multimodal medication regimen, in addition to counseling and physical therapy, will help reduce the pain.[17]

Next, the primary physician may begin non-opioid pharmacological treatment for chronic pain, understanding that it may take weeks before these medications provide relief. Medications may be complemented with alternative therapies such as biofeedback, acupuncture, or transcutaneous electric nerve stimulation[22] if available during hospitalization. A conversation about potential complementary modalities may help the patient become more engaged in treatment. More details on these modalities are available elsewhere in this book. If the initial upward titration of pain medications failed to control acute pain in the chronic pain patent, then the chronic pain service should be consulted.

MALFUNCTION OF COMMON PAIN DEVICES

Two common devices used in patients with chronic pain are intrathecal pumps (ITP) and spinal cord stimulators (SCS). Both typically are implanted by interventional pain physicians or neurosurgeons, and these physicians typically manage complications associated these devices. Primary care providers need to familiarize themselves with these devices, as they have gained popularity in the United States.[18] A detailed description of management of these devices in the hospital can be found elsewhere in this book. Here we provide a brief overview of how to manage problems that may arise in the hospitalized or outpatient setting. Adjustment of these devices typically requires support from a chronic pain service.

Intrathecal Pumps (ITP)

Complications associated with intrathecal pumps are typically related to pharmacology. The ITP is a reservoir of medications that is slowly infused into the cerebral spinal fluid (CSF) through an intrathecal catheter. The U.S. Food and Drug Administration (FDA) has approved morphine, ziconitide, and baclofen as medications that can be used in intrathecal devices. Fentanyl, hydromorphone, and bupivicaine are also agents, though not approved by the FDA, that are commonly used in intrathecal pumps. Malfunction or injury of the pump or catheter can lead to an inability of these drugs to reach the CSF. Abrupt discontinuation of opioids can cause withdrawal symptoms such as pain, tremors, tachycardia, anxiety, nausea, diarrhea, akathisia, and generalized malaise.[19] Restarting opioid pain medications and sometimes low-dose clonidine can mitigate the symptoms of withdrawal. Conversely, an overdose of medication to the CSF can cause sedation, respiratory depression, and weakness. In a select group of patients, especially those on high doses of intrathecal drugs, a granuloma can form around the tip of the intrathecal catheter. This prevents the medication from entering the CSF, causing a constellation of symptoms that can mimic a malfunctioning ITP catheter.

Spinal Cord Stimulators and Peripheral Stimulators

The spinal cord stimulator (SCS) typically stimulates an area of the body that is producing pain, such as a certain limb in complex regional pain syndrome (CRPS) or radicular pain associated with lumbosacral neuritis and chronic low back pain. The stimulator leads in the spine can migrate, leading to stimulation of regions outside the area of interest. For instance, a patient may have CRPS in the right lower extremity; however, lead migration may cause stimulation of the right thoracic area. The discomfort from the stimulation in regions outside of interest will cause a patient to report an elevated level of pain. In this case, the SCS lead may need to be electively repositioned or reprogrammed by a pain physician.

Other complications these devices can cause are bleeding and infection. Infection will present with exquisite pain and erythema at the device insertion site. Constitutional symptoms such as fever, chills, generalized malaise may also be present. The most feared infectious complication from these devices is meningitis, a situation that would require removal of the device. Bleeding will also present with pain at the device site and at times a palpable hematoma surrounding the device or neurological symptoms such as weakness if there is bleeding in the spine. It is important to note if the medication history includes anticoagulant or antiplatelet drugs.

CANCER AND PALLIATIVE CARE PAIN

Palliative care is supportive treatment of the terminally ill patient. Supportive care involves pain control, psychosocial support, promotion of spiritual health, introduction of coping and bereavement skills, and affirmation of death as a part of life. While some hospitals have supportive services such as a chaplain or grief counseling, the pain physician may also become involved in comfort measures for a dying patient.

Advanced cancer is a common terminal illness in which pain control plays a major role in palliative care. When consulting on a patient, it is important to know the type and stage of cancer as well as type of pain the patient is experiencing. Pain is a prominent feature in cancer that metastasizes to the bone, especially the spine and ribs. Nociceptive pain caused by the tumor can be treated with anti-inflammatory and opioid medications. These patients will typically require patient-controlled analgesia with a basal rate. It is important to slowly titrate the opioid medication upward to avoid excessive sedation and respiratory depression. It is common for tumor masses to impinge on nerve fibers, causing neuropathic pain. Membrane stabilizers such as gabapentin are excellent first-line agents for treating neuropathic pain; however, it may take several days or weeks before pain relief can be appreciated.[20] High doses of opioids may negatively impact a patient's quality of life.

A chronic pain service can help achieve the goal of inpatient reasonably controlled pain at the time of discharge from the hospital. This service may set up home-going patient-controlled analgesia, tunneled epidural or peripheral catheter, or an ITP trial.

Summary

It is important to understand the training and expertise of your consulting pain provider so that you may match your patient's needs with the provider's expertise. In addition, knowledge of the pain services provided by the hospital system can streamline the process of finding the appropriate services for your patient. If the initial upward titration of pain medications failed to control acute pain in chronic pain patent, then chronic pain services should be consulted.

It is essential that primary physicians are familiar with general principles of operation of implantable devices and with initial management of their common complications.

References

1. Abbott FV, Gray-Donald K, Sewitch MI, Johnston CC, Edgar L Jeans ME. The prevalence of pain in hospitalized patients: a national survey. *J Clin Anesth*. 1998;10(1):77–85.
2. Oden R. Acute post-operative pain: incidence and characteristics of pain in a sample of medical-surgical inpatients. *Pain*. 1987;30:69–78.
3. Rathmell J. The evolution of the field of pain medicine. *Reg Anesth Pain Med*. 2012;37:652–656.

4. Board Certification in an Anesthesiology Subspecialty: Pain Medicine. http://www.the-aba.org/pdf/PM_Board_Stmt.PDF

5. Emanuel LL, Richter J. The consultant and the patient–physician relationship: a trilateral deliberative model. *Arch Intern Med.* 1994;154:1785.

6. Ballard WP, Gold JP, Charlson ME. Compliance with the recommendations of medical consultants. *J Gen Intern Med.* 1986;1:220.

7. Bickley LS, Szilagyi PG. *Bates' Guide to Physical Examination and History Taking.* Philadelphia: Lippincott, Williams & Wilkins; 2002.

8. Bonica JJ. *Pain Terms and Taxonomies of Pain. The Management of Pain*, 3rd ed. Philadelphia: John Loeser; 2001.

9. Coderre TJ, Katz I, Vaccarino AL, et al. Contribution of central neuroplasticity of patho-logical pain: review of clinical and experimental evidence. *Pain.* 1993;52:259–285.

10. Willis WD, Westlund KN. Neuroanatomy of the pain system and of the pathway that mod-ulate pain. *J Clin Neurophysiol.* 1997;14:2–31.

11. Turk DC, Swanson KS, Wilson HD. The biopsychosocial model of pain and pain man-agement. In: Ebert M, Kerns RD, eds. *Behavioral and Pharmacological Pain Management.* New York: Cambridge University Press; 2011:16–43.

12. Donohoe CD. Targeted history and physical examination. In: Waldman SD, ed. *Interventional Pain Management*, 2nd ed. Philadelphia: WB Saunders; 2001:83–94.

13. Kateric S, Williams DB, Beard CM, et al. Epidemiology and clinical features of idiopathic trigeminal neuralgia and glossopharyngeal neuralgia: similarities and differences. *Neuroepidemiology.* 1991;10:276–281.

14. Turk DC, Okifuji A. Pain terms and taxonomies of pain. In: Loeser JP, Butler SH, Chapman CR, et al., eds. *Bonica's Management of Pain*, 3rd ed. Baltimore, MD: Lippincott, Williams, & Wilkins; 2001:241–254.

15. Dworkin RH, O'Connor AB, Backonja M, et al. Pharmacologic management of neuropathic pain: evidence-based recommendations. *Pain.* 2007;132:237–251.

16. Jensen MP, Turner LR, Turner JA, et al. The use of multi-item scales for pain intensity measurement in chronic pain patients. *Pain.* 1996;67:35–40.

17. Kehlet H, Dahl JB. The value of "multimodal" or "balanced" analgesia in postoperative pain treatment. *Anesth Analg.* 1993;77:1048–1056.

18. Prager J. Estimates of annual spinal cord stimulator implant rises in the United States. *Neuromodulation.* 2010;13:68–69.

19. Coffey RJ, Edgar TS, Francisco GE, et al. Abrupt withdrawal from life-threatening syn-drome. *Arch Phys Med Rehabil.* 2002;83:735–741.

20. Keskinbora K, Pekel AF, Aydinli I. Gabapentin and an opiod combination versus opi-oid alone for management of neuropathic cancer pain: a randomized open trial. *J Pain Symptom Manage.* 2007;34:183–189.

21. Walder B, Schafer M, Henzi I, Tramer MR. Efficacy and safety of patient-controlled opioids for acute postoperative pain. *Acta Anaesthesiol Scand.* 2001;45:795–804.

22. Johnson MI. Trancutaneous electrical nerve stimulation. (TENS). In: Watson I, ed. *Electrotherapy, Evidence-Based Practice*, 12th ed. Edinburgh: Churchill Livingstone; 2008:253–296.

Part II

MANAGEMENT OF CHRONIC PAIN IN SELECTED SETTINGS

8

Management of Chronic Pain in the Emergency Department

WALEED SHAH, DAJIE WANG, AND DAVID E. CUSTODIO

KEY POINTS

- Long-term success in the management of chronic pain in patients frequently presenting to the emergency department with pain requires that healthcare providers of different specialties work together as a team.
- Multidisciplinary collaboration and other factors ultimately may be more important for patient satisfaction with emergency department management of their pain than whether they receive analgesics or opioids.
- Suggestions for use of opioids in the emergency department include but are not limited to using short-acting opioids for acute pain when pain severity warrants use, using the lowest effective dose, avoiding long-acting/extended release formulations, limiting opioids to a short course, and assessing for opioid misuse and abuse.

Introduction

Pain is a major complaint in emergency medical care; nearly half of chief complaints in the emergency department (ED) concern pain. In terms of treatment, between 2001 and 2010, opioid use in EDs escalated, the use of non-opioid pain killers decreased, and yet prevalence of pain among ED patients remained constant.[1,2] This increase in opioid use may have contributed to the increased incidences of opioid overdose and misuse and as a result, limiting the amount of opioids prescribed (not administered) for patients leaving the ED.[3,4] One high-quality study found that "frequent ED visits for opioid overdose were associated with a higher likelihood of future hospitalizations and near-fatal events."[5] State-regulated monitoring programs, advanced technological solutions, as well as attempts to use poison center exposure calls, used to predict prescription opioid abuse and misuse-related ED visits, have met with variable success.[6,7] One of the major concerns of the medical community is that patient satisfaction surveys, such as the Press Ganey survey, are flawed metrics for chronic pain management in the ED setting, with potential "unintended negative consequences to patients and providers alike."[8] The authors of the study state that administrators, patients, and payors are confronted with the limitations of Press Ganey in chronic pain treatment and thus the need to develop more accurate tools.

This chapter discusses the complexity of and controversy surrounding chronic pain management in the ED.

Chronic Pain Versus Acute Pain in the Emergency Department

Pain in the ED setting can be classified into three general categories: acute pain, chronic pain, and acute on chronic pain. While medical professionals in the ED are well trained and equipped to manage acute pain or pain secondary to a medical condition, the appropriate diagnosis and treatment of chronic pain conditions remains a daunting challenge. Patients with chronic pain conditions who present to the ED with increased pain and/or new onset of pain require a different approach and thorough understanding of chronic pain and acute pain management and the keen skills of ED physicians to provide appropriate care.

Acute pain is related to an injury and generally resolves after an appropriate healing period. The duration is typically less than 3 months. It is an internal warning system that harm or damage is occurring. Those presenting with acute pain should undergo a comprehensive workup and receive appropriate care in the emergency setting. Chronic pain conditions, by contrast, serve no known purpose and have no positive benefit to the patient. Chronic pain persists even though the injury has healed. Generally, chronic pain is defined as pain persisting beyond the expected period of time for tissue healing following an injury or surgery. However, the specific time frame for an expected healing period is variable. It has been suggested that pain persisting beyond 3–6 months is chronic pain.

Patients with chronic pain conditions who present to the ED can be divided into three main categories: chronic pain, chronic pain with new onset acute pain, and a chronic pain exacerbation. Each of these patient groups will require specific management based on their disease process and the etiology of their pain. For those with exacerbations of pain or new pain complaints, it is important to conduct an evaluation in the same fashion as for an acute medical process or complication. For those patients with known chronic diseases that cause frequent pain crises, such as back pain, sickle cell disease, or pancreatitis, a preset multidisciplinary approach, discussed later in the chapter, should be in place that involves the other treating physicians. An organized plan is the best approach to preventing inadequate pain control for patients and providing appropriate support and reliable resources for ED physicians.

The choice of opioid treatment in the ED is not well understood.[9] While overall opioid doses in the ED have been linked to equianalgesic doses, in one study the median hydromorphone dosage was more than 50% higher than that of morphine. The use of hydromorphone was strongly related to opioid dependency and a diagnosis of kidney stones. Almost half of the ED providers gave reasons that did not seem to have pharmacological validity.[10] This study suggested that ED physicians and other providers "seem to prescribe 'usual' dosages of morphine and relatively higher usual dosages of hydromorphone" accompanied by "common misconceptions about opioid pharmacology." Anxiolytics, commonly used in chronic pain patients, especially, benzodiazepines, have been found to be a major component in unintentional prescription drug overdoses when combined with opioid analgesics.[11]

SHOULD CHRONIC PAIN BE MANAGED IN THE EMERGENCY DEPARTMENT?

A variety of reasons, including limited access to primary medical care and pain management care, are associated with higher self-reported rates of chronic pain in the ED patient population.[12] In many cases, the ED has replaced these services for patients.[13] Unfortunately, prescription opioid misuse is widespread among chronic pain patients presenting to the ED.[14] One study revealed improper storage and disposal of controlled substances prescribed.[15] The ED readmission rates for elderly people with chronic pain, especially those prescribed opioid analgesics, are higher than overall ED readmission rates.[16] The number of ED visits and overall alcohol- or drug-related encounters have been found to be strongly associated with use of Schedule II opioids, headache, back pain, and substance use disorders.[17] The authors suggest that it may be possible to increase the safety of chronic opioid therapy by minimizing the prescription of Schedule II opioids in these higher-risk patients. Moreover, an opinion circulating in the literature is that the ED is not the best setting for chronic pain management. However, at the same time, it is the last resort for many patients who do come to the ED and who will continue to come should their pain continue.

That is why it is important to develop a system for the ED, using a reliable multidisciplinary approach, for managing patients with chronic pain.[18] Something as unpretentious as a short consultation was found to have a significant impact on chronic pain patients using the ED as their site of choice for chronic pain care: the average number of ED admissions per patient per year dropped from 6.8 to 2.3. Substantiation of validity of their chronic pain, introduction of non-opioids, and a series of letters to patients after discharge with lists of local primary care and pain providers were enlisted to treat patients; these measures were used effectively for patients "who had no medical home."[19]

Some additional tools had been developed. Low-dose ketamine analgesia has been found to be an effective tool for treating acute pain in opioid-dependent patients in the ED.[20] In a recent randomized, double-blind, controlled trial, intravenous acetaminophen, dexketoprofen, and morphine were found to be equally effective in treating acute mechanical low back pain in the ED.[21] Physical therapy in the ED is an effective adjunct tool for management of pain.[22] A performance improvement prescribing guideline reduced opioid prescriptions for ED patients with dental pain.[23] Discharge preparation and assessment of outpatient supports, detailed discussion of medication side effects, and improved delivery of printed materials in relevant languages have also been suggested. For patients with chronic pain that is not adequately controlled, it is prudent to contact the patient's treating pain physician to formulate a short-term plan for pain control in the ED and long-term plan to minimize return visits. These approaches, when implemented, can help improve quality of care and reduce the use of opioid medication discharge prescriptions.[24]

RESTRICTING OPIOID PRESCRIPTIONS BY EMERGENCY PHYSICIANS: WOULD THIS SOLVE THE PROBLEM OF OPIOID MISUSE?

The ED is sometimes erroneously labeled a "leading source of opioid prescriptions."[2] In fact, ED providers are responsible for fewer than 5% of "immediate-release opioid prescriptions and an even smaller proportion of extended or long-acting opioid prescriptions."[2] Despite this misperception, some U.S. states have suggested that ED providers be barred from prescribing more than a 3-day supply of opioid drugs.[2] There are suggestions, however, that a 3- to 7-day supply is more appropriate for patients admitted to the ED because it will provide enough time for the patient to obtain relevant outpatient care and prevent ED readmission. Logan et al. suggest that one of the solutions is "closing corrupt pain centers and improving access to high-quality, nonemergency care will improve the care of patients with pain."[3] They advise that limiting opioid prescription by ED providers will not solve the conundrum of opioid misuse and abuse (Table 8.1).

SUBSTANCE USERS IN THE EMERGENCY DEPARTMENT

Patients who present to the ED primarily seeking narcotics continue to be a source of stress and concern for the medical community. The true prevalence of patients presenting to the ED to obtain narcotics for illegitimate use is unknown. Substance users commonly overstate their pain.[25] They tend to report more severe pain, more chronically painful conditions, more functional impairment, and more psychological and mental problems. Given the complex relationship

Table 8.1 **Opioid Prescribing in the Emergency Department**

Key Points	Comments
1. Use short-acting opioids for acute pain when pain severity warrants use.	Maximize non-opioids and nerve blocks as primary pain management.
2. Use the lowest effective dose.	High-dose and potent narcotics risk adverse events and effects.
3. Prescribe a short course of opioids.	A 1-week prescription is usually sufficient; expedite follow-up care if pain is expected to last longer than the prescription.
4. Assess for opioid misuse and abuse.	Use opioid/drug abuse risk tools, focused history-taking, lab tests, and controlled substance information databases when available.
5. Avoid long-acting/extended release formulations.	These are usually not necessary for acute or intermittent pain management. Long-acting medications should be closely managed and monitored in the follow-up setting.

Adapted from Wattana M, et al. Prescription opioid guidelines and the emergency department. *Journal of Pain and Palliative Care Pharmacotherapy,* 2013;27:155–162.

between substance use, mood disorders, and chronic pain, it has been suggested that staff be trained in identifying patients with these conditions and in facilitating appropriate referrals to psychiatric and addictive services. While some patients are malingering, one must not overlook those with legitimate "drug-seeking" behavior, such as those in a true pain crisis. The diagnosis of malingering or drug-seeking is often difficult to make because of the lack of concrete supporting evidence in the ED setting. This diagnosis should be made in the outpatient setting, with multiple evaluations performed by physicians in multiple specialties.

Some patients present to the ED requesting pain medications for other reasons, such as running out of opioid medication, having an increased need for pain medications, or losing their medications. In these situations, both physical dependence and psychological dependence on prescribed medications need to be addressed. Physical dependence is a common phenomenon among all patients taking opioids for a long period of time. It is characterized by physical withdrawal symptoms when an opioid is discontinued. These patients need to continue taking opioids until they are evaluated by their treating pain specialists in order to prevent withdrawal symptoms. One study suggested that patients with complex nociceptive, neuropathic, and myofascial pain syndromes may have a lower prevalence of substance abuse disorders than that among the general population.[26] Nonetheless, evaluation for aberrant drug-related behaviors is necessary, in addition to a routine workup. Examples of aberrant drug-related behaviors include selling prescription drugs, prescription forgery, stealing or "borrowing" drugs from others, multiple episodes of prescription loss, and repeatedly seeking prescriptions from multiple clinicians. If there is suspicion of drug-seeking behavior, the best approach is to contact the patient's pain specialist or prescribing doctor to formulate a long-term treatment plan with strategies to address drug-seeking behaviors.

Communication with the physician prescribing the controlled substances is an excellent way to verify the patient's condition, home medication regimen, and current plan of care. Currently, there is a growth of statewide prescription-monitoring programs that allow online access to confirm prescribed medications and guide patient care.[27] A detailed assessment is necessary to rule out any true medical or surgical emergencies, if there are no emergent medical issues, the best approach is to refer these patients to their treating physicians for follow-up. The treatment of acute on chronic pain in patients with a history of substance abuse is discussed in detail in Chapter 22.

PATIENTS ON OPIOID REPLACEMENT THERAPY

Buprenorphine is a partial μ-opioid agonist and a weak κ antagonist. It has been approved for office-based treatment of opioid addiction. It has a long duration of action and 25–40 times the potency of morphine.[32,33] At high doses, it has a ceiling effect that limits both the analgesic effect and respiratory depression. This reduces the level of physical dependence and withdrawal symptoms. The combination of buprenorphine and naloxone is known as suboxone.

Naloxone is added to sublingual buprenorphine to prevent intravenous abuse of buprenorphine. Buprenorphine alone is available in sublingual and intravenous formulations and as a transdermal patch for treatment of pain.[28] The primary use of buprenorphine/naloxone is for detoxification and maintenance therapy for opioid addiction. This medication has also been prescribed off-label to treat acute and chronic pain by specialists with additional training in addictionology, because of its reduced potential for abuse and favorable side effects.[29] Patients who are on buprenorphine/naloxone may eventually require additional pain medications for various medical reasons. For these patients, the best approach is multimodal analgesia with nonsteroidal anti-inflammatory drugs (NSAIDs), neuromodulators, or nerve blocks, if possible. If opioid analgesics are considered, a higher dose and more potent drug such as fentanyl may be required to overcome the competitive effect of buprenorphine. Frequent evaluation in a monitored setting is necessary in order to avoid side effects of sedation and respiratory depression in these cases (more details on management of acute pain in patients taking buprenorphine and methadone are given elsewhere in this book).

Back Pain

Back pain is one of the most frequent complaints that brings patients to the ED. While the majority of back pain patients recover within weeks, a number of these patients can suffer chronic back pain. Many structures, including the intervertebral disc, ligaments, muscles, and facet joint, can cause pain, yet some of these patients do not have a definite pain generator, which poses a challenge for physicians.

Patients with chronic back pain are typically treated by pain specialists, with injections, medications, and rehabilitation modalities. The biopsychosocial model is the basis of treatment, emphasizing the biological, psychological, and social aspect of the condition.[30] Patients with more complex pain require a multidisciplinary team that includes psychologists and psychiatrists who can address the psychological and social component of chronic pain. Despite extensive and comprehensive interventions, some patients may still present to the ED because of inadequate control of chronic pain or because of new pain. When these patients present to the ED for inadequate pain control, evaluation and monitoring of psychological and psychiatric issues, including suicidal behaviors, need to be performed, in addition to the necessary medical evaluation. If there are any indications of suicidality, prompt psychiatric consultation is prudent to prevent self-harm.

For those patients who have had recent pain interventions such as epidural or intra-articular injection, it is especially important to evaluate for infection and epidural hematoma. These complications are rare—data are limited to case reports—but they do pose a significant threat to the patient. Prompt evaluation for overt signs of infection should be conducted and imaging and laboratory tests ordered if there is any suspicion of these complications. Neurological evaluation should be thorough and repeated to evaluate and monitor such patients. Emergent surgical evaluation is necessary if epidural or joint hematoma or abscess is suspected.

Postdural Puncture Headache

Postdural puncture headaches can occur after lumbar puncture, neuraxial anesthesia, and epidural steroid injections.[35] The typical presentation is positional headache that develops within the first 48 hours of dural puncture, but it can occur later. Diagnosis is based on history, physical exam, and the postural component of headache—worse when standing, and improved when recumbent. In the absence of these features, another differential diagnosis should be sought. Most patients will improve within 5 days with conservative therapy, including bed rest, aggressive hydration, caffeine, and oral analgesics.[35,36] When conservative treatments fail, or the patient suffers severe headache with nausea and vomiting and is unable to tolerate oral medications, a pain management special-ist or anesthesiologist should be consulted for an epidural blood patch.

Sickle Cell Disease

Sickle cell disease (SCD) is a chronic, debilitating condition that is frequently encountered in the ED. This condition can be associated with chronic pain. The pain during a crisis is related to the ischemia secondary to sickle-shaped red blood cells causing vasoocclusion and decreased blood flow to distal tissues. Acute painful crises, due to vasoocclusion, are the hallmark of this disease. The pathophysiology of chronic pain associated with SCD is unclear. The assessment of chronic pain is often difficult because these patients do not present with the typical signs of sickle cell crisis. Treatment of SCD with associated chronic pain with opioid medications is common, further perplexing the physician's assess-ment, especially in the ED setting.

Acute sickle cell crisis is a common occurrence in the ED. The frequency of these attacks is variable, ranging from less than once a year to a few times per month.[37] Acute pain can occur in multiple sites, including the chest, abdomen, joints, and bone. Treatments with NSAIDs, opioids, and adequate hydration are standard and effective. However, for patients who present to the ED with exac-erbation of chronic pain, especially those on chronic opioid medications, assess-ment is more complex. Treatment is often more extensive because both the acute pain and chronic pain need to be addressed.

Most sickle cell patients do not experience chronic pain; they only have pain during a crisis. But some patients, especially elderly patients and those with recur-rent and severe painful crises, can develop chronic pain.[38] While the exact etiol-ogy of chronic pain from SCD is unclear, it has been hypothesized that repeated pain stimuli can cause abnormalities in the tissue, leading to central sensitization and chronic pain. In the clinical assessment of these patients, the physician will need to obtain detailed information about their opioid medication regimen and the frequency of crises, in addition to conducting a routine evaluation for SCD. Assessment of acute pain or acute exacerbation of chronic pain is an important part of the evaluation. In normal patients with acute pain or chronic pain with exacerbation, there are signs of sympathetic activation, such as hypertension, tachycardia, and diaphoresis. These objective sympathetic changes are absent in chronic pain patients. The typical presentation of chronic pain in SCD patients includes guarding, grimacing, and sighing. Among these signs, guarding has been found to correlate with the physician's rating of the patient's pain.[39]

For patients who present with chronic pain and signs of acute pain, treatment can be challenging due to opioid tolerance. Parenteral anti-inflammatory drugs such as ketorolac are beneficial because of their opioid-sparing effects and fast onset of analgesic effect.[40,41] Opioid medications remain the mainstay of treating these pain exacerbations. It is important to obtain a detailed history of opioid use prior to initiating any opioids in the ED. Morphine, oxycodone, hydrocodone, and fentanyl patch are commonly prescribed by pain management specialists, family doctors, and internists for chronic sickle cell pain. The choice of opioid medication and route of administration in the ED will depend on the opioid, its dosage, and the duration of the patient's opioid medication use. Intermittent intravenous injection with titration and careful monitoring is the most appropriate approach for patients on large doses and chronic use of opioids.

While patient-controlled analgesia is primarily employed in the inpatient setting to provide pain relief, this can be used in the ED setting as well. It allows a controlled amount of medication to be delivered more frequently to avoid peaks and troughs of plasma concentration.

One of the most challenging problems in treating sickle cell patients is that they present repeatedly to the ED for pain relief or pain medication. In this clinical scenario, it is important not to label these patients "drug seekers." Urine drug screening should be part of the evaluation to confirm the medications prescribed by their pain doctors and to rule out illicit drug use. Multidisciplinary pain management for these patients is the best approach for long-term care for relieving pain and improving functionality. Although this approach is not feasible in the ED setting, it is prudent to consult the patient's primary care doctor, hematologists, or physician who prescribes the opioids in order to formulate a long-term treatment plan.

Complex Regional Pain Syndrome

Complex regional pain syndrome (CRPS) typically presents as chronic pain in an extremity. The exact etiology of CRPS is unclear; it usually occurs after injury to an extremity. The severity and duration of the pain are disproportionate to the causative event. Clinical presentation is often associated with allodynia, hyperalgesia, swelling, edema, weakness, and sudomotor and vasomotor change. *Allodynia* is pain resulting from a stimulus such as light touch of the skin which would not normally provoke pain. *Hyperalgesia* is increased sensitivity to pain stimuli or enhanced intensity of pain sensation. Although uncommon, this condition can present in the face and trunk.

The incidence of CRPS is 26/100,000 life-years, the female-to-male ratio is 3.5:1. CRPS is divided into type I and type II.[42] CRPS I is chronic pain that developed without a nerve injury, and CRPS II occurs after damage to a peripheral nerve. Patients with CRPS should get treatment from a multidisciplinary team of specialists.

The current hypothesis regarding CRPS is that it consists of limb-confined inflammation and tissue hypoxia, sympathetic dysregulation, small pain fiber damage, serum autoantibodies, central sensitization, and cortical reorganization.[43] The treatments are diverse, to target presumed pathophysiological processes. The main goal of treatment is to sustain or restore functionality and to reduce pain. The best treatment approach is multidisciplinary, with pain management specialists to provide pain control, rehabilitation specialists to sustain or restore limb function, and psychiatrists or psychologists to offer psychiatric support and pain coping techniques.

Despite the extensive treatments provided by physicians from various medical specialties, CRPS patients may still present to the ED for pain flare-ups or inadequate pain control. For patients who are otherwise stable on their pain treatment regimen, their pain flare-ups can be managed by additional pain medications. Intravenous analgesics with opioids and NSAIDs may be required for patients who routinely take opioid medications. The principle of using opioids for opioid-tolerant patients is the same as that for patients without opioid tolerance. However, higher doses of opioids and individualized titration are necessary to achieve adequate pain relief and to avoid overdose.

Patients with Implanted Pain Management Devices Who Present to the Emergency Department

SPINAL CORD STIMULATORS

Spinal cord stimulation (SCS) is employed by chronic pain specialists or neurosurgeons to manage various chronic pain conditions that are refractory to conservative pain management therapies. SCS can have significant analgesic properties for a multitude of chronic pain states, including angina, ischemic limb pain, diabetic peripheral neuropathy, phantom limb pain, radiculopathy, and CRPS. These devices have electrodes that are implanted in the spinal canal to send pulsed electrical energy toward the dorsal columns of the spinal cord for pain control.[44] It was first used by Shealy in 1967 in the intrathecal space to treat cancer pain. Currently, electrodes are placed surgically or percutaneously in the epidural space and a permanent pulse generator is placed subcutaneously, usually above the iliac crest.

Chronic pain patients who have undergone SCS can present to the ED with various other medical conditions or increased pain. The status of the SCS device should be investigated as part of the initial evaluation. Modern pulse generators have a battery life from 2 to 10 years, and most recently implanted devices have rechargeable batteries. They have multiple power settings and may even be turned off, or the battery may be low if not recharged properly; both are potential causes of increased pain. Patients with an SCS device who present to the

ED with increasing pain should be questioned about the efficacy and function of their device. It may require investigation by a pain physician if the patient doesn't experience adequate stimulation in the painful area.

Complications associated with SCS include lead migration, infection, epidural hematoma, seroma, hematoma, paralysis, CSF leak, skin erosion, hardware malfunction, and battery failure.[45] Most of these complications related to SCS are not life-threatening and can be resolved by removal of the device.[45] Although uncommon, serious complications such as epidural abscess or hematoma can occur and lead to paralysis and even death. If there are any signs of infection or neurological deficit, immediate communication with the pain physician managing the device is important in order to provide appropriate intervention in a timely fashion. If the treating pain physician cannot be reached, the alternative is a neurosurgical consultation.

It is important to note that most SCS devices are not MRI compatible and thus should be removed before using this imaging modality; CT scanning and X-ray are considered safe. Currently, three companies produce SCS (Medtronic, Boston Scientific, St Jude Medical) information regarding imaging compatibility and safety, which can be found at their company websites.

TREATING PATIENTS WITH AN INTRATHECAL PUMP IN THE EMERGENCY DEPARTMENT

Systemic delivery of medications such as opioids or muscle relaxants in high doses can cause significant side effects that ultimately limit pain relief. Intrathecal delivery of opiates can offer significant pain relief with limited systemic side effects. Multiple drugs, including morphine, hydromorphone, fentanyl, local anesthetics (bupivacaine), and ziconotide, are used in various combinations to treat pain. Baclofen can be delivered intrathecally as well for the treatment of muscle spasticity and dystonia.[46]

The implantation procedure involves a catheter placed in the intrathecal space that is tunneled to a subcutaneous programmable medication pump. Complications of intrathecal drug delivery systems (IDDS) can be related to mechanical failures, infection, drug effects, catheter migration, spinal hematoma, epidural hematoma, and arachnoiditis. [47,48,49] Patents presenting to the ED with IDDS and exacerbations of their pain should have their devices investigated. A pain specialist with an appropriate investigation device should determine functionality of the pump, drug delivery settings, drug reservoir volume, battery life, and the combinations of drugs being delivered. More invasive evaluation of the device may be necessary if there is any suspicion of catheter dysfunction or breakage. Given the high concentration of medication used, small errors in pump programming can result in significant over- or under-dosing.

Most currently available IDDS and some SCS devices are MRI compatible. Those patients undergoing MRI should have their device checked afterward to ensure proper functioning of the IDDS. The infusion mechanism may stall during MRI and fail to restart, resulting in cessation of drug delivery. All patients with IDDS for baclofen intrathecal administration are at a potential risk for acute baclofen withdrawal if there is malfunction of the device.[50,51] Symptoms of baclofen withdrawal include rebound spasticity, itching, tachycardia, fever, hyperthermia, rhabdomyolysis, autonomic instability, multi-organ system failure, seizures, hallucinations, delirium, and confusion.[51] Some of these complications can be life-threatening. Prompt recognition of withdrawal and communication with the treating physician and intensivist are crucial to prevent serious complications.

When acute baclofen withdrawal is suspected, treatment should involve resuming intrathecal baclofen, when possible. Oral baclofen, unfortunately, is unreliable as a rescue medication because of its inability to achieve necessary CSF concentrations, especially in patients receiving a high dose of intrathecal baclofen. Nevertheless, oral baclofen is commonly administered in combination with benzodiazepines as adjuvant therapy.[50,51]

Summary

Despite the best efforts of physicians in multidisciplinary teams, typically consisting of pain specialists, psychologists, psychiatrists, and other specialists, some patients with chronic pain continue to present to the ED and for various reasons. These cases require that the ED physician be an active part of the multidisciplinary team. For long-term success in management of these patients' complex issues and to prevent repeated visits to the ED, healthcare providers of different specialties need to work together as a team. These factors ultimately may be more important for patient satisfaction with ED management of their pain than their receiving analgesics or opioids.[31]

References

1. Chang HY, Daubresse M, Kruszewski SP, Alexander GC. Prevalence and treatment of pain in EDs in the United States, 2000 to 2010. *Am J Emerg Med.* 2014;32(5):421–431.
2. Rosenau AM. Guidelines for opioid prescription: the devil is in the details. *Ann Intern Med.* 2013;158(11):843–844.
3. Logan J, Liu Y, Paulozzi L, Zhang K, Jones C. Opioid prescribing in emergency departments: the prevalence of potentially inappropriate prescribing and misuse. *Med Care.* 2013;51(8):646–653.
4. Brandenburg MA, Subera L, Doran-Redus A, Archer P; Oklahoma Workgroup. Opioid prescribing guidelines for Oklahoma emergency departments (ED) and urgent care clinics (UCC). *J Okla State Med Assoc.* 2013;106(10):391–397.

5. Hasegawa K, Brown DF, Tsugawa Y, Camargo CA Jr. Epidemiology of emergency department visits for opioid overdose: a population-based study. *Mayo Clin Proc.* 2014;89(4):462–471.

6. Neven DE, Sabel JC, Howell DN, Carlisle RJ. The development of the Washington State emergency department opioid prescribing guidelines. *J Med Toxicol.* 2012;8(4):353–359.

7. Davis JM, Severtson SG, Bucher-Bartelson B, Dart RC. Using poison center exposure calls to predict prescription opioid abuse and misuse-related emergency department visits. *Pharmacoepidemiol Drug Saf.* 2014;23(1):18–25.

8. Darnall BD, Schatman ME. Autonomy vs paternalism in the emergency department: the potential deleterious impact of patient satisfaction surveys. *Pain Med.* 2013;14(7):968.

9. Bounes V, Jouanjus E, Roussin A, Lapeyre-Mestre M. Acute pain management for patients under opioid maintenance treatment: what physicians do in emergency departments. *Eur J Emerg Med.* 2014;21(1):73–76.

10. O'Connor AB, Rao A. Why do emergency providers choose one opioid over another? A prospective cohort analysis. *J Opioid Manag.* 2012;8(6):403–413.

11. Jann M, Kennedy WK, Lopez G. Benzodiazepines: a major component in unintentional prescription drug overdoses with opioid analgesics. *J Pharm Pract.* 2014;27(1):5–16.

12. Hanley O, Miner J, Rockswold E, Biros M. The relationship between chronic illness, chronic pain, and socioeconomic factors in the ED. *Am J Emerg Med.* 2011;29(3):286–292.

13. Dixon WJ, Fry KA. Pain recidivists in the emergency department. *J Emerg Nurs.* 2011;37(4):350–356.

14. Beaudoin FL, Straube S, Lopez J, Mello MJ Baird J. Prescription opioid misuse among ED patients discharged with opioids. *Am J Emerg Med.* 2014;32(6):580–585.

15. Tanabe P, Paice JA, Stancati J, Fleming M. How do emergency department patients store and dispose of opioids after discharge? A pilot study. *J Emerg Nurs.* 2012;38(3):273–279.

16. Howard R, Hannaford A, Weiland T. Factors associated with re-presentation to emergency departments in elderly people with pain. *Aust Health Rev.* 2014;38(4):461–466.

17. Braden JB, Russo J, Fan MY, Edlund MJ, Martin BC, DeVries A, Sullivan MD. Emergency department visits among recipients of chronic opioid therapy. *Arch Intern Med.* 2010;170(16):1425–1432.

18. McLeod D, Nelson K. The role of the emergency department in the acute management of chronic or recurrent pain. *Australas Emerg Nurs J.* 2013;16(1):30–36.

19. Intervention reduces chronic pain visits. *ED Manag.* 2010;22(12):141–142.

20. Richards JR, Rockford RE. Low-dose ketamine analgesia: patient and physician experience in the ED. *Am J Emerg Med.* 2013;31(2):390–394.

21. Eken C, Serinken M, Elicabuk H, Uyanik E, Erdal M. Intravenous paracetamol versus dexketoprofen versus morphine in acute mechanical low back pain in the emergency department: a randomised double-blind controlled trial. *Emerg Med J.* 2014 Mar;31(3):177–181.

22. Fleming-McDonnell D, Czuppon S, Deusinger SS, Deusinger RH. Physical therapy in the emergency department: development of a novel practice venue. *Phys Ther.* 2010;90(3):420–426.

23. Fox TR, Li J, Stevens S, Tippie T. A performance improvement prescribing guideline reduces opioid prescriptions for emergency department dental pain patients. *Ann Emerg Med.* 2013;62(3):237–240.

24. Gugelmann H, Shofer FS, Meisel ZF, Perrone J. Multidisciplinary intervention decreases the use of opioid medication discharge packs from 2 urban EDs. *Am J Emerg Med.* 2013;31(9):1343–1348.

25. Neighbor ML, Dance TR, Hawk M, Kohn MA. Heightened pain perception in illicit substance-using patients in the ED: implications for management. *Am J Emerg Med.* 2011;29(1):50–56.

26. Proctor SL, Estroff TW, Empting LD, Shearer-Williams S, Hoffmann NG. Prevalence of substance use and psychiatric disorders in a highly select chronic pain population. *J Addict Med.* 2013;7(1):17–24.

27. Baehren DF, Marco CA, Droz DE, Sinha S, Callan EM, Akpunonu P. A statewide prescription monitoring program affects emergency department prescribing behaviors. *Ann Emerg Med.* 2010;56(1):19–23.

28. Davis MP. Twelve reasons for considering buprenorphine as a frontline analgesic in the management of pain. *J Support Oncol.* 2012;10(6):209–219.

29. Rosenblum A, Cruciani RA, Strain EC, et al. Sublingual buprenorphine/naloxone for chronic pain in at-risk patients: development and pilot test of a clinical protocol. *J Opioid Manag* 2012;8(6):369–382.

30. Hancock MJ, Maher CG, Laslett M, Hay E, Koes B Discussion paper: what happened to the 'bio' in the bio-psycho-social model of low back pain? *Eur Spine J.* 2011;20(12):2105–2110.

31. Schwartz TM, Tai M, Babu KM, Merchant RC. Lack of association between press Ganey emergency department patient satisfaction scores and emergency department administration of analgesic medications. *Ann Emerg Med.* 2014;64:469–481.

32. Raisch DW, et al. Opioid dependence treatment, including buprenorphine/naloxone. *The Annals of pharmacotherapy* 2002;36(2):312–321.

33. Heel RC, et al. Buprenorphine: a review of its pharmacological properties and therapeutic efficacy. *Drugs.* 1979; 17(2):81–110.

34. Boothby LA, Doering PL. Buprenorphine for the treatment of opioid dependence. *American Journal of Health-System Pharmacy.* 2007; 64(3):266–272.

35. Ahmed Ghaleb, "Postdural Puncture Headache," Anesthesiology Research and Practice, vol. 2010, Article ID 102967, 6 pages, 2010. doi:10.1155/2010/102967

36. Bezov D, Lipton RB, Ashina S. Post-Dural Puncture Headache: Part I Diagnosis, Epidemiology, Etiology, and Pathophysiology. *Headache: The Journal of Head and Face Pain.* 2010;50(7):1144–1152.

37. Vichinsky EP, Lubin BH. Sickle cell anemia and related hemoglobinopathies. *Pediatr Clin North Am.* 1980 May;27(2):429–447.

38. Mark H, Stonerock GL, Kisaalita NR, Jones S, Orringer E, Gil KM. Detecting the Emergence of Chronic Pain in Sickle Cell Disease. *J Pain Symptom Manage.* 2012 June;43(6):1082–1093.

39. Gil KM, Phillips G, Edens J, Martin NJ, Abrams M. Observation of pain behaviors during episodes of sickle cell disease pain. *Clin J Pain.* 1994 Jun;10(2):128–132.

40. Malan Jr, T. Philip, et al. Parecoxib sodium, a parenteral cyclooxygenase 2 selective inhibitor, improves morphine analgesia and is opioid-sparing following total hip arthroplasty. *Anesthesiology.* 2003;98(4):950–956.

41. Joishy SK, Walsh D. The opioid-sparing effects of intravenous ketorolac as an adjuvant analgesic in cancer pain: application in bone metastases and the opioid bowel syndrome. *Journal of Pain and Symptom Management.* 1998;16(5):334–339.

42. deMos M, De Bruijn AG, Huygen FJ, Dieleman JP, Stricker BH, Sturkenboom MC. The incidence of complex regional pain syndrome: a population-based study. *Pain.* 2007;129:1220.

43. Goebel A. Complex regional pain syndrome in adults. *Rheumatology (Oxford).* 2011 Oct;50(10):1739–1750.

44. Kumar K, Nath R, Wyant GM. Treatment of chronic pain by epidural spinal cord stimulation: a 10-year experience. *Journal of Neurosurgery.* 1991;75(3):402–407.

45. Cameron T. Safety and efficacy of spinal cord stimulation for the treatment of chronic pain: a 20-year literature review. *J Neurosurg.* 2004;100(suppl 3):254–267.

46. Haranhalli N, Anand D, Wisoff JH, Harter DH, Weiner HL, Blate M, et al. Intrathecal baclofen therapy: complication avoidance and management. *Childs Nerv Syst.* 2011;27:421–427.

47. Vender JR, et al. Identification and management of intrathecal baclofen pump complications: a comparison of pediatric and adult patients. *Journal of Neurosurgery: Pediatrics.* 2006;104(1):9–15.

48. Saltuari L, et al. Indication, efficiency and complications of intrathecal pump supported baclofen treatment in spinal spasticity. *Acta neurologica.* 1992;14(3):187–194.

49. Atli A, et al. Intrathecal opioid therapy for chronic nonmalignant pain: a retrospective cohort study with 3-year follow-up. *Pain Medicine.* 2010;11(7):1010–1016.
50. Ross JC, et al. Acute intrathecal baclofen withdrawal: a brief review of treatment options. *Neurocritical Care.* 2011;14(1):103–108.
51. Watve SV, et al. Management of acute overdose or withdrawal state in intrathecal baclofen therapy. *Spinal Cord.* 2012;50(2):107–111.

9

Management of Chronic Pain in the Intensive Care Unit

PAVAN TANKHA AND MARISA LOMANTO

KEY POINTS

- Pain is a common complaint among ICU patients. Hospitalized patients with acute or chronic decompensation of vital organ systems admitted to the intensive care unit present a challenge for the clinician, as a third to almost half of these patients will have pre-existing chronic pain conditions they are being treated for.
- Frequent assessment of pain via validated pain scales will allow safe and effective titration of pain medication in the ICU.
- Abrupt discontinuation of chronic opiates or adjuvant medications may precipitate symptoms of withdrawal.
- Critically ill patients have altered physiological and pharmacokinetic changes and, when combined with pre-existing pain medications, risk altered mental status, worsening of their clinical condition, or even respiratory failure and death.
- The ICU team is presented with a challenging task in which hemodynamic and respiratory instability combined with altered pharmacokinetics may preclude continuing a pre-existing pain management regimen. Critically ill patients may exhibit altered pharmacokinetics, and care must be taken to avoid potentially life-threatening side effects from pre-existing pain regimens.
- Pharmacological therapies include the use of NSAIDs, acetaminophen, opioids, adjuvants, muscle relaxants, and local anesthetics. In addition, intravenous infusions of dexmedetomidine, ketamine, and short-acting opioids may also prove useful. The clinician must be aware of the signs of withdrawal from opioids and benzodiazepines as well as be mindful of resuming home medications when clinically indicated.
- If clinically indicated, resuming home pain medications is warranted prior to transfer from the ICU.

Introduction

While the prevalence of chronic pain in the general population is estimated to be slightly higher than 30%, patients with chronic medical conditions such as renal failure have rates of chronic pain exceeding 50%.[1,2] The challenge of treating chronic pain in the intensive care unit is made more difficult by concomitant hemodynamic or respiratory collapse with or without altered pharmacokinetics secondary to end-organ failure. These physiological disturbances may lead to decreased medication metabolism, excretion, or both, the results of which may present as altered mental status, seizures, and respiratory failure. Scheduled, protocol-driven assessments of pain will allow the clinician to avoid the pitfalls of over- and undersedation. The goal of this chapter is to provide the reader with a conceptual overview of how chronic pain is best managed in this challenging patient population.

Before a treatment plan can be made, an assessment of the patient's pain must be obtained. The gold standard for pain assessment still remains the patient's own report. However, often, critically ill patients either have altered mental status, are sedated, or are intubated. Two behavioral pain assessments, the Behavioral Pain Scale (BPS) and the Critical-Care Pain Observation Tool (CCPOT), have been shown to be both valid and reliable in patients who are unable to communicate their pain scores to the clinician (Table 9.1 and Table 9.2). Frequent assessment of subjective pain scores allows the clinician to titrate the pain management regimen to effect.

The diagnosis of chronic pain in the ICU is beyond the scope of this chapter. However, given the prevalence of pain in the ICU population, the World Health Organization step ladder approach to managing pain may be a foundation from which to begin. Alternatively, patients may have already been established on a pharmacological regimen prior to ICU presentation. As such, nonsteroidal anti-inflammatories (NSAIDs), acetaminophen (APAP), opioids, membrane stabilizers, antidepressants, and local anesthetics are all classes of medications that must be addressed. It should be noted that patients who have been managed on long-term opioid or benzodiazepine medication regimens may present with symptoms of withdrawal if those medications have been discontinued abruptly either before or upon ICU admission.

Chronic Pain Patients with Renal Failure or Dysfunction

Renal failure may present in the ICU as either acute or chronic disease. Of note, the treatment recommendations outlined here are applicable to patients who present in either state.

Table 9.1 **Behavioral Pain Scale (Payen)**

Item	*Description*	*Score**
Facial expression	Relaxed	1
	Partially tightened (e.g., brow lowering)	2
	Fully tightened (e.g., eyelid closing)	3
	Grimacing	4
Upper limb movements	No movement	1
	Partially bent	2
	Fully bent with finger flexion	3
	Permanently retracted	4
Compliance with mechanical ventilation	Tolerating movement	1
	Coughing but tolerating ventilation for most of the time	2
	Fighting ventilator	3
	Unable to control ventilation	4

*BPS score ranges from 3 (no pain) to 12 (maximum pain).

As noted earlier, the prevalence of chronic pain in patients with chronic kidney disease (CKD) is approximately 50%.[2] Despite this large percentage of patients in pain, pharmacological management remains underutilized.[3] When these patients present to the ICU, the clinician must be acutely aware of the altered pharmacokinetics that are present. Because of these alterations either the parent drug or metabolite(s) may accumulate, resulting in potentially life-threatening respiratory failure or seizures (Table 9.3). An example of this is when morphine is metabolized into morpine-3-glucuronide and morphine-6-glucuronide. Accumulation of the former in renal failure may result in seizures; accumulation of the latter may result in respiratory failure.

Systematically approaching treatment for the patient with renal failure allows for optimal pain management while potentially avoiding adverse events. In the patient who presents with renal failure, an assessment of baseline pain via a verbal rating or the BPS/CCPOT needs to be made. Dosage adjustment of pain medications should be made based on the glomerular filtration rate (GFR) (Box 9.1). There are varied ways of calculating the GFR, but many handheld devices as well as online tools can help with this calculation (www.mdrd.com). However, if the patient is unable to take medications by mouth, intravenous therapy can be initiated. If the patient's renal status deteriorates and dialysis is required, further dosage adjustments may be indicated. When the patient is

Table 9.2 **Critical Care Pain Observation Tool (Gelinas)**

Indicator	Description		Score (Total Range 0–8)
Facial expression	No muscular tension observed	Relaxed, neutral	0
	Presence of frowning, brow lowering, orbit tightening, and levator contraction	Tense	1
	All of these facial movements plus eyelid tightly closed	Grimacing	2
Body movements	Patient does not move at all (does not necessarily mean absence of pain)	Absence of movements	0
	Slow, cautious movements, touching or rubbing the pain site, seeking attention through movements	Protection	1
	Pulling tube, attempting to sit up, moving limbs/thrashing, not following commands, striking at staff, trying to climb out of bed	Restlessness	2
Muscle tension; evaluation by passive flexion and extension of upper extremities	No resistance to passive movements	Relaxed	0
	Resistance to passive movements	Tense, rigid	1
	Strong resistance to passive movements, inability to complete them	Very tense, rigid	3
Compliance with the ventilator (intubated patients)	Alarms not activated, easy ventilation	Tolerating ventilator or movement	0
	Alarms stop spontaneously	Coughing but tolerating	1
	Asynchrony: blocking ventilation, alarms frequently activated	Fighting ventilator	2

(continued)

Table 9.2 **Continued**

Indicator	Description		Score (Total Range 0–8)
Or Vocalization (extubated patients)	Talking in normal tone or no sound	Talking in normal tone or no sound	0
	Sighing, moaning	Sighing, moaning	1
	Crying out, sobbing	Crying out, sobbing	2

able to take medications by mouth, liquid forms of gabapentin and carbamazepine are available to begin titration back to baseline levels. If possible, restarting home medication regimens based on corrected GFR is indicated prior to be transferred off the unit.

The paucity of evidence regarding pharmacological pain management in CKD lends itself to conservative treatment regimens. Given the likelihood of worsening GFR when used over an extended period of time, as well as the risk for gastrointestinal irritation, NSAIDs, if used, should be limited to no more than 5 days of use in renal failure.[4] Acetaminophen is safe in CKD and can be used as a single agent or in conjunction with other medications. Dose adjustments for chronic neuropathic pain medications, including secondary-amine tricyclic antidepressants (TCAs; e.g., amitriptyline), selective serotonin-norepinephrine reuptake inhibitors (SNRIs; e.g., venlafaxine), and the calcium channel alpha-2 delta ligand (gabapentin), should be made based on GFR, but, again, there are limited data regarding this. Though there is weak evidence to support the use of opiates for chronic pain states, patients may still be prescribed them prior to ICU admission secondary to nociceptive or neuropathic pain. With the exception of morphine, whose metabolites may result in confusion and respiratory depression, hydromorphone, oxycodone, fentanyl, and methadone are well tolerated in CKD when properly monitored.[5-7]

Gabapentin, briefly mentioned previously, deserves special attention in this subset of patients. While it has been used effectively for the treatment of neuropathic pain states, in patients with CKD it has also shown efficacy with diabetic peripheral neuropathy, restless leg syndrome, and insomnia.[8-10] And though it is widely used in those conditions, its pharmacokinetics in CKD are altered significantly, as nearly 100% of the drug is excreted in the urine. After calculation of the estimated GFR, dosing should be modified accordingly, with 600 mg TID for a GFR of 50–79 to 300 mg daily for GFR <15.

Table 9.3 Effects of Drugs Used to Treat Chronic Pain in Patients with Chronic Kidney Disease (CKD)

Medication	% Parent Drug Excreted in Urine	Dialyzed	Hepatic Metabolism	Active Metabolites	Comments
Acetaminophen	5	Yes	Yes	No	Single dose >10 g can cause hepatic and renal toxicity
Ibuprofen	1	Yes	Yes	No	Does not accumulate in CKD nor is dose adjustment required
Naproxen	<1	No	Yes	No	Not recommended for CKD
Meloxicam	Minimal	No	Yes	No	If used in mild CKD, 7.5 mg is preferred
Celecoxib	<3	No	Yes	No	Not recommended for CKD; 50% dose reduction in hepatic impairment
Gabapentin	100	Yes	No	No	Dose modifications based on GFR required to avoid side effects
Pregabalin	99	No	No	No	Case reports suggest Na+ and water retention may precipitate congestive heart failure
Amitriptyline	<5%	No	Yes	Yes	Active metabolite is nortriptyline
Duloxetine	<1	No	Yes	No	Caution required with coexisting renal, liver disease
Venlafaxine	5	No	Yes	Yes	Dose reduction required with renal and hepatic insufficiency
Tramadol	30	Yes	Yes	Yes	Re-dose after dialysis
Codeine	Varies 3–15	No	Yes	Yes	Multiple active metabolites; avoid in CKD
Morphine	10	Yes	Yes	Yes	Avoid in CKD, as active and inactive metabolites can rapidly accumulate
Hydromorphone	6	Yes	Yes	No	Inactive metabolite may cause agitation and neuroexcitation
Fentanyl	5	No	Yes	No	Recommend lower dose in moderate/severe CKD
Oxycodone	19	Yes	Yes	Yes	Weak active metabolite
Methadone	Varies 15–60	No	Yes	No	Safe in CKD with close monitoring
Buprenorphine	<5	Yes	Yes	No	Sudden discontinuation can precipitate withdrawal
Ketamine	4	No	Yes	Yes	No dose adjustments necessary

> *Box 9.1* **Calculation of Glomerular Filtration Rate (GFR)**
>
> $$GFR = 186.3 \times (\text{serum creatinine})^{-1.154} \times (\text{age})^{-0.203}$$
> $$\times\ 0.742 \text{ (if female)}$$
> $$\times\ 1.210 \text{ (if African American)}$$

Advanced Liver Disease and Cirrhosis

The pharmacokinetics of analgesic medications is highly dependent on hepatic and renal function. Many analgesics are largely metabolized by the liver, and adverse effects in advanced liver disease are frequent and include hepatic encephalopathy, acute renal failure, and gastrointestinal bleeding.[11] The ability of the liver to process drugs depends on hepatic blood flow, hepatic enzyme capacity, and plasma protein binding, all of which may be affected by liver disease. Chronic liver disease is associated with variable and non-uniform reductions in drug metabolism, depending on the severity of disease. For example, hepatic glucuronidation is thought to be less affected than CYP450 oxidation in mild to moderate liver disease; however, it can be significantly impaired in advanced cirrhosis. While the Child-Pugh score may be used to assess the severity of liver dysfunction, it cannot quantitate the ability of the liver to metabolize specific drugs.[12] Patients with cirrhosis also often have impaired renal function. Therefore, analgesics that undergo predominant renal elimination may also require dose reduction in patients with advanced liver disease (Table 9.3). These individuals often have reduced muscle mass with a resultant decrease in creatinine production and may therefore have impaired renal function despite a normal creatinine level.[11] GFR (Box 9.1) or creatinine clearance (Box 9.2) should be calculated to better estimate the dosing of drugs that have predominantly renal elimination.[11,13] We recommend referring to readily available drug dosing guides for specific analgesic dosing regimens in hepatic and renal impairment.

NSAIDs are indicated for the treatment of mild to moderate pain. They are predominantly metabolized by hepatic CYP and most are heavily protein-bound. Reduced metabolism and increased bioavailability in cirrhosis result in increased drug serum levels. NSAIDs may be tolerated in patients with mild liver disease but should be avoided in cirrhotics with portal hypertension due to the increased risk of hepatorenal syndrome caused by prostaglandin reduction in renal perfusion and GFR. NSAIDs may also increase the risk of mucosal bleeding in these patients, who are already at risk due to pre-existing thrombocytopenia and coagulopathy.[11]

Box 9.2 **Calculation of Creatinine Clearance**

Estimated Creatinine Clearance (mL/min):

(Cockcroft and Gault equation)

$$CrCl = (140 - age) \times IBW / (Scr \times 72) (\times 0.85 \text{ for females})$$

Estimated Ideal body weight (kg)

Males: IBW = 50 kg + 2.3 kg for each inch over 5 feet

Females: IBW = 45.5 kg + 2.3 kg for each inch over 5 feet

Acetaminophen is indicated for the treatment of mild to moderate pain. It has minimal anti-inflammatory properties and at recommended doses is not associated with GI side effects or bleeding. APAP-induced hepatotoxicity is caused by altered CYP metabolism in conjunction with depleted glutathione stores, resulting in production of the hepatotoxic intermediate, *N*-acetyl-p-benzoquinone imine (NAPQI).[11] While glutathione stores are depleted in chronic alcohol (ETOH) consumption and malnutrition, they are not critically depleted in cirrhotics who are taking recommended doses of APAP.[11,14] In addition, although the half-life of oral APAP in cirrhotics is double that of healthy controls, hepatic and renal injury are rare when the dose is limited to <4 g/day.[15,16] On the basis of the available data, expert opinion for long-term (>14 days) APAP use in cirrhotics who are not actively drinking ETOH is for reduced dosing at 2–3 g/day.[14] In addition, while 3–4 g/day may appear safe for single or short-term dosing in cirrhotics who are not actively drinking, new FDA guidelines recommend a maximum dose of 2–3 g/day. In those who continue to drink mild to moderate amounts of ETOH, most hepatologists recommend <2 g/day for both short- and long-term administration.[11]

Opioids are indicated for the treatment of severe pain. The liver is the primary site for opioid metabolism and, as a result, individuals with advanced liver disease have decreased drug clearance and/or increased bioavailability, leading to drug accumulation, especially with repeated administration. Although glucuronidation is thought to be less affected by cirrhosis than CYP oxidation, studies have shown that the half-life of morphine may be double that of healthy individuals.[11,12,17,18] Other opioids have also been shown to have increased bioavailability and prolonged half-life. In addition, certain opioids, such as codeine, hydrocodone, and oxycodone, require conversion via CYP to morphine, hydromorphone, and oxymorphone, respectively, for a portion of their analgesic effect. Tramadol is also a prodrug that requires CYP conversion to desmethyltramadol.

In these patients, decreased drug metabolism may lead to variable serum levels and altered analgesic response.[11,12,17] Meperidine, which is highly protein-bound, is metabolized largely by CYP to normeperidine, a metabolite with CNS toxicity. It should be avoided in patients with liver disease, particularly in the setting of concomitant renal dysfunction.[11] Methadone and fentanyl, both highly protein-bound, also require reduced dosing; however, their metabolism via CYP does not produce toxic metabolites and they may be better tolerated.[11] Hydromorphone, which is minimally protein-bound and undergoes glucuronidation, may require dose reduction in liver disease but is safe to use in renal failure.[11] Methadone has high oral bioavailability and low hepatic extraction and undergoes significant hepatic metabolism; however, usual methadone maintenance doses appear to be safe in patients with advanced liver disease.[11,17,19] Nonetheless, methadone should be avoided in patients who are actively drinking ETOH because it inhibits methadone metabolism, leading to elevated plasma levels.[11,19] Patients with cirrhosis have a high prevalence of concomitant renal disease, and most opioids will require dose adjustment based on GFR. Hydromorphone and fentanyl appear to be least affected by renal dysfunction. The neurotoxic metabolite of morphine is poorly excreted in renal insufficiency and dose reduction or avoidance is recommended. Tramadol, which undergoes glucuronidation with CYP oxidation, may be used in low doses in cirrhotics; further dose reduction may be needed in renal failure. Tramadol is known to lower the seizure threshold and should likely be avoided in patients with seizure disorder.[11] Opioids commonly precipitate hepatic encephalopathy and their use should be avoided in patients with cirrhosis, particularly those with portal hypertension and pre-existing encephalopathy.[11,16]

Tricyclic antidepressants (TCAs) are effective in the treatment of neuropathic pain. TCAs undergo extensive hepatic biotransformation largely via CYP and subsequent renal elimination. Dose reduction is therefore required in the setting of liver disease. It is prudent to initiate treatment at a low dose in order to minimize side effects, such as sedation and anticholinergic effects of dry mouth, blurry vision, tachycardia, and orthostatic hypotension. It is also important to avoid intestinal stasis, as this can precipitate hepatic encephalopathy. The less potent TCAs, such as nortriptyline and desipramine, may have fewer associated side effects.[11]

SNRIs are used to treat neuropathic pain states and fibromyalgia syndrome. The metabolism of venlafaxine and duloxetine is primarily hepatic via CYP and the majority of the metabolites are renally excreted.[20–22] It is recommended that the venlafaxine dose be reduced by 50% in liver disease. Milnacipran is metabolized in the liver, also apparently exclusive of the CYP system, with the majority of drug excreted by the kidneys left unchanged. There is no dose adjustment required in mild to moderate liver disease, but caution is recommended in end-stage liver disease.[20,23]

Anticonvulsants are used in the treatment of neuropathic pain. Most anticonvulsants are metabolized by the liver via CYP and excreted renally, requiring reduced dosing in cirrhotic patients. Carbamazepine should be avoided, as it has been reported to cause hepatotoxicity in the general population and may precipitate a rapid deterioration in cirrhotics.[11,24] Gabapentin, which is not metabolized by the liver or bound to plasma proteins, may be preferable in patients with cirrhosis. However, it is excreted by the kidneys and its dose should be reduced in renal failure. Its potential side effects include sedation, nausea, and dizziness.[11] Pregabalin is also not metabolized by the liver; however, there is a case report of acute hepatotoxicity in a healthy 61-year-old male that was attributed to pregabalin.[11,25]

Diazepam is a benzodiazepine (BDZ) with muscle-relaxant properties occasionally used to alleviate pain caused by muscle spasm. It can be administered orally or intravenously. It is extensively metabolized by the liver and has several active metabolites, which are excreted renally. The elimination half-life and active metabolites are increased in advanced liver disease, and dose reduction is necessary.

Dexmedetomidine (DEX) is a centrally acting, selective alpha-2-adrenoceptor agonist that has sedative and analgesic properties, with minimal effect on respiration at clinically effective doses.[26] It has an analgesic ceiling effect at doses >0.5 mcg/kg, and can be coadministered with other analgesics such as opioids for analgesic-sparing effects and to minimize opioid side effects.[26-28] DEX is believed to provide analgesia via stimulation of spinal cord alpha-2-adrenoceptors, thereby reducing transmission of impulses in nociceptive pathways.[26,29-32] DEX also stimulates central vasomotor center alpha-2 adrenoreceptors, causing a reduction in central sympathetic outflow with resultant bradycardia and hypotension.[26,33] A biphasic cardiovascular response is seen with administration of DEX. During administration of the initial bolus dose, there is a transient increase in blood pressure (BP) with a reflex decrease in heart rate (HR), approximately 5 to 10 minutes in duration. This effect can be attenuated by eliminating or slowing the bolus dose. This is then followed by a 10%–20% reduction in BP and a stabilization of the HR, below baseline value with subsequent continuous infusion.[27,34-36] DEX is highly protein-bound with negligible displacement by fentanyl, ketorolac, and lidocaine, drugs commonly used in the ICU.[27] It is extensively metabolized in the liver via glucuronidation and CYP, and a dose reduction is likely needed in those with liver dysfunction.[27] The majority of metabolites are excreted by the kidneys; however, its pharmacokinetics does not change with renal failure. Dose reduction does not appear to be necessary in patients with renal failure, although there is a theoretical possibility of metabolite accumulation given the high degree of renal metabolite clearance.[26,27]

Ketamine, an NMDA receptor antagonist, is particularly useful in neuropathic pain states. It is a powerful analgesic with limited respiratory side effects at clinically relevant doses. It is typically administered in a subanesthetic dose as an intravenous infusion. Ketamine undergoes extensive hepatic metabolism by CYP, and one of the metabolites, norketamine, has approximately one-sixth the potency of ketamine. Therefore, significant liver disease with a reduction in hepatic blood flow will require dose reduction. The majority of ketamine is excreted by the kidneys, mostly as metabolites. There are three case reports of liver enzyme abnormalities that occurred following repeat infusions of the more active enantiomer (S)-(+)-ketamine for the treatment of chronic pain; however, they resolved after cessation of treatment.[37]

Local anesthetics are often administered as continuous infusions, as a component of peripheral or neuraxial regional analgesia. They are also formulated for topical administration. Local anesthetics are comprised of two classes, esters and amides, and they follow different metabolic pathways. Amide local anesthetics, such as lidocaine, bupivacaine, and ropivacaine, are primarily metabolized by hepatic CYP and the metabolites excreted by the kidney. Ester local anesthetics, such as chloroprocaine, undergo rapid hydrolysis by plasma pseudocholinesterase, producing metabolites that are also renally excreted. End-stage liver disease, with impaired hepatic blood flow or ability to produce pseudocholinesterase, will lead to an elevated plasma level of local anesthetic and a subsequent need for dose reduction.

In summary, there is a lack of prospective studies and evidence-based guidelines for the use of analgesics in patients with advanced liver disease. The care of these patients must be individualized and additional factors, such as nutritional status and renal function, considered. In general, many analgesics may be used in reduced doses in patients with chronic liver disease without cirrhosis. In those with cirrhosis, use of NSAIDs and opioids should be avoided because of the increased risk for acute renal failure and hepatic encephalopathy, respectively. Duloxetine has been associated with hepatic injury and should be avoided. Monitoring for toxicity and adverse events is necessary.

Respiratory Failure

Patients may present in acute respiratory failure secondary to either hypoxic or hypercarbic etiologies. Given that this is a medical emergency, stabilizing the patient's respiratory status must take precedence during the initial evaluation. Depending on the etiology of the respiratory failure, low-dose opiates may be beneficial for symptomatic relief of dyspnea.[38] Chronic respiratory failure may present to the ICU with an acute decompensation in respiratory status or may coexist with another admission diagnosis. The incidence of chronic pain in patients with pre-existing respiratory pathologies ranges from 21% to 28%.[39] Unlike renal and liver failure, there are very few pharmacological modifications that need to be made for these patients. Indeed, hypoventilation and respiratory depression are major concerns in these patients, but evidence suggests that a controlled opiate titration will avoid these side effects.[40]

It may be necessary to intubate these patients, given their tenuous respiratory status, and, as such, they may be kept NPO. Intravenous therapies include acetaminophen, ketorolac, gabapentin, carbamazepine, multiple opiates, as well as infusions of ketamine and dexmetetomidine. Ketamine, an NMDA receptor antagonist, is regarded as a third-line agent when other more conventional therapies have not been successful. Indeed, there are a number of untoward effects, including nausea/vomiting, confusion, and hallucinations, as well as contraindications to its use, including pulmonary hypertension. However, infusions of subanesthetic doses have been shown to be moderately effective for multiple pain states and should be considered when other modalities have either failed or are not options.[41] Dexmedetomidine, a selective centrally acting alpha-2 agonist, has been shown to be effective as a sole agent for analgesia at doses of 0.5 mcg/kg.[42] Special care must be taken in the ICU, as it is completely metabolized by the liver, and those metabolites, which are thought to be inactive, are predominantly excreted through the renal system.[43] As such, dose modifications need to be made and the agent titrated to proper effect.

Cardiovascular Collapse and Sepsis

While previous sections involved specific organ systems, issues with the cardiovascular system have the potential to involve the entire body. Altered hemodynamics can result in acute renal and/or liver failure, while cardiac dysfunction may precipitate respiratory failure. There is a wide spectrum of disease states that patients can present with, including acute myocardial infarction, congestive heart failure, and sepsis, all of which require alterations of previously described pain management strategies. Often these patients will need mechanical ventilation, which can require added support for anxiety as well as pre-existing pain.

There are multiple challenges in treating chronic pain in this population. NSAIDs, which are normally first-line agents for musculoskeletal pain, can cause an accumulation of sodium and water, precipitating congestive heart failure.[44] The same concern exists when initiating pregabalin; reports have shown acute decompensation in congestive heart failure.[45,46] Due to hemodynamic collapse in sepsis, initiating pain management is dictated by both cardiovascular stability and the previously mentioned validated pain scales (Table 9.1, 9.2,). Given the dynamic nature of cardiovascular collapse, short-acting intravenous agents, which can be titrated to hemodynamic as well as pain measures, are recommended. Upon clinical stability and extubation, resuming pre-existing chronic pain medications, with special caution for these agents, is warranted.

Summary

Pain is a common complaint among ICU patients. The ICU physician is presented with a difficult task in which hemodynamic and respiratory instability combined with altered pharmacokinetics may preclude continuing a pre-existing pain management regimen. After careful and systematic evaluation using validated pain assessments, which will allow careful titration of medications while avoiding excessive sedation, a treatment plan can be designed that allows the patient to remain comfortable during this time. Pharmacological therapies include the use of NSAIDs, acetaminophen, opioids, adjuvants, muscle relaxants, and local anesthetics. In addition, intravenous infusions of dexmedetomidine, ketamine, and short-acting opioids may prove useful. The clinician must be aware of signs of withdrawal from opioids and benzodiazepines as well as be mindful of resuming home medications when clinically indicated.

References

1. Johannes CB, Le TK, Zhou X, Johnston JA, Dworkin RH. The prevalence of chornic pain in United States adults: results of an Internet-based survey. *J Pain*. 2010;11:1230–1239.
2. Davison SN. Pain in hemodialysis patients: prevalence, cause, severity, and management. *Am J Kidney Dis*. 2003;42(6):1239–1247.
3. Bailie GR, Mason NA, Bragg-Grasham JL, Gillespie BW, Young EW. Analgesic prescription patterns among hemodialysis patients in the DOPPS: potential for under prescription. *Kidney Int*. 2004;65:2419–2425.
4. Bajwa ZH, Gupta S, Warfield CA, et al. Pain management in polycystic kidney disease. *Kidney Int*. 2001;60:287–313.
5. Davison SN, Mayo PR. Pain management in chronic kidney disease: the pharmacokinetics and pharmacodynamics of hydromorphone and hydromorphone-3-glucoronide in hemodialysis patients. *J Opioid Manag*. 2008;4:335–336.
6. Kaiko R, Benziger D, Cheng C, Hou Y, Grandy R. Clinical pharmacokinetics of controlled-release oxycodone in renal imparment. *Clin Pharmacol Ther*. 1996;59:130.
7. Dean M. Opioids in renal failure and dialysis patients. *J Pain Symptom Manage*. 2004;28(5):497–504.
8. Backnoja M, Beydoun A, Edwards KR, et al. Gabapentin for the symptomatic treatment of painful neuropathy in patients with diabetes mellitus: a randomized controlled trial. *JAMA*. 1998;280:1831–1836.
9. Thorp ML, Morris CD, Bagby SP. A crossover study of gabapentin in treatment of restless legs syndrome amoung hemodialysis patients. *Am J Kidney Dis*. 2001;38:104–108.
10. Lo HS, Yang, CM, Lo HG, et al. Treatment effects of gabapentin for primary insomnia. *Clin Neuropharmacol*. 2010;33:84–90.
11. Chandok C, Watt K. Pain management in the cirrhotic patient: the clinical challenge. *Mayo Clin Proc*. 2010;85(5):451–458.
12. Verbeeck RK. Pharmacokinetics and dosage adjustment in patients with hepatic dysfunction. *Eur J Clin Pharmacol*. 2008;64(12):1147–1161.
13. Cockcroft DW, Gault MH. Prediction of creatinine clearance from serum creatinine. *Nephron*. 1976;16(1):31–41.
14. Benson GD, Koff RS, Tolman KG. The therapeutic use of acetaminophen in patients with liver disease. *Am J Ther*. 2005;12(2);133–141.

15. Villeneuve JP, Raymond G, Bruneau J, et al. Pharmacokinetics and metabolism of acetaminophen in normal, alcoholic and cirrhotic patients. *Gastroenterol Clin Biol.* 1983;7(11):898–902.

16. Hirschfield GM, Kumagi T, Heathcote EJ. Preventive hepatology: minimizing symptoms and optimizing care. *Liver Int.* 2008;28(7);922–934.

17. Tegeder I, Lotsch J, Geisslinger G. Pharmacokinetics of opioids in liver disease. *Clin Pharmacokinet.* 1999;37(1):17–40.

18. Hasselstrom J, Eriksson S, Persson A, et al. The metabolism and bioavailability of morphine in patients with severe liver disease. *Br J Clin Pharmacol.* 1990;29(3):289–297.

19. Novick DM, Kreek MJ, Fanizza AM, et al. Methadone disposition in patients with chronic liver disease. *Clin Pharmacol Ther.* 1981;30(3);353–362.

20. Shelton RC. Serotonin norepinephrine reuptake inhibitirs: similarities and differences. *Primary Psychiatry.* 2009;16(Suppl 4):25–35.

21. Effexor XR (package insert). Philadelphia, PA: Wyeth Pharmaceuticals; 2008.

22. Cymbalta (package insert). Indianapolis, IN: Eli Lily and Company; 2007.

23. Ixel (package insert). Paris: Pierre Fabre Medicamant; 2003.

24. Harvey JN. Update on treatments for neuropathic pain. *J Pain Palliat Care Pharmacother.* 2008;22(1):54–57.

25. Einarsdottir S, Bjornsson E. Pregabalin as a probable cause of acute liver injury. *Eur J Gastroenterol Hepatol.* 2008;20(10):1049.

26. Tse I, Zhao H, Ma D. Organoprotective effects of dexmedetomidine: from bench to bedside. *J Perioper Sci.* 2014;1(3):1–15.

27. Gertler R, Brown HC, Mitchell DH, et al. Dexmedetomidine: a novel sedative-analgesic agent. *Proc (Bayl Univ Med Cent).* 2001;14:13–21.

28. Jaakola ML, Salonen M, Lehtinen R, et al. The analgesic action of dexmedetomidine—a novel alpha 2-adrenoceptor agonist—in healthy volunteers. *Pain* 1991;46:281–285.

29. Huang Y, Stamer WD, Anthony TL, at al. Expression of alpha 2 adrenergic receptor subtypes in prenatal rat spinal cord. *Dev Brain Res.* 2002;133(2):93–104.

30. Savola MK, Savola JM. Adrenoceptor subtype predominates also in the neonatal rat spinal cord. *Dev Brain Res.* 1996;94(1):106–108.

31. Fairbanks CA, Stone LS, Kitto KF, at al. Alpha 2C-adrenergic receptors mediate spinal analgesia and adrenergic-opioid synergy. *J Pharmacol Exp Ther.* 2002;300(1):282–290.

32. Stone S, Broberger C, Vulchanova L, et al. Differential distribution of alpha 2A and alpha 2C adrenergic receptor immunoreactivity in the rat spinal cord. *J Neurosci.* 1998;18(15);5928–5937.

33. Ebert TJ, Hall JE, Barney JA, et al. The effects of increasing plasma concentrations of dexmedetomidine in humans. *Anesthesiology.* 2000;93(2):382–394.

34. Dyck JB, Maze M, Haack C, et al. The pharmacokinetics and hemodynamic effects of intravenous and intramuscular dexmedetomidine hydrochloride in adult human volunteers. *Anesthesiology.* 1993;78:813–820.

35. Bloor BC, Ward DS, Belleville JP, et al. Effects of intravenous dexmedetomidine in humans. II. Hemodynamic changes. *Anesthesiology.* 1992;77:1134–1142.

36. Hall JE, Uhrich TD, Barney JA, et al. Sedative, amnestic, and analgesic properties of small-dose dexmedetomidine infusions. *Anesth Analg.* 2000;90:699–705.

37. Sear, JW. Ketamine hepatotoxicity in chronic pain management: another example of unexpected toxicity or a predicted result from previous clinical and preclinical data. *Pain* 2011(commentary);152 (9):1946–1947.

38. Booth S, Kelly MJ, Cox NP, et al. Does oxygen help dyspnea in patients with cancer? *Am J Respir Crit Care Med.* 1996;153:1515–1518.

39. SUPPORT principal investigators. A controlled trial to improve care for seriously ill hospitalized patients: the Study to Understand Prognoses and Preferences for Outcomes and Risks of Treatments (SUPPORT). *JAMA.* 1995;274(20),1591–1598.

40. Clemens KE, Klaschik E. Effect of hydromorphone on ventilation in palliative care patients with dyspnea. *Supp Care Cancer.* 2008;16:93–99.

41. Hocking G, Cousins MJ. Ketamine in chronic pain management: an evidence-based review. *Anesth Analg.* 2003;97(6):1730–1739.
42. Jaakola ML, Salonen M, Lehtinen R, Scheinin H. The analgesic action of dexmedetomidine—a novel alpha 2-adrenoceptor agonist—in healthy volunteers. *Pain.* 1991;46:281–285
43. Abbott Labaratories. Precedex. Dexmedetomidine hydrochloride injection prescribing information. Abbott Labaratories, USA, 2000
44. Bleumink GS, Feenstra J, Strukenboom MC, et al. Nonsteroidal anti-inflammatory drugs and heart failure. *Drugs.* 2003;63(6):525–534.
45. Gallagher R, Apostle N. Peripheral edema with pregabalin. *CMAJ.* 2013;185:e506.
46. Fong T, Lee A. Pregabalin-associated heart failure decompensation in a patient with a history of stage I heart failure. *Ann Pharmcother.* 2014;48(8):1077–1081.

10

Chronic Pain Patients in the Labor and Delivery Unit

DMITRI SOUZDALNITSKI, SYED ALI, AND DENIS SNEGOVSKIKH

KEY POINTS

- Chronic pain is a common comorbidity in pregnancy, which may affect maternal and fetal outcomes.
- Labor and delivery analgesia and postpartum pain management must be specifically tailored for patients with chronic pain, a history of opioid dependence, or a history of substance abuse.
- Sudden discontinuation of maintenance treatment (buprenorphine or methadone) or use of partial opioid agonist-antagonists, commonly used in other parturients, may cause intolerable pain or acute withdrawal. This in turn may contribute to preterm labor, fetal abnormalities, or fetal demise.
- Use of opioid agonist-antagonist drugs (nalbuphine, butorphanol, pentazocine and others) and even tramadol should be avoided in patients receiving maintenance opioid therapy (except buprenorphine), as these substances may provoke acute withdrawal. For the same reason, buprenorphine should not be given to a parturient who takes methadone.
- These patients typically have a lower pain threshold and require administration of higher doses of opioids, which subsequently may compromise patient and fetal or newborn safety.
- A special plan of neonatal care and breastfeeding is important during hospital admission of opioid-dependent patients.
- Parturients with an implanted spinal cord stimulator (SCS) or intrathecal pain pump (ITP) require special attention from healthcare providers. Familiarity with the SCS lead or the ITP catheter position is important. Therefore, it is important to obtain fluoroscopic images taken *prior* to pregnancy to avoid damage to these leads, especially where they enter the epidural space in the lumbar region. Peripartum ultrasonography may be helpful in identifying the lead or catheter position if fluoroscopic images are not available.

Introduction

Chronic pain affects one-third of the general population. Chronic pain is also a common comorbidity during pregnancy. The prevalence of low-back, leg, and pelvic pain during pregnancy is very high, ranging from 42% to 71%.[1] While the overall incidence of back pain during pregnancy alone is reported by up to 4 in 5 of women, this pain commonly resolves postpartum.[2] A history of chronic musculoskeletal and pelvic pain *prior* to pregnancy are associated with preterm labor and other untoward obstetrical events, including low birth weight and neonatal intensive care unit admission.[3,4] Lower education level, depression younger age, obesity, sleep deprivation, and later stages of pregnancy were associated with a higher probability of reporting pain during pregnancy. Most women manage their pain during pregnancy without opioids. However, a number of women (as high as 21% in some studies), have used opioids for pain control or recreational purposes, including heroin use or misuse of prescription opioids. About 5% of pregnant women reported recreational drug use in the past month.[5] The high prevalence of prescription (including buprenorphine and methadone) or recreational drug use during pregnancy requires hospital staff to be cognizant of related problems and realize that labor and delivery analgesia and postpartum pain management is significantly different in patients with chronic pain, or women with history of opioid dependence, or history of substance comparing to the routine regular labor and delivery.[6] Hospital staff should be familiar with proper management strategies during the peripartum period in these patients.

Most commonly used pain medications can cross the placenta. With the mother's use of these drugs, there is a sixfold increase in obstetrical problems (parturient bleeding, including abruptio placentae, preterm labor, fetal malpresentation, growth retardation, toxemia, distress, fetal death, intrauterine aspiration of meconium, and others). Repeated exposure of the fetus and placenta to opioids is thought to be the cause of these abnormalities. There are additional problems associated with the injection of drugs, including increased risk of abscess at the injection site, sepsis and septic shock, endocarditis, infectious arthritis, osteomyelitis, hepatitis B or C, and contracting human immunodeficiency virus (HIV). Neonatal problems include opioid withdrawal, slow growth, microcephaly, neurological and behavioral problems, and a spike in neonatal mortality, and there is a 74-fold increase in sudden infant death syndrome.[7] At the same time, a sudden discontinuation of maintenance treatment (buprenorphine or methadone) or use of partial opioid agonist-antagonists may cause intolerable pain or acute withdrawal. This can be associated with preterm labor, fetal abnormalities, or even fetal demise.[8] Since these patients typically have a lower pain threshold, they require higher opioid doses. While this strategy may improve immediate patient satisfaction, it may compromise patient and fetal/newborn safety. There are also special considerations to bear in mind when treating patients with implanted pain management devices.

Peripartum Analgesia in Opioid-Dependent Women

There are no guidelines and recommendations based on high-level evidence for management of peripartum pain in opioid-dependent patients. The following are typical concerns related to the peripartum anesthetic management of pain in the patient with current or former opioid dependence:

- Risk of relapse of addiction, due to use of opioids for peripartum analgesia
- Risk of maternal withdrawal
- Inadequate pain control due to tolerance to the opioid effect or due to opioid-induced hyperalgesia
- The possibility of developing complications related to exacerbation of pre-existing medical conditions frequently associated with opioid dependence, such as bacterial and viral infection, liver disorder, depression, and withdrawal from other concomitantly used illicit drugs

There is no evidence to support the concern about recurrence of addiction after use of opioid-based peripartum analgesia. Patients should receive adequate analgesia during the peripartum period because poorly controlled pain is a main reason for drug-seeking behavior and recurrence of addiction.

Maternal withdrawal can trigger preterm labor and fetal demise and thus must be avoided.[9] Methadone and buprenorphine maintenance therapy may prevent development of maternal withdrawal. The MOTHER study prospectively compared safety and effectiveness of buprenorphine versus methadone maintenance therapy during pregnancy. It demonstrated some advantages of buprenorphine treatment for neonatal outcome (less severe neonatal abstinence syndrome, better neurobehavioral function) but more frequent self-discontinuation of therapy (33% versus 18%) compared to mothers treated with methadone.[10]

Use of naloxone and opioid agonist-antagonist drugs (nalbuphine, butorphanol, pentazocine, among others) and even tramadol should be avoided in patients receiving maintenance opioid therapy (except buprenorphine), as these substances may provoke acute withdrawal.[5]

Two pathophysiologically different phenomena of opioid tolerance (decreased sensitivity of anti-nociceptive system) and opioid-induced hyperalgesia (increased sensitivity of pro-nociceptive system) result in the same clinical outcome: significantly elevated doses of opioids are needed to adequately control pain during the peripartum period. It has been suggested that, compared to opioid-naïve patients, opioid-dependent patients may need 2 to 4 times higher doses of opioids to achieve adequate pain control. For patients on opioid maintenance therapy, treatment with a maintenance dosage of methadone, buprenorphine, extended-release morphine, or intrathecal morphine should not be interrupted.[9] Analgesia for a vaginal delivery can be successfully achieved by adding standard neuraxial analgesia to opioid maintenance therapy.

Pain control after cesarean section is more problematic. Most authors suggest that continuing maintenance therapy does not provide adequate analgesia for labor.[11,12] Additional doses of oral or intravenous methadone can be used for parturients on a methadone maintenance program. Some clinicians suggest that a single bolus of intravenous methadone may be a relatively safe option for analgesia after caesarean delivery because of its fast onset and long, extended effect. Others recommend dividing the total daily dose equally into three or four doses to achieve better analgesia.[13] One study showed that intraoperative methadone combined with postoperative intravenous patient-controlled analgesia (PCA) with fentanyl or morphine had a significant opioid-sparing effect in these patients postoperatively.[11]

Conversion of oral to parenteral dosage of opioids and from one opioid to another is challenging because of the difference in recommended ratio. It varies between clinicians' and pharmaceuticals' recommendations, and between different authors. It also depends on the direction of conversion, present comorbidities, and other medications used by the patient. Young to calculate the first dose of the chosen opioid. Correction of subsequent doses should be performed individually, based on clinical response.

There is a theoretical concern about the inability to provide adequate analgesia for parturients treated with buprenorphine because of its partial μ-opioid receptor agonist effect and ceiling analgesic effect. In a prospective study comparing 63 buprenorphine-treated parturients with healthy control patients, it was demonstrated that there was no difference between the two groups in pain and opioid requirements during vaginal delivery.[14] Among women treated with buprenorphine, there was a 47% increase in need for opioids after cesarean section, which is similar to the previously reported elevated opioid requirement among parturients on methadone maintenance therapy. For two patients in buprenorphine group, adequate pain control was achieved only after patient-controlled epidural analgesia was used.

At the same time, one should remember that the standard dose of neuraxial opioids in opioid-dependent patients neither prevents opioid withdrawal nor provides adequate perioperative analgesia.[15] It has been suggested that doubling or tripling the standard dose of neuraxial opioids may be necessary to achieve acceptable neuraxial analgesia in opioid-dependent patients.[16] Fentanyl PCA may be a preferable option in management of postoperative pain in a parturient taking buprenorphine because of higher fentanyl affinity to μ-receptors than that of buprenorphine.

These patients need to be closely monitored for respiratory depression. In one study, during the postoperative period moderate sedation was observed significantly more frequently (50% versus 19%) among an opioid-dependent group of patients than in the control group. The postoperative pain score was also higher in the opioid-dependent group.[17]

The safety and effectiveness of adding non-opioid analgesics to opioid therapy for post-cesarean patients have not been studied extensively. Intravenous acetaminophen has been demonstrated to have good analgesic effect during the first stage of labor[18] and after surgical interventions.[19] Preoperative administration of 600 mg of oral gabapentin significantly reduced pain score after cesarean delivery performed under standard (bupivacaine/fentanyl/morphine) spinal anesthesia among opioid-naïve patients.[20] Similar results were reported in another double-blind controlled study.[21] Premedication with 4 mcg/kg of oral clonidine reduced post-cesarean use of morphine PCA among opioid-naive patients.[22] Among opioid-naive patients, post-cesarean analgesia did not decrease pain after addition of 10 mg intravenous ketamine.[23] According to some authors, ultrasound-guided transversus abdominus plane block may be beneficial for post-cesarean pain control among opioid-dependent patients, while other authors have not found this to be beneficial.[9,24]

Additional means of providing pain relief in the peripartum period may include use of a labor ball and special postpartum exercises,[25,26] administration of other adjuncts (ketorolac[27] and other nonsteroidal anti-inflammatory medications, nitrous oxide inhalation, magnesium sulfate intrathecally),[28] acupuncture,[29] aromatherapy, massage,[30] music and other complimentary/alternative medicine therapies,[31] transcutaneous electrical stimulation,[32] trigger point injections,[33,34] and immersion in warm water during the first stage of labor. Sterile water injected intracutaneously or subcutaneously in lumbar paravertebral areas helped with pain control and reduced the incidence of cesarean deliveries.[35]

While neonatal care is outside the scope of this chapter, it is important to keep in mind that the neonatology team staff needs to be informed as early as possible of all fetuses who may have been exposed to opioids or illicit substances. These newborns should be monitored for neonatal abstinence syndrome—preferably in intensive care settings. Patients should be advised that some levels of methadone and buprenorphine are found in breast milk regardless of maternal dose, but breastfeeding is not contraindicated.

All chronic pain parturients should have access to psychosocial and chaplain support services. They should also receive comprehensive postpartum care, including addiction medicine specialists if indicated.

Peripartum Management of Patients with Implanted Pain Management Devices

LABOR AND POSTPARTUM ANALGESIA IN PARTURIENTS WITH SPINAL CORD SIMULATION

Spinal cord stimulation (SCS) is a neuromodulation technique commonly used to treat patients with intractable neuropathic pain. Being a woman of childbearing age is not a contraindication for the SCS implant. Women of childbearing age should be tested for pregnancy before SCS implantation. The impact of SCS on the pregnancy and the fetus remains unknown and women considering an SCS implant should be informed of this. Some of these patients may become pregnant after they become SCS recipients. The plan of prenatal care in these cases should be made individually after thoroughly weighing the possible risks and benefits and considering alternative options. There are multiple successful cases of labor, delivery, and postpartum analgesia among patients with SCS implants.[36] Fluoroscopic images of the spine taken *prior* to pregnancy that show the location of SCS leads are usually available for patients with an SCS implant. Familiarity with the leads' position in the spine may help to avoid damage to these leads, especially where they enter the epidural space in the lumbar region. Some advocate that patients with SCS have images of leads' position in their possession so that they can be used in case of obstetrical emergency.[37]

The lumbar SCS leads are typically inserted somewhere between T12 and upper lumbar interspaces, and end in the epidural space in the middle to lower thoracic levels. The leads are fixed to a lumbar spinous process or its ligaments, and then connected with the generator, which is usually located in the patient's buttock or paravertebrally in the lumbar area. The cervical SCS leads are typically inserted somewhere between C7 und upper thoracic interspace, and end in the epidural space somewhere at the middle to upper cervical level. The leads are commonly fixed to a lumbar spinous process or its ligaments and then followed to the generator, which is located in ether the chest or the buttock. One case report on use of epidural anesthesia during labor in a patient with a cervical SCS implanted prior to pregnancy described acceptable analgesia using a standard Tuohy needle technique; she had intractable pain in the right upper extremity secondary to chronic regional pain syndrome. The patient stated that her affected hand felt at ease and pleasantly warm. Her labor and delivery continued without incident. The SCS was active throughout the entire labor period and delivery. The patient noted that the painful feeling in her right hand returned to baseline postpartum.[38]

LABOR AND POSTPARTUM ANALGESIA IN PARTURIENTS WITH AN INTRATHECAL PUMP

Intrathecal infusion of morphine or ziconotide are the FDA-approved, favorable treatment options for patients with chronic intractable pain who have failed conventional pain management including medications, physical therapy, and interventions. It is a sustainable option for childbearing-age women.

Management of the intrathecal pump (ITP) during labor and postpartum presents a number of considerations the hospital team should be aware of. Current practice indicates that conventional approaches to labor and delivery analgesia, including non-neuraxial techniques as well as spinal, epidural, or combined techniques, are commonly used for patients with an ITP. One report describes a nulliparous patient with severe abdominal pain secondary to pancreatitis managed with morphine administered through an ITP for 4 years prior to hospital admission during labor. The team had planned to escalate the dose of intrathecal morphine, but the patient presented with acute preterm labor. The attempt to use intravenous PCA with fentanyl was not successful. As a result, epidural bupivacaine analgesia was initiated and produced adequate analgesia. The authors conclude that the ITP does not prevent the use of neuraxial analgesia during labor.[39]

If no images of the catheter are available, ultrasound-assisted epidural or spinal analgesia may be used. Ultrasonography can be used to detect the location of the ITP catheter or SCS lead.[40] Use of an ITP for acute pain, including during labor and delivery, is generally not advisable. We recommend maintaining the baseline ITP dose and using *additional* labor and delivery analgesia as well as postpartum pain control with conventional techniques. Management of acute pain in patients with an ITP is discussed further elsewhere in this book.

It is important to discuss the risks of the ITP failure (dislodgement, dislocation) during the antenatal period. The possibility of escalating the dose of intrathecal medicine and its subsequent maternal and fetal effects, including neonatal opioid withdrawal, should be discussed. With careful planning of prenatal care as well as labor, delivery, and postpartum pain control the risks can be minimized.

Summary

Special attention is needed when treating parturients with chronic pain who are on maintenance opioid treatment or using an implanted pain management device because these factors may affect both maternal and fetal outcomes. Sudden discontinuation of opioids or administration of partial opioid agonist-antagonists may produce intolerable pain or acute withdrawal and result in preterm labor, fetal abnormalities, or even fetal demise. Higher opioid doses are typically required for better patient satisfaction with peripartum analgesia but may negatively affect the patient or newborn. Therefore, an individualized plan of peripartum care is of great importance.

References

1. Kovacs FM, Garcia E, Royuela A, González L, Abraira V; Spanish Back Pain Research Network. Prevalence and factors associated with low back pain and pelvic girdle pain

during pregnancy: a multicenter study conducted in the Spanish National Health Service. *Spine (Phila Pa 1976)*. 2012;37(17):1516–1533.

2. Sabino J, Grauer JN. Pregnancy and low back pain. *Curr Rev Musculoskelet Med.* 2008;1(2):137–141.

3. Bayram C, Osmanağaoğlu MA, Aran T, Güven S, Bozkaya H. The effect of chronic pelvic pain scoring on pre-term delivery rate. *J Obstet Gynaecol.* 2013;33(1):32–37.

4. Mallen CD, Peat G, Thomas E, Croft PR. Is chronic musculoskeletal pain in adulthood related to factors at birth? A population-based case-control study of young adults. *Eur J Epidemiol.* 2006;21(3):237–243.

5. ACOG Committee on Health Care for Underserved Women; American Society of Addiction Medicine. ACOG Committee Opinion No. 524: Opioid abuse, dependence, and addiction in pregnancy. *Obstet Gynecol.* 2012;119(5):1070–1076.

6. Gopman S. Prenatal and postpartum care of women with substance use disorders. *Obstet Gynecol Clin North Am.* 2014;41(2):213–228.

7. Minozzi S, Amato L, Bellisario C, Ferri M, Davoli M. Maintenance agonist treatments for opiate-dependent pregnant women. *Cochrane Database Syst Rev.* 2013;12:CD006318.

8. Arunogiri S1, Foo L, Frei M, Lubman DI. Managing opioid dependence in pregnancy—a general practice perspective. *Aust Fam Physician.* 2013;42(10):713–716.

9. Young JL, Lockhart EM, Baysinger CL. Anesthetic and obstetric management of the opioid dependent parturient. *Intern Anesth Clin.* 2014;52:67–85.

10. Jones HE, Fischer G, Heil SH, et al. Maternal Opioid Treatment: Human Experimental Research (MOTHER)—approach, issues and lessons learned. *Addiction.* 2012;107(Suppl 1):28–35.

11. Jones HE, O'Grady K, Dahne J, et al. Management of acute postpartum pain in patients maintained on methadone or buprenorphine during pregnancy. *Am J Drug Alcohol Abuse.* 2009;35:151–156.

12. Kaltenbach K, Berghella V, Finnegan L. Opioid dependence during pregnancy. Effects and management. *Obstet Gynecol Clin North Am.* 1998;25:139–151.

13. Alford DP, Compton P, Samet JH. Acute pain management for patients receiving maintenance methadone or buprenorphine therapy. *Ann Intern Med.* 2006;144:127–134.

14. Meyer M, Paranya G, Keefer Norris A, Howard D. Intrapartum and postpartum analgesia for women maintained on buprenorphine during pregnancy. *Eur J Pain.* 2010;14(9):939–943.

15. Mitra S, Sinatra RS. Perioperative management of acute pain in the opioid-dependent patient. *Anesthesiology.* 2004;101:212–227.

16. de Leon-Casasola OA, Lema MJ. Epidural bupivacaine/sufentanil therapy for postoperative pain control in patients tolerant to opioid and unresponsive to epidural bupivacaine/morphine. *Anesthesiology.* 1994;80:303–309.

17. Rapp SE1, Ready LB, Nessly ML. Acute pain management in patients with prior opioid consumption: a case-controlled retrospective review. *Pain.* 1995;61(2):195–201.

18. Elbohoty AE, et al. Intravenous infusion of paracetamol versus pethidine as an intrapartum analgesic in the first stage of labor. *Int J Gynaecol Obstet.* 2012;118:7–10.

19. Jahr JS, Lee VK. Intravenous acetaminophen. *Anesthesiol Clin.* 2010;28(4):619–645.

20. Moore A, Costello J, Wieczorek P, Shah V, Taddio A, Carvalho JC. Gabapentin improves postcesarean delivery pain management: a randomized, placebo-controlled trial. *Anesth Analg.* 2011;112(1):167–173.

21. Najafi Anaraki A, Mirzaei K. The effect of gabapentin versus intrathecal fentanyl on postoperative pain and morphine consumption in cesarean delivery: a prospective, randomized, double-blind study. *Arch Gynecol Obstet.* 2014;290(1):47–52.

22. Yanagidate F, Hamaya Y, Dohi S. Clonidine premedication reduces maternal requirement for intravenous morphine after cesarean delivery without affecting newborn's outcome. *Reg Anesth Pain Med.* 2001;26(5):461–467.

23. Bauchat JR, et al. Low-dose ketamine with multimodal postcesarean delivery analgesia: a randomized controlled trial. *Int J Obstet Anesth.* 2012;20:30–39.

24. McKeen DM, George RB, Boyd JC, Allen VM, Pink A. Transversus abdominis plane block does not improve early or late pain outcomes after cesarean delivery: a randomized controlled trial. *Can J Anaesth.* 2014;61(7):631–640.

25. Leung RW, Li JF, Leung MK, et al. Efficacy of birth ball exercises on labor pain management. *Hong Kong Med J.* 2013;19(5):393–399.

26. Nascimento SL, Surita FG, Cecatti JG. Physical exercise during pregnancy: a systematic review. *Curr Opin Obstet Gynecol.* 2012;24(6):387–394.

27. Todd G, John A, Vacchiano C, Pellegrini J. Intradermal ketorolac for reduction of epidural back pain. *J Obstet Anesth.* 2002;11(2):100–104.

28. Morrison AP, Hunter JM, Halpern SH, Banerjee A. Effect of intrathecal magnesium in the presence or absence of local anaesthetic with and without lipophilic opioids: a systematic review and meta-analysis. *Br J Anaesth.* 2013;110(5):702–712.

29. Borup L, Wurlitzer W, Hedegaard M, Kesmodel US, Hvidman L. Acupuncture as pain relief during delivery: a randomized controlled trial. *Birth.* 2009;36(1):5–12.

30. Dhany AL, Mitchell T, Foy C. Aromatherapy and massage intrapartum service impact on use of analgesia and anesthesia in women in labor: a retrospective case note analysis. *J Altern Complement Med.* 2012;18(10):932–938.

31. Wang SM, DeZinno P, Fermo L, et al. Complementary and alternative medicine for low-back pain in pregnancy: a cross-sectional survey. *J Altern Complement Med.* 2005;11(3):459–464.

32. van der Spank JT, Cambier DC, De Paepe HM, Danneels LA, Witvrouw EE, Beerens L. Pain relief in labour by transcutaneous electrical nerve stimulation (TENS). *Arch Gynecol Obstet.* 2000;264(3):131–136.

33. Gómez-Ríos M, Paech MJ. Postoperative analgesia with transversus abdominis plane catheter infusions of levobupivacaine after major gynecological and obstetrical surgery. A case series. *Rev Esp Anestesiol Reanim.* 2014;pii:S0034-9356(14)00115-7.

34. Tsen LC, Camann WR. Trigger point injections for myofascial pain during epidural analgesia for labor. *Reg Anesth.* 1997;22(5):466–468.

35. Rooks JP. Labor pain management other than neuraxial: what do we know and where do we go next? *Birth.* 2012;39(4):318–322.

36. Fedoroff IC, Blackwell E, Malysh L, McDonald WN, Boyd M. Spinal cord stimulation in pregnancy: a literature review. *Neuromodulation.* 2012;15(6):537–541.

37. Patel S, Das S, Stedman RB. Urgent cesarean section in a patient with a spinal cord stimulator: implications for surgery and anesthesia. *Ochsner J.* 2014;14(1):131–134.

38. Hanson JL, Goodman EJ. Labor epidural placement in a woman with a cervical spinal cord stimulator. *Int J Obstet Anesth.* 2006;15(3):246–249.

39. Byrd LM, Jadoon B, Lieberman I, Johnston T. Chronic pain and obstetric management of a patient with tuberous sclerosis. *Pain Med.* 2007;8(2):199–203.

40. Badve M, Shah T, Jones-Ivy S, Vallejo MC. Ultrasound guided epidural analgesia for labor in a patient with an intrathecal baclofen pump. *Int J Obstet Anesth.* 2011;20(4):370–372.

11

Management of Chronic Pain in Patients in the Pediatric Unit

ORVIL LOUIS AYALA AND ALEXANDRA SZABOVA

KEY POINTS

- Hospitalization can be a source of great stress for children with a history of chronic pain and often manifests complex interactions between the child, parents, illness, their pain and healthcare providers.
- The child with pre-existing chronic pain and the family may become overwhelmed, especially if the pain does not have or is out of proportion to medical or anatomical reasons. The interplay of psychosocial and medical factors may engulf the patient's and the family's coping abilities, at which time the threshold for decompensating may decrease.
- Understanding the underlying problems is the crucial first step in successful treatment. The role of the physician is to recognize not only the underlying medical reasons for pain but also the other factors that may be contributing to the pain and negating successful treatments.
- Emphasis on diagnosing and managing chronic pain in children admitted to the hospital using a multimodal approach is key to successfully treating this patient population.
- These patients require a bit more time than average, and a calm, understanding demeanor and a willingness to educate the patient and family while ensuring the patient's safety can be rewarding and result in good outcomes.

Introduction

Chronic pain continues to be a worldwide issue, and some investigators estimate that as many as 20%–35% of the world's children and adolescents are affected.[1,2] Psychosocial factors play a major role in onset, maintenance, and flare-ups of pain. The presentation of various pain complaints sometimes can be dramatic. It is a priority to rule out any "red flags"—signs of serious or life-threatening disease or injury. It is also important to understand that once the red flags have been ruled out and medical treatment has been initiated, the focus should turn to teaching the patient to cope with pain effectively and rehabilitating the patient to improve function. Opioids have a very limited role in the treatment of chronic pain in children and generally are weaned off or discontinued. Instead, a spectrum of adjunct medications have been used, but given the side effects and pediatric patients' dislike of taking medications in general, their role is limited.

Some of the most common conditions experienced by this patient population are highlighted in Box 11.1. A more detailed discussion of each follows.

Abdominal Pain

Pediatric patients hospitalized for abdominal pain represent a challenging and sometimes frustrating patient population. Management is straightforward in cases of acute pancreatitis or flare-up of inflammatory bowel disease (IBD), as laboratory and imaging testing aid the diagnosis. The analgesic treatment of these conditions is multimodal. In addition to treating the illness, analgesics include intravenous acetaminophen (for IBD and pancreatitis patients), ketorolac (for pancreatitis patients unless there is a concern for hemorrhage), and parenteral opioids (if NPO or in severe cases). In patients with IBD, the concern for

---

Box 11.1 **Common Conditions Experienced in Children with Chronic Pain**

Abdominal pain
Musculoskeletal pain/back pain
Chronic regional pain syndrome (CRPS)
Headache
Chest pain
Chronic illness
• Sickle cell pain
• Epidermolysis bullosa
• Cystic fibrosis
Cancer-related pain

Modified from Suresh S, McClain BC, Tarbell S. Chronic pain management in children. In: Benzon HT, Wu CL, Rathmell JP, et al., eds. *Raj's Practical Management of Pain*, 4th ed. Philadelphia, PA: Mosby Elsevier, 2008; 343.

toxic megacolon induced by opioid administration is theoretical, given the availability of improved disease-specific therapies. Mixed opioid agonist-antagonists such as butorphanol and nalbuphine affect gut motility to a lesser degree and can be used as first-line treatment, although escalation to a μ-opioid agonist may be needed. If used, opioids should be limited to the shortest possible duration. Patients with underlying "organic" disease who have symptoms that are either out of proportion or atypical are particularly challenging to treat (10%–15% of patients have both IBD and functional gastrointestinal disorders [FGID], discussed later in the chapter). In these cases, close collaboration with the gastroenterology consulting service is crucial to establish reasonable diagnostic workup to address any red flags (see Box 11.2). Once the red flags have been taken care of, the concept of FGID should be introduced and a multidisciplinary treatment approach instituted. The idea of FGIDs may be difficult for patients and families to grasp, so continuing education is often needed (see Box 11.3, Box 11.4A, and Box 11.4B for details).

The treatment of FGIDs includes medications, psychological interventions, and dietary changes. The establishment of realistic goals is one of the most important components of treatment, and emphasizing return of function rather than complete elimination of pain is a key. Tricyclic antidepressants (TCAs) such as amitriptyline, nortriptyline, or doxepin have been extensively used for FGID-related pain. However, overall evidence in pediatric patients is poor, though evidence exists for use of amitriptyline in adults with FGIDs.[3-5] Another

---

Box 11.2 **Alarm Symptoms, Signs, and Features in Children and Adolescents with Noncyclic Abdominal Pain—Related Functional Gastrointestinal Disorders**

Persistent right upper or right lower quadrant pain
Pain that wakes the child from sleep
Dysphagia
Arthritis
Persistent vomiting
Perirectal disease
Gastrointestinal blood loss
Involuntary weight loss
Nocturnal diarrhea
Deceleration of linear growth
Family history of inflammatory bowel disease, celiac disease, or peptic
    ulcer disease
Delayed puberty
Unexplained fever

Box 11.3 Classification of Pediatric Functional Gastrointestinal Disorders

H. Functional disorders: children and adolescents
H1. Vomiting and aerophagia
H1a. Adolescent rumination syndrome
H1b. Cyclic vomiting syndrome
H1c. Aerophagia
H2. Abdominal pain–related FGIDs
H2a. Functional dyspepsia
H2b. Irritable bowel syndrome
H2c. Abdominal migraine
H2d. Childhood functional abdominal pain
H2d1. Childhood functional abdominal pain syndrome
H3. Constipation and incontinence
H3a. Functional constipation
H3b. Nonretentive fecal incontinence

---

drug group used in adult patients with an irritable bowel syndrome (subtype of FGID) is anticonvulsants (e.g., gabapentin and pregabalin).[6] The rationale for use in children with chronic abdominal pain has been extrapolated from adult-patient experience. Symptomatically, bulking agents, antispasmodics, or antidepressants may be added.[7] Peppermint oil capsules have found some success in improving the quality of life for patients with FGID.[8] Pediatric patients with FGID need cognitive behavioral therapy for developing coping skills, as well as biofeedback and relaxation techniques. It is important to have all team members on "the same page," sending a consistent message to the patient and family, to prevent unnecessary escalation of testing.

Box 11.4A Diagnostic Criteria* for Childhood Functional Abdominal Pain

Must include *all* of the following:

1. Episodic or continuous abdominal pain
2. Insufficient criteria for other FGIDs
3. No evidence of an inflammatory, anatomic, metabolic, or neoplastic process that explains the subject's symptoms

---

*Criteria fulfilled at least once per week for at least 2 months before diagnosis.

Box 11.4B **Diagnostic Criteria* for Childhood Functional
Abdominal Pain Syndrome**

Must include childhood functional abdominal pain at least 25% of the time
and one or more of the following:

1. Some loss of daily functioning
2. Additional somatic symptoms such as headache, limb pain, or difficulty
   sleeping

---

*Criteria fulfilled at least once per week for at least 2 months before diagnosis.

On occasion, patients spend weeks and months in the hospital while their
workup and treatment progress. We have found benefit in creating a daily schedule
for the patient that reflects normal daily functioning with a set wake-up time and
time for schoolwork, physical therapy, work with psychologists, and any other routine activities. The emphasis is placed on the least possible disruption for medical
interventions and testing. Out-of-bed time, ambulation, and visits to an activity
center and play rooms are encouraged in order to assist functional rehabilitation
and support healthy lifestyle habits. The goal is to make the transition from hospital to home and school environments smooth and less stressful[9] (Figure 11.1).

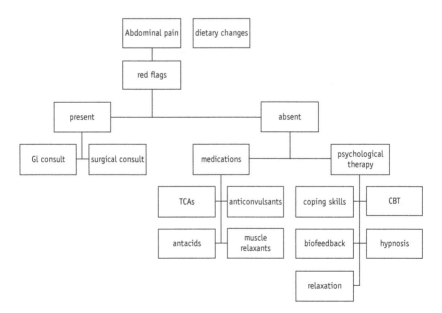

Figure 11.1 Algorithm for managing abdominal pain. CBT, cognitive behaviorial
therapy.

Chest Pain

Chest pain is a fairly uncommon source of pain in the pediatric patient popula-tion.[10,11] In most cases, it is of non-cardiac origin and associated with benign or self-limited conditions (Table 11.1.)[12-14] If a detailed history and physical exam, and limited testing (ECG and chest X-ray) suggest a cardiac component, referral to a pediatric cardiologist is warranted. Chest pain of non-cardiac ori-gin is usually managed by providing the patient with reassurance, counseling, non-steroidal anti-inflammatory drugs (NSAIDs), and regional nerve blocks[13,15] (Figure 11.2).

Sickle Cell–Related Pain

Sickle cell disease (SCD) is a hereditary disorder that affects millions of people worldwide and approximately 100,000 Americans. It is characterized by chronic hemolytic anemia and complications that are mostly related to tissue ischemia secondary to vaso-occlusion.[16] Acute chest is the most severe and potentially life-threatening complication with a mortality rate of 10%. Episodes of vaso-occlusion are often predictable (triggered by fever, dehydration, excessive heat or cold exposure, hypoxemia), recurrent, and painful. They may account for mul-tiple emergency department visits and hospital admissions.[16] Stress as a trigger of pain flare-up needs to be high on a differential diagnoses list, especially if laboratory markers are not significantly different from the patient's baseline. Similarly, discerning whether a pain flare is related to vaso-occlusion or to a flare of chronic musculoskeletal pain may present a challenge. Pain may range from mild to severe, lasting from several hours to several days, often necessitating the use of opioids.

Children with SCD have been historically undertreated despite the recogni-tion that pain is a common feature in this disease.[16] Treatment advances, such as use of prophylactic hydroxyurea, apheresis, and monthly transfusion therapy,

Table 11.1 **Chest Pain in the Pediatric Population (Non-cardiac Origin)**

Costochondritis	*Trauma*
Tietze's syndrome	Hypermobility syndrome
Myofascial pain syndrome	Herpes zoster

Modified from Suresh S, Shah R. Chronic pain management in children and adolescents. In Benzon HT, Raja S, Liu SS et al., eds. *Essentials of Pain Medicine*, 3rd ed. Philadelphia, PA: Elsevier Saunders, 2011; 403–403.[33]

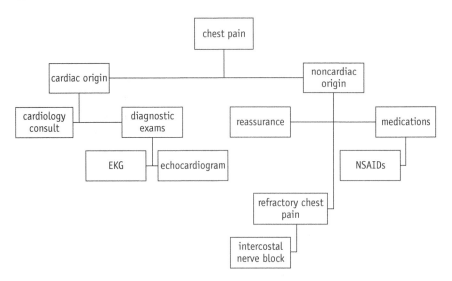

Figure 11.2 Algorithm for managing chest pain.

have helped to decrease the morbidity in children with SCD.[17] Compliance with a home regimen remains problematic, as often children come from underprivileged families with little social support. Communicating with the hematologists involved in patients' care, who often have long-standing patient–physician relationships, can foster understanding of the severity of the patient's disease and psychosocial background.

Severe vaso-occlusive episodes require IV patient-controlled analgesia (PCA), where available. Good outcomes (e.g., shorter hospital stay, less opioid use, the same readmission rate) have been obtained when PCAs were managed by hospitalists as compared to hematologists, mainly due to ordering continuous infusions less frequently and using oral long-acting opioids more regularly.[18] Children with SCD are usually managed by a medical team and are provided with rehydration, rest, antibiotics if indicated, hydroxyurea, transfusion therapy, and analgesia (e.g., acetaminophen, NSAIDs, opioids). Functional rehabilitation is crucial but sometimes very challenging; while patients are hospitalized, psychological, behavioral, and aggressive physical therapy must be part of the treatment plan, ideally to continue after hospital discharge, on an outpatient basis.[16]

Epidermolysis Bullosa (EB)-Related Pain

EB is a rare inherited skin fragility disorder characterized by blister formation of the skin and mucosa. It is estimated to affect about 1 child out of every 20,000 births.[19] EB presents a spectrum of disease, from the mildest to the most severe and disabling condition. Patients with the most severe EB tend to suffer from constant daily pain. Its etiology is often a combination of somatic and neuro-pathic pain and intractable pruritus. Far from being just a dermatological condition, sources of EB pain include skin, bones, gastrointestinal (GI) tract, joints, and eyes. With improved wound care, treatment of infection, and aggressive nutritional support, patients with a severe form of EB survive to mid-adulthood, though the rate of onset of squamous cell carcinoma is 90% by age 55 years.[20] As they age and mature, many individuals become increasingly anxious and depressed, adding another layer of complexity to care.

Management of this population presents many challenges and requires a multidisciplinary approach (e.g., dermatologist, pain specialist, gastroenterologist, surgeons, dentist, nutritionist, physical and occupational therapists, and psychologist). For patients with severe forms of EB, use of the WHO analgesic ladder works well. Pain treatment may need to be started early in life (newborn period) with acetaminophen and NSAIDS and escalated to opioids around pre-school age, as needed, and titrated to effect. Long-acting opioids may be needed in early teens or adolescents, though esophageal strictures can prohibit pill-swallowing. For non-healing, painful, smaller wounds, topical morphine gel can be applied. When hospitalized, patients come in for treatment of infections, nutritional support, and aggressive skin care.

Use of opioids presents a double-edge sword, more so for EB patients than non-EB children and adolescents, as opioids negatively affect already marginal GI function and motility. There is no cure for EB, and most therapies are supportive or at early stages of clinical applications. Given the multiple organ systems affected, the painfulness of many health care requirements (e.g., bandage changes), and the sheer amount of time needed for care at home, cognitive behavioral therapy early in life, learning pain coping skills, and adding counseling for anxiety and depression may be of great benefit to this patient population.

Headache in Children

Headaches are a common symptom that may affect up to 90% of children between the ages of 6 and 18 years of age.[1,2] Children who suffer from frequent chronic headaches experience a decrease in their quality of life, as headaches affect daily activities (e.g., school, participating in social events).[21] Headaches may be divided into three major categories. *Primary headaches* include migraine (with and without aura), tension type, cluster headaches, and trigeminal autonomic cephalalgias. *Secondary headaches* are attributed to head and neck traumas, vascular and nonvascular intracranial disorders, infection, psychiatric disorders, or substance use or its withdrawal (such as medication overuse headaches).[22] While most of these disorders are infrequent in children, medication overuse headaches are more often encountered in children. *Tertiary headaches*, such as cranial neuralgias, or other central causes of facial pain are rare in children.

Table 11.2 **Red Flags of Headaches in Children**

Headaches that awaken patient from sleep	Headaches with persistent fevers
Persistent vomiting	Changes in personality
Posttraumatic headaches	Sudden onset of severe headache ("worst headache of my life")
History of malignancy	Young age (without family history of headaches)
Meningeal signs	Headaches with focal neurologic complaints

Modified from Kashikar-Zuck S, Zafar M, Barnett KA, et al. Quality of life and emotional functioning in youth with chronic migraine and juvenile fibromyalgia. *Clin J Pain.* 2013; 29(12):1066–1072.[21]

In most cases, chronic headaches are benign and tend to run in families.[22] Migraines and tension-type headaches are the most common types of headaches in the pediatric population. In the absence of focal neurological findings, diagnostic studies (e.g., CT scan or MRI) are not typically recommended. The presence of "red flags" may merit further evaluation to rule out a life-threatening condition (see Table 11.2 for details).

Migraine headache management includes a two-step pharmacological approach as part of multidisciplinary care. Infrequent headaches (<5 times/month) can be treated solely by abortive treatment. Acetaminophen, ibuprofen, sumatriptan, ketorolac, and prochlorperazine can all be used with reasonable efficacy.[23] For refractory migraine headaches, dihydroergotamine can be administered in the emergency room or in the hospital.[24] For frequent, disabling headaches, patients may be candidates for prophylactic therapy. Amitriptyline or topiramate may be considered.[25] Due to the high level of disability in headache patients, cognitive behavioral therapy is a priority; it can include biofeedback and relaxation techniques.[21] Regional nerve blocks (e.g., trigeminal or occipital nerve block) have been used in adult patients and sporadically used in pediatric and adolescent patients with intractable migraine[26,27] (Figure 11.3).

Back Pain in Children

Back pain is surprisingly common in the pediatric population, with up to 50% of 16-year-olds reporting having had back pain.[28] As is true for all pain conditions, a detailed history and physical examination will determine the majority of diagnoses and guide the need for further evaluation. For adults, the American Pain Society guidelines do not recommend routine imaging studies for back pain.[29]

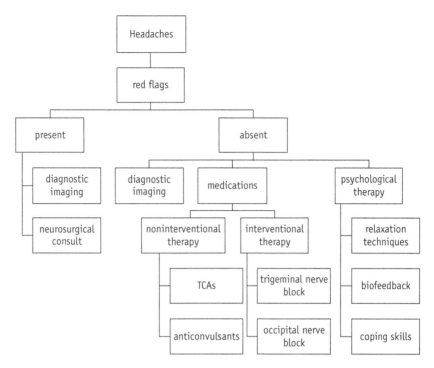

Figure 11.3 Algorithm of managing headaches.

In children, however, back pain is a more compelling reason to pursue imaging, to rule out serious underlying pathologies (e.g., tumors or infections). Certainly, "red flags" for back pain (Box 11.5) indicate strong reasons to pursue advanced imaging or blood work.

The etiology of back pain in children is diverse. Athletes are prone to spondylolysis or listhesis (acquired due to repetitive microtrauma, or congenital).

Box 11.5 **Back Pain Red Flags**

Night sweats
Unexplained fever
Weight loss
Night pain
Constant pain
Stool incontinence or constipation
Urinary retention or incontinence
Neurological changes in lower extremities (e.g., difficulty walking, foot drop, weakness, loss of reflexes, sensory changes)

Pain is triggered and becomes magnified by intense physical activity. Disk herniation is much less frequent, and scoliosis rarely causes significant pain. Back pain in children may also be referred from other sites, such as muscle strains, urinary tract infections, nephrolithiasis, endometriosis, and viral infections.[30] Nephrolithiasis can cause referred back pain and reflex muscle spasm that can be refractory to treatment, requiring a complex regimen of muscle relaxants, transcutaneous electrical nerve stimulation (TENS), and mobilization/physical therapy. Other causes of pain can be detected during physical examination— for example, a hairy patch, suggesting intraspinal anomalies; abnormal skin markings—café au lait spots—suggesting neurofibromatosis; asymmetry, suggesting scoliosis; or limb length discrepancy.[30]

For pediatric patients in acute pain in the hospital, while workup is in progress, opioids, muscle relaxants, acetaminophen, and NSAIDs can be used, as needed. Once the cause is identified and treated, the patient should be weaned off opioids. Physical therapy must be involved, as well as psychology for pain coping skill training. A TENS unit is a great tool to use for back pain (as well as abdominal pain and CRPS). About 20% of pediatric patients with back pain have nonspecific pain—pain that lacks an underlying etiology and tends to be magnified by stress. These patients need to work with counselors on stress management and address underlying anxiety disorders or depression on an outpatient basis; getting started on this program while an inpatient is efficient[31] (Figure 11.4).

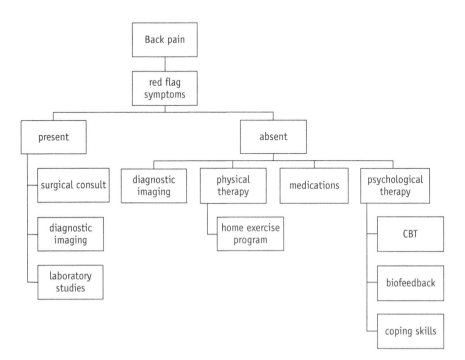

Figure 11.4 Algorithm for managing back pain. CBT, cognitive behaviorial therapy.

Complex Regional Pain Syndrome in Children

In hospital settings, patients occasionally may present in various stages of complex regional pain syndrome (CRPS). Sometimes, onset correlates with surgical trauma or trauma related to an accident. Less frequently, patients are admitted with pain flare-up, being unable to cope effectively or to continue outpatient therapies. Lastly, patients with active or remote CRPS are admitted for unrelated reasons.

There are two major categories of CRPS (e.g., type 1 and type 2), and they differ only in the presence or absence of a documented nerve injury. Pain is an obligatory sign and may be accompanied by hyperalgesia or allodynia as well as motor disturbances. There must be evidence or a history of edema, changes to skin blood flow, or abnormal sudomotor activity in the region of pain at some point in time but not necessarily at the at time of diagnosis. CRPS may also cause loss of joint mobility, atrophy, and weakness of the involved extremity, as well as lead to decreased nail and hair growth.

Clinically, it is important to take a detailed history and physical exam, as early diagnosis and treatment are extremely important for restoration of normal function and prevention of long-term disability caused by delayed diagnosis and treatment.[32]

Treatment of CRPS in children is complex and requires a multidisciplinary approach, with a focus on the psychological and physical aspects of the disease. The mainstay of treatment in CRPS is physical therapy; emphasis is directed at restoring function to the affected part of the body. Psychological treatment used in conjunction with physical therapy includes cognitive behavioral therapy with emphasis on acquiring effective pain coping skills. It may incorporate biofeedback or hypnosis, guided imagery, or distraction techniques. The excruciating pain may become a hurdle and impede the patient's active participation in the physical therapy program. Pharmacological treatment may help facilitate physical therapy and includes acetaminophen, NSAIDS, TCAs (e.g., amitriptyline, nortriptyline), anticonvulsants (e.g., gabapentin, pregabalin), and opioids.[33] In refractory cases, interventional therapy may provide additional relief and an opportunity to tolerate and make advances in physical therapy. Interventional therapies may include epidural analgesia, intrathecal analgesia, IV regional analgesia, sympathetic chain blocks, and peripheral nerve analgesia.[34,35]

In refractory cases of CRPS or any chronic pain condition, when a child is severely disabled by pain, we consider transfer to an inpatient chronic pediatric pain rehabilitation program. These programs are limited in number. Generally, they provide 2–3 weeks of intense physical and psychological therapies as well as complementary and alternative therapies. They focus on building up physical stamina and effective coping skills to resume a normal, age-appropriate, healthy lifestyle[36] (Figure 11.5).

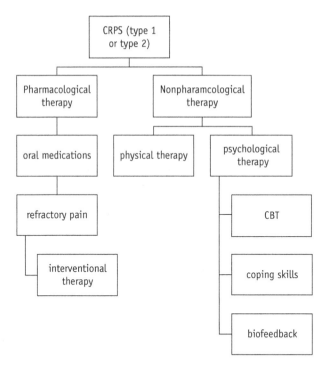

Figure 11.5 Algorithm for managing complex regional pain syndrome (CRPS).

Perioperative Pain Management in Children with Chronic Pain

Central sensitization is a set of processes within the central nervous system that amplifies the intensity of painful stimuli, increasing the area from which the painful stimulation is felt far beyond the site of initial insult. This process may tend to make new pain more intense than expected and lead to a flare-up of pre-existing chronic pain, even if the surgery site is not related to the site of chronic pain. Thus, preoperative planning that encompasses good communication and a team approach may lead to better success in perioperative pain management. In patients with chronic pain conditions, it is recommended that home medications be continued to help mitigate patients' pain throughout the perioperative period.

Opioids are the cornerstone of analgesia and are the most commonly pre-scribed medications used to treat moderate and severe acute pain in the pediatric population. However, in the presence of chronic pain conditions, central sensitization, and in certain cases, opioid tolerance, and rarely opioid-induced hyperalgesia, may present difficulties in appropriate dosing calculation. Thus, a multimodal approach that implements various techniques and pharmacological options and reduces the emphasis of opioids is the best way to adequately treat this patient population in the perioperative period.

Regional and neuraxial blocks are some of the techniques in the toolbox of multimodal analgesia that may be used safely in anesthetized pediatric patients and that may significantly reduce pain. The use of gabapentin and pregabalin prophylactically preoperatively has also been found to be effective at decreasing the incidence of acute postsurgical pain and the development of chronic postsurgical pain in adults and children.[37,38] The intraoperative use of acetaminophen and NSAIDs has yielded some positive results in children, although authors caution that such reports may have potential publication bias.[39] Complementary and alternative medicine (massage, healing touch), child-life interventions, music therapy, and visits to an activity center (or play room) while in the hospital are added tools in multimodal analgesia, often available for pediatric patients and their families.

Weaning Opioids in Children with Chronic Opioid Exposure

Children with complex medical problems may become exposed to opioids or benzodiazepines during hospitalizations when there is a need for prolonged sedation in the intensive care unit setting in an attempt to mitigate stress response and pain. This practice places the children at risk for dependency and withdrawal if medications are stopped abruptly. Addiction, per se, is rare. Withdrawal from opioids is unpleasant and can be destabilizing to a patient who cannot tolerate uncontrolled sympathetic nervous system activity. Seizures from benzodiazepine withdrawal can be life-threatening.

The mainstay of opioid weaning in children is an individualized, stepwise approach. Regular assessments for signs of opioid withdrawal (e.g., anxiety, agitation, grimacing, insomnia, increased muscle tone, vomiting, tachycardia, sweating, hypertension, abdominal pain, and diarrhea) must be done regularly. There are standardized withdrawal scales available (e.g., WATS) that can be used to organize assessment of the weaning process.[40] Several pharmacological techniques may be used to treat or prevent opioid withdrawal and may include methadone, buprenorphine, clonidine, and gabapentin.[41] Methadone is a great analgesic used commonly for opioid withdrawal. A methadone weaning protocol is highlighted in Table 11.3, but has to be individualized to reflect duration of patient opioid exposure and the total dose of opioid used prior to weaning. The longer the exposure and the higher the doses, the slower the wean should be, to minimize withdrawal.

Recommendations for Dosing Medications in the Pediatric Population

The following tables are recommended doses of commonly prescribed medications in the pediatric population (Table 11.4, Table 11.5, Table 11.6, Table 11.7, Table 11.8).

Table 11.3 **Methadone Opioid-Weaning Protocol**

Short-Term Protocol (7–14 days)	Long-Term Protocol (>14 days)
Use 1-hour dose of opioid to convert to methadone	Use 1-hour dose of opioid to convert to methadone
Day 1: give methadone PO every 6 hours for 24 hours	Day 1: give methadone PO every 6 hours for 24 hours
Day 2: reduce methadone by 20%, give PO every 8 hours for 24 hours	Day 2: give methadone, change to PO every 6 hours for 24 hours
Day 3: reduce methadone by 20%, give PO every 8 hours for 24 hours	Day 3: reduce methadone by 20%, give PO every 6 hours for 48 hours
Day 4: reduce methadone by 20%, give PO every 12 hours for 24 hours	Day 5: reduce methadone by 20%, give PO every 8 hours for 48 hours
Day 5: reduce methadone by 20%, give PO every 24 hours for 24 hours	Day 7: reduce methadone by 20%, give PO every 12 hours for 48 hours
Day 6: stop methadone	Day 9: reduce methadone by 20%, give PO every 24 hours for 48 hours
	Day 11: stop methadone

Modified from Robertson RC, Darsey E, Fortenberry JD, et al. Evaluation of an opiate-weaning protocol using methadone in pediatric intensive care unit patients. *Pediatr Crit Care Med.* 2000;1(2):19–23.

Table 11.4 **Pediatric Dosing for NSAIDs**

Medication	Route	Dose	Dosing Interval	Maximum Daily Dose for Patient
Ibuprofen	PO	8–10 mg/kg	Every 6 hours	**<60 kg patient:** 40 mg/kg/day **>60 kg patient:** 2400 mg/day
Ketorolac	IV	0.25–0.5 mg/kg	Every 6 hours	**<60 kg patient:** 2 mg/kg/day **>60 kg patient:** 120 mg/day

Modified from Birmingham PK. Pediatric postoperative pain. In: Benzon H, et al., eds. *Essentials of Pain Medicine,* 3rd ed. Philadelphia, PA: Saunders, 2011, 238–242.[41]

Table 11.5 **Pediatric Dosing for Opioids**

Medication	Equianalgesic Doses	Typical IV Starting Dose		Typical Oral Starting Dose	
		<50 kg	>50 kg	<50 kg	>50 kg
Morphine	PO: 30mg IV: 10 mg	0.1 mg/kg every 2–4 hours Infusion: 0.01–0.02 mg/kg/h	5–10 mg every 3–4 hours Infusion: 1.5 mg/h	0.3 mg/kg every 3–4 hours	15–20 mg every 3–4 hours
Hydromor-phone	PO: 6–8 mg IV: 1.5–2 mg	0.015 mg/kg every 3–4 hours Infusion: 0.006 mg/kg/h	1–1.5 mg every 3–4 hours Infusion: 0.3 mg/h	0.04–0.08 mg/kg every 3–4 hours	2–4 mg every 3–4 hours
Oxycodone	PO: 15–20 mg IV: N/A	N/A	N/A	0.1–0.2 mg/kg every 3-4 hours	5–10 mg every 3–4 hours
Methadone	PO: 10–20 mg IV: 10mg	0.1 mg/kg every 4–8 hours	5–8 mg every 4–8 hour	0.1–0.2 mg/kg every 4-8 hours	5–10 mg every 4–8 hours
Fentanyl	PO: N/A IV: 100 mcg (0.1 mg)	0.5-1.5 mcg/kg every 1–2 hours Infusion: 0.5–2.0 mcg/kg/h	25–75 mcg/kg every 1–2 hours Infusion: 25–100 mcg/h	N/A	N/A

Modified from Berde CB, et al. Analgesics for the treatment of pain in children. *N Engl J Med.* 2002;347:1094–1103.

Table 11.6 **Pediatric Dosing for Epidural Infusions**

Medication	Loading Dose	Concentration of Solution	Infusion limits
Bupivacaine	2.5–3 mg/kg	0.0625–0.1%	0.2–0.4 mg/kg/h
Ropivacaine	2.5–3 mg/kg	0.1–0.2%	0.2–0.4 mg/kg/h
Fentanyl	1–2 mcg/kg	2–5 mcg/mL	0.5–2 mcg/kg/h
Morphine	10–30 mcg/kg	5–10 mcg/mL	1–5 mcg/kg/h
Hydromorphone	2–6 mcg/kg	2–5 mcg/mL	1–2.5 mcg/kg/h
Clonidine	1–2 mcg/kg	0.5–2 mcg/mL	0.1–0.5 mcg/kg/h

Modified from Birmingham PK. Pediatric postoperative pain. In: Benzon H, et al., eds. *Essentials of Pain Medicine*, 3rd ed. Philadelphia, PA: Saunders, 2011, 238–242.[41]

Table 11.7 Pediatric Dosing for Acetaminophen

Route	Age	Dose	Interval	Maximum daily dose
IV	1 month–24 months	7.5–10 mg/kg	Every 6 hours as needed	40 mg/kg/day
	2–12 years	15 mg/kg	Every 6 hours as needed	75 mg/kg/day or 3750 mg/day
	>12 years <50 kg >50 kg	15 mg/kg 12.5 mg/kg 1000 mg 650 mg	Every 6 hours Every 4 hours Every 6 hours Every 4 hours	Max 750 mg/dose or 75 mg/kg/day Max 1000 mg per dose or 4000 mg/day
PO		10–15 mg/kg	Every 4–6 hours as needed	Not to exceed 5 doses/day; not to exceed 4000 mg/day
Rectal		10–20 mg/kg	Every 4–6 hours as needed	Not to exceed 5 doses/day

Modified from Cincinnati Children's Hospital Medical Center Pain Service Medication Dosing Guide, 2009 (courtesy of David Moore, MD). Use with caution in hepatic impairment. If creatinine clearance <10 mL/min, dose every 8 hours.

Table 11.8 Pediatric Dosing for Commonly Prescribed Adjuvants

Medication	Dose	Adjuvant Quality	Class of Medication
Gabapentin	5 mg/kg PO (Max: 300 mg) Day 2: 5 mg/kg BID Day 3: 5 mg/kg TID	Neuropathic pain	Anticonvulsant
Pregabalin	25 mg po bid, increase by 25 mg every 7 days up to 150 mg po	Neuropathic pain	Anticonvulsant
Amitriptyline	0.25–1 mg/kg PO qHs	Neuropathic pain	Antidepressant
Diazepam	0.05–0.1 mg/kg PO q4h–q6h; 0.03 mg/kg IV q4h–q6h	Muscle relaxant; anxiolytic	Anxiolytic
Clonidine	1–2 mcg/kg epidurally; 3–5 mcg/kg PO; 0.1–0.3 mg/day transdermally	Analgesia; sedative	Alpha-2 agonist
Ketamine	0.5–2 mg/kg IV; 6–10 mg/kg PO	Analgesic effects	NMDA-antagonist
Metho-carbamol	15 mg/kg (max: 1000 mg) IV/PO q6h	Reduces muscle spasm which may cause pain	Muscle relaxant

Modified from Cincinnati Children's Hospital Medical Center Pain Service Medication Dosing Guide, 2009 (courtesy of David Moore, MD).

Summary

The complexity of caring for children with chronic pain reflects both the physiological and psychosocial factors that often lead to frustration of both families and healthcare workers. The interplay of psychosocial and medical factors may engulf the patient's and family's coping abilities, at which time the threshold for decompensating may decrease. The role of the physician is not to recognize not only the underlying medical reasons for pain but also the other factors that may be contributing to the pain and negating successful treatments. Emphasis on diagnosing and managing these patients using a multimodal approach is key to successfully treating this patient population. These patients require a bit more time than average. A calm, understanding demeanor and a willingness to educate the patient and family while ensuring the patient's safety can be rewarding and result in good outcomes.

References

1. King S, Chambers CT, Huguet A, et al. The epidemiology of chronic pain in children and adolescents revisited: a systematic review. *Pain*. 2011:152(12):2729–2738.
2. Stanford EA, Chambers CT, Biesanz JC, Chen E. The frequency, trajectories and predictors of adolescent recurrent pain: a population-based approach. *Pain*. 2008;138(1):11–21.
3. Kaminski A, Kamper A, Thaler K, Chapman A, Gartlehner G. Antidepressants for the treatment of abdominal pain-related functional gastrointestinal disorders in children and adolescents. *Cochrane Database Syst Rev*. 2011;7:CD008013.
4. Teitelbaum JE, Arora R. Long-term efficacy of low-dose tricyclic antidepressants for children with functional gastrointestinal disorders. *J Pediatr Gastroenterol Nutr*. 2011;53(3):260–264.
5. Rahimi R, Nikfar S, Rezaie A, Abdollahi M. Efficacy of tricyclic antidepressants in irritable bowel syndrome: a meta-analysis. *World J Gastroenterol*. 2009:15(13):1548–1553.
6. Trinkley KE, Nahata MC. Treatment of irritable bowel syndrome. *J Clin Pharm Ther*. 2011;36(3):275–282.
7. Cochrane Database of Systematic Reviews: Plain Language Summaries. Bulking agents, antispasmodics and antidepressants for the treatment of irritable bowel syndrome. http://www.ncbi.nlm.nih.gov/pubmedhealth/PMH0012078/
8. Merat S, Khalili S, Mostajabi P, et al. The effect of enteric-coated, delayed-release peppermint oil on irritable bowel syndrome. *Dig Dis Sci*. 2010;55(5):1385–1390.
9. Rasquin A, Di Lorenzo C, Forbes D, et al. Childhood functional gastrointestinal disorders: child/adolescent. *Gastroenterology*. 2006;130(5):1527–1537.
10. Eslick GD. Epidemiology and risk factors of pediatric chest pain: a systematic review. *Pediatr Clin North Am*. 2010;57(6):1211–1219.
11. Eslick GD, Selbst SM. Pediatric chest pain. Preface. *Pediatr Clin North Am*. 2010;57(6):xiii–xiv.
12. Cico SJ, Paris CA, Woodward GA. Miscellaneous causes of pediatric chest pain. *Pediatr Clin North Am*. 2010;57(6):1397–1406.
13. McDonnell CJ, White KS, Assessment and treatment of psychological factors in pediatric chest pain. *Pediatr Clin North Am*. 2010;57(6):1235–1260.
14. Thull-Freedman J. Evaluation of chest pain in the pediatric patient. *Med Clin North Am*. 2010;94(2):327–347.

15. White KS. Assessment and treatment of psychological causes of chest pain. *Med Clin North Am.* 2010;94(2):291–318.
16. Stinson J, Naser B. Pain management in children with sickle cell disease. *Paediatr Drugs.* 2003;5(4):229–241.
17. Wethers DL. Sickle cell disease in childhood: Part II. Diagnosis and treatment of major complications and recent advances in treatment. *Am Fam Physician.* 2000;62(6):1309–1314.
18. Shah N, et al. Differences in pain management between hematologists and hospitalists caring for patients with sickle cell disease hospitalized for vasoocclusive crisis. *Clin J Pain.* 2013.
19. What is EB? The Dystrophic Epidermolysis Bullosa Research Association of America. 2013. http://www.debra.org/whatiseb. Accessed November 1, 2013.]
20. Fine JD, Johnson LB, Weiner M, Li KP, Suchindran C. Epidermolysis bullosa and the risk of life-threatening cancers: the National EB Registry experience, 1986-2006. *J Am Acad Dermatol.* 2009;60(2):203–211.
21. Kashikar-Zuck S, Zafar M, Barnett KA, et al. Quality of life and emotional functioning in youth with chronic migraine and juvenile fibromyalgia. *Clin J Pain.* 2013;29(12):1066–1072.
22. International Headache Society. IHS Classification ICHD-II. http://ihs-classification.org/en/. Accessed December 19, 2013].
23. Damen L, Bruijn JK, Verhagen AP, et al., Symptomatic treatment of migraine in children: a systematic review of medication trials. *Pediatrics.* 2005;116(2):e295–e302.
24. Kabbouche MA, Powers SW, Segers A, et al., Inpatient treatment of status migraine with dihydroergotamine in children and adolescents. *Headache.* 2009;49(1):106–109.
25. Hershey AD, Powers SW, Coffey CS, et al., Childhood and Adolescent Migraine Prevention (CHAMP) study: a double-blinded, placebo-controlled, comparative effectiveness study of amitriptyline, topiramate, and placebo in the prevention of childhood and adolescent migraine. *Headache.* 2013;53(5):799–816.
26. Ashkenazi A, Levin M. Greater occipital nerve block for migraine and other headaches: is it useful? *Curr Pain Headache Rep.* 2007;11(3):231–235.
27. Saracco MG, Valfrè W, Cavallini M, Aguggia M. Greater occipital nerve block in chronic migraine. *Neurol Sci.* 2010;31(Suppl 1):S179–S180.
28. Jones MA, Stratton G, Reilly T, Unnithan VB. A school-based survey of recurrent non-specific low-back pain prevalence and consequences in children. *Health Educ Res.* 2004;19(3):284–289.
29. Chou R, Qaseem A, Snow V, et al., Diagnosis and treatment of low back pain: a joint clinical practice guideline from the American College of Physicians and the American Pain Society. *Ann Intern Med.* 2007;147(7):478–491.
30. Bernstein RM, Cozen H. Evaluation of back pain in children and adolescents. *Am Fam Physician.* 2007;76(11):1669–1676.
31. Chou R, Huffman LH; American Pain Society; American College of Physicians. Nonpharmacologic therapies for acute and chronic low back pain: a review of the evidence for an American Pain Society/American College of Physicians clinical practice guideline. *Ann Intern Med.* 2007;147(7):492–504.
32. Harden RN, Bruehl S, Perez RS, et al., Validation of proposed diagnostic criteria (the "Budapest Criteria") for complex regional pain syndrome. *Pain.* 2010;150(2):268–274.
33. Suresh S, S.R. In: Benzon RS, Liu HT, et al., eds. *Essentials of Pain Medicine.* Philadelphia: Elsevier Saunders; 2011.
34. Dadure C, Motais F, Ricard C, et al. Continuous peripheral nerve blocks at home for treatment of recurrent complex regional pain syndrome I in children. *Anesthesiology.* 2005;102(2):387–391.
35. Meier PM, Zurakowski D, Berde CB, Sethna NF. Lumbar sympathetic blockade in children with complex regional pain syndromes: a double blind placebo-controlled crossover trial. *Anesthesiology.* 2009;111(2):372–380.

36. Logan DE, Carpino EA, Chiang G, et al., A day-hospital approach to treatment of pediatric complex regional pain syndrome: initial functional outcomes. *Clin J Pain*. 2012;28(9):766–774.

37. Sihoe AD, Lee TW, Wan IY, Thung KH, Yim AP. The use of gabapentin for post-operative and post-traumatic pain in thoracic surgery patients. *Eur J Cardiothorac Surg*. 2006;29(5):795–799.

38. Rusy LM, Hainsworth KR, Nelson TJ, et al. Gabapentin use in pediatric spinal fusion patients: a randomized, double-blind, controlled trial. *Anesth Analg*. 2010;110(5):1393–1398.

39. Michelet D, Andreu-Gallien J, Bensalah T, et al. A meta-analysis of the use of nonsteroidal antiinflammatory drugs for pediatric postoperative pain. *Anesth Analg*. 2012;114(2):393–406.

40. Franck LS, Harris SK, Soetenga DJ, Amling JK, Curley MA. The Withdrawal Assessment Tool-1 (WAT-1): an assessment instrument for monitoring opioid and benzodiazepine withdrawal symptoms in pediatric patients. *Pediatr Crit Care Med*. 2008;9(6):573–580.

41. PK, B. In: Benzone H, Raja SR, Fishman SM, et al., eds. *Essentials of Pain Medicine*, 3rd ed. Philadelphia: Saunders, 2011.

12

Management of Chronic Pain in the Geriatric Unit

BRUCE VROOMAN AND KATHY TRAVNICEK

KEY POINTS

- The elderly have a higher prevalence and incidence of pain that tends to be persistent and multifactorial in nature.
- Persistent pain is not an inevitable part of aging and should be treated with nonpharmacological and pharmacological methods with goals of increasing function, improving sleep, and helping mood.
- Hospital staff and nurses must know how to assess and monitor pain and must provide appropriate therapy for their geriatric patients during their admission.
- Physicians should do everything possible to provide appropriate pain relief in the elderly population in the hospital setting and need to recognize barriers to effective pain management.

Introduction

The prevalence of pain is high in the geriatric population given the association of pain with conditions including arthritis, cancer, fractures, and joint and spinal degeneration.[1] There is little to no robust scientific evidence to guide one in managing pain in geriatric patients. Due to stringent selection criteria in randomized controlled trials, frail elderly patients with multiple comorbidities and complex health issues are frequently either excluded or inadequately represented.[2-4] In addition, pain is an underrecognized and suboptimally treated symptom in this population.[5] Untreated pain clearly has a negative impact on a patient's quality of life. This can result in depression, social isolation, cognitive impairment, immobility, and sleep disturbances.[5-7] Pain is less reported by the elderly because of the common belief that pain is inevitable and a normal part of aging, and that their physician already knows that they have pain and is treating this. They may be particularly concerned about the cost of treatment or insurance coverage and they do not want to be a "bother." Some physicians may fear that their geriatric patients may become addicted when, in fact, this concern is often unjustified. They may understandably be concerned as well about the significant side effects of many medications because geriatric patients are at a higher risk for them.[8–10]

For pain management to be effective in the elderly, physicians and allied healthcare providers should be skilled in pain assessment and knowledgeable of the types of pain. In addition, they may be capable of recognizing the importance of a holistic, interdisciplinary team approach to care and knowledgeable of both pharmacological and nonpharmacological approaches to pain management. This chapter aims to guide healthcare providers to better recognize, assess, and manage pain in the geriatric population in the hospital setting.

Depending on the source in the literature, the following terms may have a variety of definitions. *Elderly* has been defined as the chronological age of 65 years or older with two subgroups—*early elderly* refers to patients ages 65–74 years, and *late elderly* are age 75 years and older.[11] The WHO divides the groups into "old" people aged over 60 and the "very old," or people over the age of 80. Interestingly, the age 65 was deemed as "elderly" first in Germany as the age one could participate in a national pension plan.[12] There is no general agreement on the age at which a person becomes elderly. The use of chronological age to mark the beginning of old age assumes equivalence with biological age. However, it is generally accepted that these two are not necessarily synonymous.

Physiological Changes

There are multiples changes that occur in normal aging, and they all contribute to a reduced ability of the individual to respond to stress. The clinician must be aware of specific age-related physiological changes in order to understand normal aging as compared to active disease. These changes significantly influence the response to treatments and potential complications. It is also important to know that there are wide individual differences in rate of aging and that different organ systems age at different rates.[13,14] The changes in renal, cardiac, hepatic, and gastrointestinal systems and in body composition all affect pharmacokinetics and pharmacodynamics. *Pharmacokinetics* refers to the time course of when a drug is absorbed, distributed, metabolized, and then excreted. The changes include renal and hepatic clearance reductions and the increases in volume of distribution of lipid-soluble drugs. *Pharmacodynamics* refers to the relationship of drug concentration at the site of action and the resulting effect. These changes involve altered sensitivity to several drug classes, which, in the elderly, is usually increased. The age-related changes that affect pharmacokinetics and pharmaco-dynamics that are important to know for pain management in the elderly are shown in Table 12.1.[15,16]

The impacts of aging on pharmacokinetics are particularly important. Age-related physiological and morphological changes influence drug disposition. Age-related decreases in gastric acid secretion, gastrointestinal motility, and blood flow may alter drug absorption, but no significant age-related change in drug absorption has been observed in studies to date. With aging, the percentage of body fat increases and that of total body water decreases. Therefore, water-soluble (hydrophilic) drugs have higher peak plasma levels in the elderly, while lipid-soluble (lipophilic) drugs have an increased volume of distribution in the elderly. Age-dependent decrease in the serum albumin concentration influences drug protein binding potency. Age-related reduction in liver size, hepatic blood flow, and hepatic drug-metabolizing enzyme activity decreases the hepatic drug clearance. The decreases in renal blood flow, glomerular filtration rate (GFR), and tubular secretion have a considerable impact on the renal clearance of drugs. Nervous system changes make patients more sensitive to medications such as benzodiazepines. Elderly patients also have an altered response to pain and increased pain perception when noxious stimuli are present.[16] Finally, the effect of aging on the respiratory system should be noted. Elderly patients have a decreased sensation of dyspnea and diminished ventilatory response to hypoxia and hypercapnia, making them more vulnerable to ventilatory failure during high-demand states. Thus, elderly patients who are smokers and have pulmonary conditions such as COPD, asthma, or obstructive sleep apnea are at risk when opioids are needed.[17]

Assessment of Pain in the Elderly

There are multiple complexities in assessing pain in the elderly. An accurate assessment is critical for the determining the correct treatment, and barriers must be recognized and addressed. Patient-related barriers will cause patients to downplay their pain or be unable to report it. Physicians and nurses may have similar misconceptions about pain, such as it being a part of aging. They also have been known to underestimate an elderly patient's pain and suffering. It is vital that there be a multidisciplinary approach in assessment and treatment of pain. This team includes the patient, the patient's caregivers, the primary medical or surgical team, a pain physician and other consultants, nursing, nursing aids, and physical and occupational therapies. If mental health issues are a concern, a psychologist or psychiatrist should be added to the team.[18]

A detailed history and physical examination should be performed and include all elements—medical, surgical, family, and social histories; allergies;

Table 12.1 **Physiological Changes and Consequences, Common Comorbid Issues, and Medication Effects in the Elderly**

System	Physiological Changes	Physiological Consequences	Common Comorbid Issues	Medication Effects
General	Increased body fat Decreased body water	Increased volume of distribution for lipophilic medications Increased plasma concentration of hydrophilic medications	Frailty Decreased blood volume due to diuretics	Lipophilic drugs—lidocaine, fentanyl—increased duration of effect Water-soluble drugs—morphine—more toxicity
Cardiac	Decreased cardiac index	Rapid, higher medication peak		Increased risk of toxicity
Respiratory	Reduced thoracic expansion Reduced ventilation		COPD, OSA	Higher risk of respiratory depression (opioids)
Gastro-intestinal	Altered secretions Decreased blood flow Altered motility Altered absorptive surface	Altered absorption Altered bioavailability Altered transit time Altered absorption	Disorders that alter GI pH Surgically altered anatomy Malnutrition	Unpredictable oral bioavailability
Hepatic	Reduced blood flow Decreased hepatic enzymes Decreased protein synthesis Decreased regeneration rate	Decreased metabolism up to 40% Decreased serum albumin Phase 1 reactions (oxidation, hydrolysis, reduction) more affected than phase 2 (conjugation) Decline in cytochrome P-450 function	Cirrhosis Hepatitis Tumors may disrupt oxidation but not usually conjugation	Increased risk of toxicity Increase amount of free drug availability (morphine, fentanyl, tramadol, buprenorphine)
Renal	Decreased renal blood flow Reduced GFR	Decreased excretion	Chronic kidney disease	Increased risk of toxicity (gabapentin, NSAIDS, morphine oxycodone)
Nervous	Decreased cerebral blood flow Neuronal loss/atrophy Decreased synthesis of neurotransmitters Decreased opioid receptor density	Decreased descending inhibitory pain control Altered pain processing	Dementia Stroke Vascular disease	More susceptible to sedation due to increased sensitivity to centrally acting drugs

COPD, chronic obstructive pulmonary disease; OSA, obstructive sleep apnea.

medications taken at home and in the hospital; and review of systems with cognitive and depression screening. Important questions to ask are the following: What was the reason for admission? Is there a history of chronic pain and, if so, due to what condition? Are there new pains? How are they different from their chronic condition? One must review the location of pain, intensity, aggravating and relieving factors, and impact on mood, sleep, and function. It is important to identify the patient's prior functional status at baseline and what changes have occurred lately and why. This includes assessing activities of daily living (bathing, bowel and bladder management, dressing upper and lower body, feeding self by setting up food and bringing it to the mouth, functional mobility, personal hygiene and grooming, and toilet hygiene) and instrumental activities of daily living (housekeeping, taking medications as prescribed, managing finances, shopping for groceries or clothing, use of telephone or other form of communication, driving or use of other transportation within the community, cooking). One should ask about their exercise regimen, hobbies and leisurely activities, a history of falls, living arrangements and how the home is set up, as well as what family, social, and psychological support systems are in place. Finally, it is prudent to ask about the patient's knowledge, attitudes, and beliefs regarding pain and its management. Being aware of the patient's thoughts is very important, because they reflect expression of pain and what management options one will choose (Box 12.1).

Pain can be assessed in three ways: direct patient questioning, behavioral observations, and caregiver or others reports. The self-report of pain can be used for patients with the preserved ability to communicate. Ultimately, it is the patient's self-reporting of pain that is the most accurate and reliable evidence. The visual analogue scale is commonly used, but one must be careful as the elderly may have difficulty using this scale. Pain measurement tools used should depend on the individual patient. Other scales that may be better are the "faces" pain scale, verbal descriptor scale, present pain intensity, or global pain assessment. These are quick to use but only measure pain intensity. The McGill Pain Questionnaire is more detailed; it can be used to assess sensory, affective, evaluative, and miscellaneous components of pain.[6,8,9,18]

The International Association for the Study of Pain defines pain as "an unpleasant sensory and emotional experience associated with actual or potential tissue damage or described in terms of such damage." There is a note attached to the definition indicating that inability to communicate should in no way be taken to imply that the individual experiences no pain.[19-21] Many elderly people have cognitive, hearing, or visual impairments; in the United States alone, more than 50% of nursing home residents have cognitive decline or dementia.[22,23] These impairments make the assessment of pain challenging.

Box 12.1 **Checklist: Assessment of Geriatric Patients
in the Hospital Setting**

1. Complete history and physical examination, with focus most concerning pain.
2. Review pain location, intensity, character, exacerbating and alleviating factors, and impact on mood, sleep, and function.
3. Rely on caregivers reports, particularly for elderly patients with cognitive impairment and communication disorders.
4. Review activities of daily living (ADLs; bathing, dressing, toileting, transfers, feeding, and continence) and instrumental ADLs (use of phone, travel, shopping, food preparation, housework, laundry, taking medicine, handling finances).
5. Assess for atypical manifestations of pain, such as changes in function, gait, withdrawn or agitated behavior, or increased confusion.
6. Use standard geriatric assessment tools to evaluate function, affect, cognition, gait, and psychosocial issues.
7. Screen for cognitive impairment.
8. Screen for depression.
9. Assess gait and balance.
10. Screen for sensory depression to examine basic visual and auditory function.

Other things to think about when performing the above:
- What is the patient's coping response for stress or pain, including the presence or absence of psychiatric disorders such as depression, anxiety, or psychosis?
- What are the family expectations and beliefs concerning pain, stress, and the patient's current medical status?
- What are the patient's knowledge and expectations of and preferences for pain management methods and for receiving information about pain management?
- What is the patient's attitude toward use of opioids, anxiolytics, or other medications?

Pathological changes in dementia seriously affect the ability of those with advanced stages of disease to communicate pain. Damage to the central nervous system affects memory, language, and higher-order cognitive processing necessary to communicate the pain experience. Yet, despite changes in central nervous system functioning, persons with dementia still experience pain sensation to a degree similar to that of cognitively intact older adults.[24-27] Pathological changes associated with dementia affect the interpretation of the pain stimulus and the affective response to that sensation.[25-27] Differences in pain processing have been noted in distinct types of dementia.[28] Although self-report of pain is often possible for those with mild to moderate cognitive impairment, as dementia progresses, the ability to self-report decreases and eventually is no longer possible.[29]

In the absence of self-reporting, observing behavior is a valid approach to assessing pain. The American Geriatrics Society has guidelines on common pain behaviors that may indicate pain.[30] Correlations have been found between behavioral pain scores and self-reported pain intensity; however, pain behaviors are not specific to pain intensity and in some cases indicate other sources of distress.[10,31,32] Examples of pain behaviors include facial expressions, verbalizations, body movements, changes in interpersonal interactions, changes in activity patterns or routines, and mental status changes. These are potential pain indicators in older persons with dementia.[31,32] Some behaviors are common and typically considered to be pain related (facial grimacing, moaning, groaning, rubbing a body part), but others are less obvious (agitation, restlessness, irritability, confusion, combativeness, changes in appetite or usual activities) and require follow-up evaluation.[9,31,32]

It remains unclear which behaviors are most often associated with pain in patients with dementia, although research is ongoing in this area. The American Geriatric Society's indicators of pain or a nonverbal pain assessment tool that is appropriate, valid, and reliable for use with this population is the best option for assessing pain in these patients. Behavioral observation should occur during activity whenever possible, because pain may be minimal or absent at rest. Vital sign changes are not an accurate reflection of pain in persons with or without dementia.[33]

PAIN CLASSIFICATION

Pain is generally classified into one of two broad categories: nociceptive or neuropathic pain. Analgesics such as opioids, acetaminophen, and nonsteroidal anti-inflammatory drugs (NSAIDs) are known to be more effective for nociceptive pain. Adjuvant medications, including antiepileptics and antidepressants, are more helpful in treating neuropathic pain. One should determine the particular type of pain prior to prescribing first-line medications. Musculoskeletal (lumbar spinal stenosis, degenerative disk disease, osteoarthritis, fractures) and neurological disorders (postherpetic neuralgia, trigeminal neuralgia, diabetic neuropathy, fibromyalgia) are the most common causes of pain and should be given priority in the assessment process. "Mixed" pain resulting from cancer is usually a combination of nociceptive and neuropathic pain that may be addressed with one or more agent (Table 12.2).

Table 12.2 **Common Chronic Geriatric Pain Diseases**

Common Chronic Geriatric Pain Diseases	Type of Pain
Cancer	Mixed
Angina	Nociceptive
Rheumatological	Nociceptive
Postherpetic neuralgia	Neuropathic
Temporal arteritis	Nociceptive
Peripheral neuropathy	Neuropathic
Trigeminal neuralgia	Neuropathic
Peripheral vascular disease	Neuropathic
Ischemia	Nociceptive

Treatment of Acute on Chronic Pain in the Elderly

The American Geriatrics Society Panel published the first set of guidelines on managing chronic pain in the elderly in 1998, with an updated version in 2009.[31] According to these guidelines, treatments may be considered to be nonpharmacological or pharmacological interventions. After a thorough assessment and correct diagnosis, the goals of treatment should be outlined with the patient. These are to reduce the severity of pain, though elimination of pain is usually not expected. It can be expected to improve a patient's function, mood, and sleep patterns. Noncompliance is known to be due to poor physician–patient communication, cost, medications chosen, number of medications, and insurance coverage.[34] For these reasons, one should review the plan with the patient and or caregivers and make sure they are educated appropriately. In addition, selection of treatment will be guided by the patient's comorbidities, current medications, and possible drug interactions, as well as preferences.

NONPHARMACOLOGICAL INTERVENTIONS

A first consideration is preventing patients from hurting themselves, such as from falls. Among older adults (those 65 or older), falls are the leading cause of death due to injury. They are also the most common cause of nonfatal injuries and hospital admissions for trauma.[35] Most fractures among older adults are caused by falls and frequently involve the spine, hip, forearm, leg, ankle, pelvis, upper arm, or hand.[35,36] Patients' hospital rooms should have adequate lighting, low-level beds, easily accessible call buttons, and bed alarms. Occasionally there may need to be a sitter with the patient. There should also be appropriate staffing to monitor these patients with frequent checks and reorienting. Hospitals typically have fall prevention programs in place.[37]

Box 12.2 **Checklist: Nonpharmacological Management in the Elderly**

• It is a means of avoiding adverse drug reactions.
• Consider cognitive-behavioral therapy as a means of education and for enhancing coping skills and pain prevention.
• Recognize the role of exercise as a means of pain management to maintain and enhance functioning and avoid deconditioning.
• Heat, cold, transcutaneous electrical nerve stimulation (TENS), and massage therapy
• Acupuncture
• Appreciate the spiritual aspects of pain and provide counseling or refer patient to a member of the clergy.

Nonpharmacological management and rehabilitation are essential components to a comprehensive multidisciplinary pain management plan (Box 12.2). This will help with pain but also improves coping and function. The rehabilitative aspect of pain management is to have the patient live as independently as possible by helping them adapt to and compensate for any loss of physical, psychological, or social functioning. Other important objectives of rehabilitation include stabilizing the primary disorder, preventing secondary injuries and complications, and decreasing pain via a multidisciplinary approach with a physiatrist and physical and occupational therapists. Pain-relieving modalities used are ice, heat, transcutaneous electrical nerve stimulation (TENS) units, and massage. Some patients benefit and prefer other nonpharmacological options, such as acupuncture, low-velocity osteopathic manipulation, and certain supplements. In addition, since pain is a complex sensory and emotional experience, psychological measures have to be added to a pain management program. Psychological measures should be addressed by a trained cognitive behavioral therapist who may use a structured approach to teaching coping skills. For many patients there is a spiritual aspect to persistent pain. Enlisting support of clergy or a chaplain may also be very beneficial and stress-relieving.[38-44]

SPECIFICS OF PHARMACOLOGICAL TREATMENT IN THE ELDERLY

Even though older adults have a significantly increased risk of adverse reactions to pharmacological agents, medications are still the principal treatment modality for pain. The multidimensional nature of pain, polypharmacy treatment of other comorbidities, and the lack of evidence-based guidelines make this population difficult to manage at times. The best approach is to develop a simple, individualized, patient-centered management plan after a comprehensive pain assessment. After the etiology of pain has been identified, there are several pharmacological agents with multiple delivery routes (oral, intravascular, intramuscular, rectal, sublingual, transdermal) that can be trialed. Medications can be started lower than or at the lowest effective dose, followed by a gradual and slow titration to prevent adverse side effects or overdosing. With opioids, there should be adequate intervals between the escalations of medication during titration. These intervals relate to the expected half-life of the medication used.[31,42,45–49]

Prevention, anticipation, and management of adverse side effects should all be taken into consideration by the physician when prescribing medications in this population. Use of high-dose opioids, NSAID agents, and tricyclic antidepressants should be avoided in elderly patients. High-dose opioids may cause adverse effects in most patients. Long-term use of NSAIDs is associated with renal dysfunction, gastrointestinal bleeding, and cardiac dysfunction. Tricyclic antidepressants may cause anticholinergic side effects, cognitive impairment, and cardiac dysfunction.[30] Pain medications can be classified according to three broad categories: nonopioid analgesics, opioid analgesics, and adjuvant medications. Our recommendations that follow are based on the 2009 updated guidelines published by the American Geriatric Society.[31]

Non-Opioid Analgesics

This class includes acetaminophen and all NSAIDs; these medications are well understood and discussed in detail elsewhere in this book. Acetaminophen should be considered initial and ongoing pharmacotherapy in the treatment of persistent pain, particularly musculoskeletal pain. It can be very effective and has a reasonable safety profile (high quality of evidence, strong recommendation). The absolute contraindications are liver failure. The relative contraindications and precautions are hepatic insufficiency and chronic alcohol abuse or dependence. The maximum daily recommended dosages of 4 g per 24 hours should not be exceeded. The patient and family have to be educated on hidden sources of acetaminophen such as from combination pills.

Nonselective NSAIDs and cyclooxygenase-2 (COX-2) selective inhibitors may be considered rarely, and with extreme caution, in highly selected individuals.[34] The absolute contraindications to these medications are current active peptic ulcer disease, chronic kidney disease, and heart failure. Precautions and relative contraindications are uncontrolled hypertension, *Helicobacter pylori,* history of peptic ulcer disease, and concomitant use of corticosteroids or selective serotonin reuptake inhibitors (SSRIs). Older persons taking nonselective NSAIDs or a COX-2 selective inhibitor with aspirin should use a proton pump inhibitor or misoprostol for gastrointestinal protection. Patients should not take more than one nonselective NSAID or COX-2 selective inhibitor together. Patients taking aspirin for cardioprophylaxis should not use ibuprofen. Patients taking nonselective NSAIDs and COX-2 selective inhibitors should be routinely assessed for gastrointestinal and renal toxicity, hypertension, heart failure, and other drug–drug and drug–disease interactions.[31,50,51]

Opioid Analgesics in the Elderly

Elderly patients with moderate to severe pain, pain-related functional impairment, or diminished quality of life because of pain may be considered for a short-term course of opioid therapy in order to facilitate their rehabilitation after hospital admission. First, one must determine whether the patient is opioid-naïve or opioid-tolerant. The pain history needs to be reviewed to confirm that the patient has had an adequate trial of non-opioid treatments. One must also pay attention to the dosage and duration of treatment. Some patients may report treatment failure when they have not had an adequate therapeutic trial. The currently prescribed opioid, dosage, and duration of treatment are important to determine if the patient is opioid-tolerant, as defined by the FDA. Of particular relevance is any information regarding past opioid treatment, including adherence, adverse reactions, and outcomes, as previous opioid treatment failure may argue against undertaking additional trials.

Opioid-naive elderly patients have a higher risk of serious adverse effects. The risk of respiratory depression can be significant if opioids are not slowly titrated, and this risk is heightened in patients who are opioid-naïve.[48,52] Some formulations are inappropriate and may be quite dangerous when used for treatment initiation. For example, transdermal fentanyl patches carry a black box warning against their use in opioid-naïve patients. Because of the high drug concentration and rate of delivery, this formulation can cause severe respiratory depression in this subset of patient.[53]

Opioid-tolerant patients have a much lower risk of sedation and will tolerate faster titrations at higher dosages. True addiction in the elderly is uncommon, and the possibility of addiction should not be used as justification for under-treatment of pain.[31,54]

Most opioids are available in fast-acting and long-acting formulation. Fast-acting opioids should be used for intermittent pain, such as with therapies and exercise, or for breakthrough pain. The long-acting formulations are for continuous pain and usually provide 8–12 hours of analgesia through sustained-release drug delivery systems. Fentanyl patches last longer and are usually changed every 72 hours. Methadone, which is limited by its pharmacodynamic profile, is relatively unpredictable, and its use in elderly persons with non-cancer pain is generally not advisable. Only clinicians well- versed in the use and risks of methadone should initiate it and then titrate it cautiously.[31,45,48]

When long-acting opioid preparations are prescribed, breakthrough pain should be anticipated, assessed, and treated, using short-acting immediate-release opioid medications. These patients should be reassessed for ongoing attainment of therapeutic goals (improved sleep, mood, and function), adverse effects, and safe and responsible medication use.[31,46] Depending on the situation, generally a fast-acting opioid should be started at the lowest effective dose and allowed to titrate slowly. Prescribers should check the opioid product package inserts for starting doses in opioid-naïve patients and use the minimum titration intervals.[31,48,52,55] Titration to a new dose should not occur until after drug plasma levels have reached steady state, which is approximately five half-lives, which is longer for long-acting than for short-acting opioids.[48]

Current guidelines are available to help ensure patient safety when a physician is converting treatment to a new opioid. Using an equianalgesic table one can calculate the 24-hour requirement of the current opioid and reduce the initial dose of new opioid by 25%–50%. This is done to negate an "incomplete cross-tolerance" among opioids. In high-risk patients (elderly, renal-impaired, cognitively impaired), the dose should be further reduced by another 15%–30%. These guidelines do not apply for methadone, for which the initial reduction of dose should be 75%–90%.[45,49]

The metabolism of hydromorphone, oxycodone, and methadone is directly dependent on liver function, while elimination of morphine depends on renal function. Thus, fentanyl could be a preferential opioid in liver dysfunction, while methadone and fentanyl are the agents of choice for opioid-tolerant patients with impaired renal function.[51,53,56,57] Morphine, oxymorphone, hydromorphone, and hydrocodone should be used with caution in patients with hepatic and renal impairment.[56,57]

Meperidine and high-dose tramadol (>200 mg/day) should be avoided in elderly patients, secondary to the risk that accumulation of their metabolites could lead to undesired side effects.[31] Early in a patient's management, long-acting opioid formulations should be avoided, secondary to their altered metabolism, presence of polypharmacy, and increased risk of side effects. For chronic pain management, long-acting opioids are reasonable choices, while fast-acting formulations are used for breakthrough pain.

Common opioid-induced side effects are constipation, sedation, nausea, endocrine dysfunction, and altered cognition. The only adverse effect that rarely resolves is constipation, necessitating its treatment. In addition to treatment with specific medications, side effects can be also managed with dose reduction, a change in route of administration, or change to a different opioid preparation. After excluding bowel obstruction, one can treat this with over-the-counter laxatives.[58,59]

Adjuvants

Adjuvants are pharmacological agents that were primarily developed for indications other than analgesia. Several medications belong to this group, including antidepressants, antiepileptics, corticosteroids, local anesthetics, alpha-2 adrenergic agonists, baclofen, *N*-methyl-d-aspartate receptor agonists, and calcitonin. They are commonly used in conjunction with other analgesics for persistent and refractory pain, but some are first-line therapy for neuropathic pain.

All patients with neuropathic pain are candidates for adjuvant analgesics, for which there is no to little risk of addiction. Antiepileptics (gabapentin, pregabalin, lamotrigine, levetiracetam, tiagabine, topiramate) are effective agents for treatment of the neuropathic component of pain. Titration should be done very slowly, as all of these agents can produce mild sedation. With the exception of lamotrigine and tiagabine, all antiepileptic dosages should be adjusted on the basis of renal function. Gabapentin, pregabalin, and levetiracetam are better choices for patients with hepatic dysfunction and preserved renal function. However, they will need to be renally dosed if renal dysfunction exists.[60,61]

Patients with fibromyalgia and other types of refractory-persistent pain may be candidates for certain adjuvant analgesics (back pain, headache, diffuse bone pain, temporomandibular disorder). These agents may be used alone, but often their effects are enhanced when used in combination with other pain analgesics.

As with other medications, therapy should begin with the lowest possible dose and increase slowly on the basis of response and side effects. Some agents have a delayed onset of action such that the therapeutic benefits are slow to develop. For example, gabapentin may require 2 to 3 weeks for the onset of efficacy. An adequate therapeutic trial should be conducted before discontinuation of a seemingly ineffective treatment.

Long-term systemic corticosteroids should be reserved for patients with pain-associated inflammatory disorders or metastatic bone pain. Topical over-the-counter creams can be used for mostly myofascial or musculoskeletal pain. Creams or ointments compounded at a pharmacy may consist of medications such as ketamine, gabapentin, clonidine, and local anesthetics to treat certain neuropathic pain conditions. Many other agents for specific pain syndromes may require caution in use in older persons and merit further research (glucosamine chondroitin, cannabinoids, botulinum toxin, alpha-2 adrenergic agonists, calcitonin, vitamin D, bisphosphonates, ketamine).

Summary

Pain is a complex phenomenon in which an individual's memories, expectations, and emotions modify the pain experience. The elderly have a higher prevalence and incidence of pain that tends to be persistent and multifactorial in nature. Persistent pain is not an inevitable part of aging and should be treated with nonpharmacological and pharmacological methods with goals of increasing function, improving sleep, and helping mood. Physicians can provide appropriate pain relief in this population, but they need to acknowledge certain barriers to effective pain management, understand how to assess and monitor pain, and provide appropriate therapy for their geriatric patients.

References

1. Hemle RD, Gibson SJ. Pain in older people. In Crombie IK, ed. *Epidemiology of Pain*. Seattle, WA: IASP Press; 1999:103–112.
2. Body CM, Darer J, Boult C, et al. Clinical practice guidelines and quality of care for older patients with multiple comorbid diseases. *JAMA*. 2005;294:716–724.
3. Zyczkowska J, Szczerbinska K, Jantzi MR, Hirdes JP. Pain among the oldest old in community and institutional settings. *Pain*. 2007;129:167–176.
4. Van Spall HGC, Toren A, Kiss A, Fowler RA. Eligibility criteria of randomized controlled trials published in high-impact general medical journals, a systematic sampling review. *JAMA*. 2007;297:1233–1240.
5. Under-treatment of pain in older adults: an application of beneficence. *Nursing Ethics*. 2012;19(6):800–809.
6. Rastogi R, Meek BD. Management of chronic pain in elderly, frail patients: finding a suitable, personalized method of control. *Clin Interv Aging*. 2013;8:37–46.
7. Moore HMA, Justins D. Treating acute pain in hospital. *BMJ*. 1997;314(7093):1531–1535.
8. Ciampe de Andrade D, Vieira de Faria JW, Caramelli P, Alvarenga L, Galhardon R, Siqueira SRD, Yeng LT, Teixeira MJ. The assessment and management of pain in the demented and non-demented elderly patient. *Arq Neuropsiquiatr*. 2011;69(2-B):387–394.
9. Herr KA, Garand L. Assessment and measurement of pain in older adults. *Clin Geriatr Med*. 2001;17(3):457-vi.
10. Herr K, Coyne PH, McCaffery M, Manworren R, Merkel S. Pain assessment in the patient unable to self-report: position statement with clinical practice recommendations. *Pain Manage Nurs*. 2011;12(4):230–250.
11. Orimo H, Ito H, Suzuki T, Araki A, Hosoi T, Sawabe M. Reviewing the definition of "elderly." *Geriatr Gerontol Int*. 2006;6(3):149–158.
12. Parry J. Network of cities tackles age-old problems. *Bull WHO*. 2010;88(6). http://www.who.int/bulletin/volumes/88/6/10-020610/en/
13. Braddom, RL. *Physical Medicine and Rehabilitation*, 3rd ed. Philadelphia: Saunders Elsevier; 2007:1415–1428.
14. Delisa JA, et al. *Physical Medicine and Rehabilitation Principles and Practice*, 4th ed. Philadelphia: Lippincott Williams & Wilkins; 2005:1531–1556.
15. American Society of Health-System Pharmacists. Introduction to pharmacokinetics and pharmacodynamics. Chapter 1. http://www.ashp.org/DocLibrary/Bookstore/P2418-Chapter1.aspx
16. Mangoni AA, Jackson SHD. Age-related changes in pharmacokinetics and pharmacodynamics: basic principles and practical applications. *Br J Clin Pharmacol*. 2004;57:6–14.
17. Sharma G, Goddwin J. Effect of aging on respiratory system physiology and immunology. *Clin Interv Aging*. 2006;1(3):253–260.
18. Benzon HT, et al. *Raj's Practical Management of Pain*, 4th ed. Philadelphia: Mosby Elsevier; 2008:557–563.
19. DeWaters T, Faut-Callahan M, McCann JJ, Paice JA, Fogg L, Hollinger-Smith L, Sikorski K, Stanaitis H. Comparison of self-reported pain and the PAINAD scale in hospitalized cognitively impaired and intact older adults after hip fracture surgery. *Orthop Nurs*. 2008;27(1):21–28.
20. Merskey H, Bogduk N. *Classification of Chronic Pain*. Seattle: IASP Press; 1994.
21. International Association for the Study of Pain. Pain terms. Seattle: The Association; 2005. http://www.iasp-pain.org/terms-p.html#Pain.
22. Farrell MJ, Katz B, Helme RD. The impact of dementia on the pain experience. *Pain*. 1996;67:7–15.
23. Karp JF. Shega JW. Morone NE. Weiner DK. Advances in understanding the mechanisms and management of persistent pain in older adults. *Br J Anaesth*. 2008;101(1):111–120.

24. Scherder E, Herr K, Pickering G, Gibson S, Benedetti F, Lautenbacher S. Pain in dementia. *Pain*. 2009;145(3):276–278.
25. Kunz M, Mylius V, Schepelmann K, Lautenbacher S. Effects of age and mild cognitive impairment on the pain response system. *Gerontology*. 2009;55:254–260.
26. Reynolds KS, Hanson LC, DeVellis RF, Henderson M, Steinhauser KE. Disparities in pain management between cognitively intact and cognitive impaired nursing home residents. *J Pain Sympt Manage*. 2008;35(4):388–396.
27. Scherder E, Herr K, Pickering G, Gibson S, Benedetti F, Lautenbacher S. Pain in dementia. *Pain*. 2009;145(3):276–278.
28. Carlino E, Benedetti F, Rainero I, Asteggiano G, Cappa G, Tarenzi L, Vighetti S, Pollo A. Pain perception and tolerance in patients with frontotemporal dementia. *Pain*. 2010;151(3):783–789.
29. Pesonen A, Kauppila T, Tarkkila P, Sutela A, Niinistö L, Rosenberg PH. Evaluation of easily applicable pain measurement tools for the assessment of pain in demented patients. *Acta Anaesthesiol Scand*. 2009;53:657–664.
30. Rose VL. Guidelines from the American Geriatric Society target management of chronic pain in older persons. *Am Fam Physician*. 1998;58(5):1213–1215.
31. American Geriatrics Society Panel on the Pharmacological Management of Persistent Pain in Older Persons. Pharmacological management of persistent pain in older persons. *J Am Geriatr Soc*. 2009;57(8):1331–1346.
32. Hadjistavropoulos T, Dever Fitzgerald T, Marchildon GP. Practice guidelines for assessing pain in older persons with dementia residing in long-term care facilities. *Physiother Can*. 2010;62:104–113.
33. Kunz M, Mylius V, Scharmann S, Schepelman K, Lautenbacher S. Influence of dementia on multiple components of pain. *Eur J Pain*. 2009;13:317–325.
34. Balkrishnan R. Predictors of medication adherence in the elderly. *Clin Ther*. 1998;20(4):764–771.
35. Stevens JA, Dellinger AM. Motor vehicle and fall related deaths among older Americans 1990–98: sex, race, and ethnic disparities. *Injury Prevention*. 2002;8:272–275.
36. Hornbrook MC, Stevens VJ, Wingfield DJ, Hollis JF, Greenlick MR, Ory MG. Preventing falls among community–dwelling older persons: results from a randomized trial. *Gerontologist*. 1994:34(1):16–23.
37. Dykes PC, Carroll DL, Hurley A, et al. Fall prevention in acute care hospitals. A random-ized trial. *JAMA*. 2010;304(17):1912–1918.
38. Morone NE, Greco CM. Mind-body interventions for chronic pain in older adults: a struc-tured review. *Pain Med*. 2007;8:359–375.
39. Weiner DK, Ernst E. Complementary and alternative approaches to the treatment of per-sistent musculoskeletal pain. *Clin J Pain*. 2004;20:244–255.
40. Wright A, Sluka KA. Nonpharmacological treatments for musculoskeletal pain. *Clin J Pain*. 2001;17(1):33–46.
41. Kerns RD, Otis JD, Marcus KS. Cognitive-behavioral therapy for chronic pain in the elderly. *Clin Geriatr Med*. 2001;17(3):503–523.
42. Cavalieri TA. Pain management in the elderly. *J Am Osteopath Assoc*. 2002;102:481–485.
43. Wright A, Sluka KA. Nonpharmacological treatments for musculoskeletal pain. *Clin J Pain*. 2001;17(1):33–46.
44. Kerns RD, Otis JD, Marcus KS. Cognitive-behavioral therapy for chronic pain in the elderly. *Clin Geriatr Med*. 2001;17(3):503–523.
45. Huang AR, Mallet L. Prescribing opioids in older people. *Maturitas*. 2013;74(2):123–129.
46. American Geriatrics Society updated Beers criteria for potentially inappropriate medication use in older adults. The AGS 2012 update expert panel. *J Am Geriatr Soc*. 60(4):616–631.
47. Derby S, Chin J, Portenoy RK. Systemic opioid therapy for chronic cancer pain: practi-cal guidelines for converting drugs and routes of administration. *CNS Drugs*. 1998;9(2)(11):99–109.

48. Fine PG, Mahajan G, McPherson ML. Long-acting opioids and short-acting opioids: appropriate use in chronic pain management. *Pain Med.* 2009;10(Suppl 2):S79–S88.

49. Chou R, Fanciullo GJ, Fine PG, et al. American Pain Society–American Academy of Pain Medicine Opioids Guidelines Panel Clinical guidelines for the use of chronic opioid therapy in chronic noncancer pain. *J Pain.* 2009;10(2):113–130.

50. Mason L, Moore RA, Edwards JE, Derry S, McQuay HJ. Topical NSAIDs for chronic musculoskeletal pain: systematic review and meta-analysis. *BMC Musculoskelet Disord.* 2004;5:28.

51. Cavalieri TA. Managing pain in geriatric patients. *J Am Osteopath Assoc.* 2007;107(Suppl 4):ES10–ES16.

52. Portenoy RK, Lesage P. Management of cancer pain. *Lancet.* 1999;353(9165):1695–1700.

53. Duragesic (transdermal fentanyl). Package Insert. Titusville, NJ: Ortho-McNeil-Janssen Pharmaceuticals, Inc.; 2008.

54. Forman WB. Opioid analgesic drugs in the elderly. *Clin Geriatr Med.* 1996;12(3):489–500.

55. U.S. Food and Drug Administration. Blueprint for Prescriber Education for Extended-Release and Long-Acting Opioid Analgesics. www.fda.gov/downloads/Drugs/DrugSafety/PostmarketDrugSafetyInformationforPatientsandProviders/UCM311290.pdf.

56. Dean M. Opioids in renal failure and dialysis patients. *J Pain Symptom Manage.* 2004;28(5):497–504.

57. Bosilkovska M, Walder B, Besson M, Daali Y, Desmeules J. Analgesics in patient with hepatic impairment: pharmacology and clinical implications. *Drugs.* 2012;72(12):1645–1669.

58. Harris JD. Management of expected and unexpected opioid-related side effects. *Clin J Pain.* 2008;24(Suppl 10):S8–S13.

59. Katz N, Mazer N. The impact of opioids on the endocrine system. *Clin J Pain.* 2009;25(2):170–175.

60. Ahmed SN, Siddiqi ZA. Antiepileptic drugs and liver disease. *Seizure.* 2006;15(3):156–164.

61. Israni RK, Kasbekar N, Haynes K, Berns JS. Use of antiepileptic drugs in patients with kidney disease. *Semin Dialysis.* 2006;19(5):408–416.

13

Management of Chronic Pain in the Palliative Care Unit

JENNIFER DROST, DANIELLE INGRAM, AND MELISSA SOLTIS

KEY POINTS

- Palliative care is a specialty in which a team of physicians, nurses, and other healthcare providers manages pain and symptoms for patients with serious and life-limiting illnesses.
- Medical treatments advance every day, leading to increased survival in many chronic diseases, including cancer. There is now a need for expertise in treating chronic pain in cancer survivors in the hospital setting.
- The palliative care interdisciplinary team addresses chronic pain in the hospital setting and includes social workers, chaplains, mental health specialists, and massage therapists, among others

---

Introduction

Palliative care is focused on providing patients with severe illnesses and their families with relief from the symptoms of illness, including, but not limited to, pain.[1] Palliative care providers and teams recognize that patients with life-threatening and life-limiting illnesses suffer from a variety of symptoms that are difficult to manage. Palliative care teams assess and treat patients in a variety of settings, from nursing homes to acute care hospitals. Identifying patients in the hospital setting who might benefit from a palliative care consult is challenging. Traditionally, patients with metastatic or recurrent cancer first come to mind for consult. However, patients with advanced-stage lung, heart, or renal disease, stroke or other illness with poor prognosis, functional decline, or uncontrolled pain and symptoms may be appropriate for palliative care consultation or admittance to the palliative care unit.[2] The Center to Advance Palliative Care reviewed consultation triggers from the literature and developed recommendations for referral during the hospitalization (Box 13.1). The palliative care team provides an example of the benefits of a interdisciplinary team in managing chronic pain.

Box 13.1 **Recommendations for Palliative Care Consultation in the Acute Care Hospital**

Consider consultation if the patient has any of the basic disease processes listed here and two other criteria.

BASIC DISEASE PROCESS

Cancer (metastatic or recurrent)

Advanced lung disease (oxygen dependent, symptomatic despite treatment)

Advanced cardiac disease (severe valvular disease, reduced ejection fraction <25%, New York Heart Association Class III–IV)

End-stage renal disease

Acute severe stroke (significant functional decline, encephalopathy, dysphagia)

Other life-threatening or life-limiting illness

COMORBIDITIES

Liver disease

Moderate pulmonary, cardiac, renal disease impacting quality of life or functional ability

FUNCTIONAL STATUS

Inability to carry out work activities

Inability to manage instrumental activities of daily living

Inability to manage basic activities of daily living due to disease process

Bed-bound and dependent on others

OTHER

Not a candidate for therapy or has chosen to forgo curative therapy

Has unacceptable level of pain for more than a day

Has uncontrolled symptoms, including nausea, vomiting

Has uncontrolled psychosocial or spiritual issues

Frequent emergency department visits or hospitalization

Has prolonged length of stay without evidence of improvement

Has poor prognosis

───────────

Based on Identifying patients in need of a palliative care assessment in the hospital setting: a consensus report from the Center to Advance Palliative Care. 2011.[2]

Chronic Pain in Cancer Survivors

Each year, approximately 1.5 million people in the United States are diagnosed with cancer.[3] Early detection of cancer and emerging treatment strategies have led to an increase in cancer survivorship. The National Comprehensive Cancer Network (NCCN) defines a survivor as someone who has completed initial treatment and has no evidence of active disease, is living with disease but is not in terminal stages, or has had cancer in the past. There were an estimated 13.7 million cancer survivors in 2012,[4] with the majority being alive more than 5 years after diagnosis.[3] Forty to fifty percent of cancer survivors are living with chronic pain,[4] particularly patients with breast cancer, head and neck cancer, or a history of amputation.[5] Patients may experience cancer-related pain from tumor burden due to location, growth, or compression and displacement of surrounding structures. Alternatively, they may also have pain related to treatments, including chemotherapy, radiation, and surgery.

Hospitalized Patients with Multicomorbid Conditions: Why Palliative Care?

Patients with chronic medical conditions have similar patterns of chronic pain prevalence. National Health and Nutrition Examination Survey (NHANES) data estimate that 5.1 million adults are living with heart failure.[6] Studies suggest that 40% of these patients have severe pain most days of the week, leading to functional limitations and disablility.[7,8] Likewise, each year 750,000 people suffer a stroke, resulting in physical, cognitive, and functional impairments.[6] Ten percent will develop chronic pain syndromes.[9] In patients receiving hemodialysis for end-stage renal disease, 50% have chronic pain.[10] While advancing age, functional decline, and debility play a role in the development of chronic pain in these situations, the mechanism and etiology of pain are complex and poorly understood. Patients with chronic medical conditions often require complex medication regimens, and therapy for pain symptoms poses challenges related to tolerance and polypharmacy. Psychological, physical, spiritual, and social factors also contribute to pain perception and tolerance for many of these individuals.

Chronic pain in patients with advanced illnesses is often multifaceted and requires evaluation and treatment from an interdisciplinary team (IDT).[1] Multiple studies, particularly of children, have demonstrated the benefit of the IDT, such as the palliative care team, in managing chronic pain. Cancer survivors with chronic pain, as a growing population of patients, present a new challenge in chronic pain management. Likewise, evidence-based treatment of chronic medical conditions increases survivorship. However, patients with multiple comorbidities remain at high risk for hospital admission. Exacerbation of illnesses may also contribute to worsening of chronic pain syndromes. Hospitalized patients with multicomorbid conditions may benefit from evaluation by the palliative care team and admittance to the palliative care unit given the complex and multifaceted nature of patients' pain (Box 13.2).

The concept of total pain, as first described by Dame Cicely Saunders, is a concept that addresses suffering in those with severe illness that embraces not only the physical symptoms but also the social, spiritual, and psychological aspects of an individual's struggles.[11,12] The concept recognizes that the perception and management of an individual's chronic pain may be affected not only by the disease process but also by anxiety and anger, interpersonal relationships and self-perception, and spiritual needs and values. Total pain is important to consider, as cancer survivors struggle with pain, disability, anxiety, depression, and fear

---

Box 13.2 **Clinical Situation**

Patty is a 59-year-old female with a complex medical history including metastatic lung cancer, oxygen-dependent chronic obstructive pulmonary disease, systolic heart failure, depression, and anxiety. During her course of treatment she developed complaints of back and right-sided chest pain. Despite months of aggressive treatment for her lung cancer, she continued to complain of pain requiring the use of opioid and adjuvant analgesics to maintain her functional status.

Despite therapy, her pain had become worse. Her medications were titrated in the palliative care clinic but are unable to control her pain. She was admitted to the palliative care unit for symptom management and control of her pain.

Upon arrival, Patty described severe, right-sided back pain that was sharp and wrapping around her chest wall to the sternum. She reported that this pain was getting worse, and though her current medications were "somewhat helpful," nothing provided adequate relief. She was tearful and had multiple complaints, including severe fatigue, decreased appetite, and worries about not having further life-prolonging treatment options. On examination, paraspinal musculature was tender to palpation at discrete thoracic levels. The physician reviewed recent computed tomography, which did not demonstrate metastatic disease related to her pain complaints.

The help of the pharmacist was enlisted. The patient was on several medications to control her comorbidities, so the pharmacist evaluated the home medication list to assess for drug interactions and safety of various pain medications. The patient was started on an appropriate dose of methadone along with as-needed medications. Topical lidocaine was also applied to her paraspinal musculature.

Almost immediately Patty acknowledged improvement in her back pain. When the nurse was in her room to administer medications and apply the topical lidocaine, Patty admitted that she had very little support at home and was having more difficulty keeping up with her housework and activities. She lived on her own, and her adult daughter lived several hours away. After evaluating Patty's financial resources, the social worker referred her to local supports to provide homemaking activities, in hopes of easing the pain and anxiety she suffered.

Patty reported to the palliative care team that while she held a belief in a "higher power," she had never been one who went to religious services regularly or had a faith-based community. She appreciated the support of meeting with the chaplain, however. During that discussion she expressed worries and concerns about the meaning of her worsening pain. She was also trying to find meaning in her life now that she was unable to continue her community involvement. She admitted to feeling lonely and isolated.

After a few days Patty's pain was under good control and she was ready to return home. She left with prescriptions for new medications, home nursing to assist with medication management, along with an appointment with a local agency to arrange for housekeeping services. She also reconnected with her community groups, who committed to visiting with her at home a few times a week.

of recurrence (Box 13.3). Even patients who have achieved cancer cure or remission may have ongoing needs related to their diagnosis that complicate the resolution of their pain. New or changing pain must be thoroughly evaluated to rule out cancer recurrence or progression.[13] Survivors may be hypervigilant and more aware of acute somatic symptoms. It is thought that inadequate treatment of acute cancer-related pain increases the risk of future chronic pain syndromes.[14] They also face changes in interpersonal perceptions at home and at work, which may affect coping with life-changing events.[15] As with non-cancer-related pain, the primary mode of treatment is with medications, including opioids. Cognitive behavioral therapies,[14] massage,[4] and involvement of IDTs are effective adjuvant modalities in managing total pain.

Though the component members of the IDT on the palliative care unit will vary, the core participants include specialist doctors and advance practice nurses, social workers, chaplains, and bedside nurses. Additional team members may include mental health providers, pharmacists, physical and occupational therapists, allied health providers, including massage or alternative health therapists, and volunteers. Each team member offers unique insight to assess and treat different aspects of the pain (Figure 13.1).

Box 13.3 **Causes of Chronic Pain in Cancer Survivors**

Phantom limb pain after amputation

Radiation-induced plexopathy

Chemotherapy-induced neuropathy

Postsurgical pain from thoracotomy, mastectomy, head and neck surgery

Side effects of steroids, including avascular necrosis and osteoporotic fractures

Jaw osteonecrosis

Pain related to aromatase inhibitor use

Anxiety, depression, and fear of recurrence

The Palliative Care Interdisciplinary Team

PHYSICIAN/ADVANCE PRACTICE NURSE

Palliative care physicians and practitioners have a unique role in the assessment and treatment of pain. The first step, and standard of care, is a thorough history of the patient's pain—location, duration, quality, severity, and aggravating and alleviating factors. The goal of this assessment is to identify the etiology and mechanism of pain.[1] Often, multimodal treatment in addition to opioid pain relievers is necessary. In accordance with the World Health Organization pain treatment ladder, non-opioid analgesics, including acetaminophen and

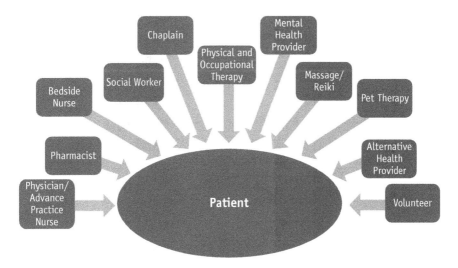

Figure 13.1 The interdisciplinary team: providers at work to assess and manage pain and related symptoms.

nonsteroidal anti-inflammatories (NSAIDs), are commonly used prior or in addition to opioid pain relievers.[16] Adjuvant medications, though originally for non-pain indications, have been shown to offer analgesic benefits in some patients. These medications can improve function without increasing opioid doses and side effects. Common adjuvants include steroids, tricyclic antidepressants, antiepileptics, and NMDA receptor antagonists. These diverse medications may address symptoms associated with bone pain, neuropathic pain, or bowel obstructions (Figure 13.2).[16]

Procedural interventions are often used in palliative care to alleviate pain. The palliative care team works closely with pain management and anesthesiology, interventional radiology, surgery, and radiation oncology. Somatic nerve blocks, trigger point injections, and spinal analgesia may be employed for nociceptive pain complaints that are inadequately treated with oral medication or when medication side effects or interactions limit further use.[17] Vertebroplasty or spinal cord and brain stimulator implantation also provide benefit in selected patients. Percutaneous gastrostomy and diverting colostomy may alleviate pain associated with obstructive gastrointestinal tumors.[18] Radiation therapy to

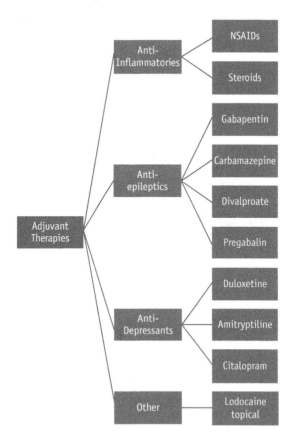

Figure 13.2 Adjuvant pain medications used in palliative care.[16]

metastases in bone, epidural space, spinal cord, and brain has been shown to reduce pain and improve function for patients on the palliative care unit.[19,20]

PHARMACIST

The pharmacist plays an integral and vital role on the palliative care team. Studies suggest that involvement of pharmacists in chronic pain management decreases pain severity and improves quality of life.[21,22] Clinical pharmacists in the hospital setting often provide direct patient and caregiver education regarding medication use, risks, and side effects.[23] The pharmacist on the team also provides expertise in medication management, including pharmacodynamics and kinetics, drug–drug or drug–host interactions, and adverse drug events. As well, chronic pain in cancer survivors may be related to previous chemotherapy or radiation treatments. The pharmacist can offer unique strategies for pain control in relation to specific treatment effects.

BEDSIDE NURSING

The palliative care unit offers specialized and dedicated nursing care to patients who are severely ill. The bedside nurse frequently assesses symptoms, administers medications, and monitors treatment effects. The nurse provides ongoing evaluation of medication adherence and understanding. As well, the bedside nurse educates patients and families regarding both pharmacological and nonpharmacological treatment of pain. The nurse plays an invaluable role in the assessment of effectiveness of medications, and sometime patients and families will provide more detailed information and feedback to the nurse than to other team members.

SOCIAL WORKER

The social worker is integral to the palliative care team and serves several functions in both evaluation and treatment of chronic pain. Often patients' poor social, financial, or emotional support contributes to poorly controlled pain. Research suggests that social isolation, environmental stressors, and coping skills affect perception and adjustment to pain.[24,25] The social worker evaluates the psychosocial mediators of pain and makes recommendations to better support the patient. Social workers play a unique role in the treatment of pain in cancer survivors and those with chronic medical illnesses through validation of symptoms and active listening techniques.

CHAPLAIN

The multifaceted concept of total pain allows for consideration of spiritual or existential suffering and its impact on an individual's perception of physical pain. Patients with cancer, as well as cancer survivors, may seek to find meaning in their diagnosis and symptoms. Likewise, patients with chronic medical conditions often seek meaning in their suffering of pain and illness.[26] Many patients find comfort in spirituality. Indeed, patients with cancer are some of the most frequent users of chaplain services in the hospital setting, and they frequently discuss pain issues with the chaplain.[27] Spiritual well-being has been correlated with decreased pain, fatigue, and depression in cancer patients.[28] The hospital chaplain offers expertise in the realm of spirituality, faith, and meaning. Inclusion of the chaplain in the palliative care team allows for the tailoring of services and supports for individual patients.

MENTAL HEALTH SPECIALISTS

Mental health providers, including psychiatrists, psychologists, and counselors, provide assessment and interventions aimed at the interaction between emotion and cognition and pain perception and integration.[24,29] Though wide variations in prevalence exist in the literature, mental health disorders are common among cancer survivors. Depressive symptoms are present in up to half and anxiety in up to one-quarter of survivors. Similarly, depression is common among patients with chronic medical illnesses. One-third of patients experience depression after stroke.[6] Depression and anxiety may alter the perception of pain and the ability of an individual to cope with pain. Inclusion of mental health providers on the palliative care unit and interdisciplinary team is essential for management of patients with chronic pain.

ALLIED AND ALTERNATIVE HEALTH

At least one-third of cancer survivors have used complementary health approaches in the last year.[30] In patients with chronic medical conditions, up to 50% may use complementary health techniques including massage, biofeedback, relaxation techniques, and herbal supplements.[31] Massage therapy has been shown to aid palliative care patients in the reduction of pain in up to 75% of cases.[32] Other modalities, including Reiki, aromatherapy, and acupuncture, may offer benefit to patients. An internal study conducted at Summa Health System, Akron City Hospital (unpublished work, Ruggieri, 2013) demonstrated that patients admitted to the palliative care unit who participated in holistic therapy including Reiki, aromatherapy, and reflexology experienced reduction in pain severity. Half of patients reported a 50% or more improvement in their pain. Many palliative care units also employ pet therapy animals. Anecdotal evidence suggests that animal-assisted therapy is effective for the relief of pain.[33] The role of alternative health and roles of other elements of the IDT are provided in Table 13.1).

Table 13.1 **Roles of the Palliative Care Interdisciplinary Team**

Physician/advance practice nurse	History and physical examination
	Evaluation and testing
	Specialist symptom management
	Ongoing evaluation for procedural interventions
	Multimodal treatment strategies
	Education and support of patient and family
Bedside nurse	Frequent bedside evaluation of pain and symptoms
	Medication administration
	Ongoing education and support
	Assessment of adherence to medication regimen and ability to take medications
Social worker	Social assessment of needs and caregiving
	Financial assessment and ability to afford medications and services
Chaplain	Spiritual assessment and beliefs about pain and symptoms
	Prayer
Pharmacist	Detailed assessment of medications, interactions, side effects
	Recommendations for adjuvant medications
	Dosing and titration of medications
Physical and occupational therapies	Functional assessment
	Range of motion and mobility
	Discharge planning
Mental health provider	Counseling and medication management for depression and anxiety
	Coping strategies
	Cognitive-behavioral therapies
	Relaxation therapy, guided imagery, stress management
Alternative health Providers	Massage therapy
	Reiki
	Music therapy
	Art therapy
	Pet therapy
	Aromatherapy
	Acupuncture
Volunteers	Counseling and support services
	Transportation
	Companionship
Other	Specialist medical providers for expertise and procedural assessment (pain management physicians, anesthesiology, radiation oncology)
	Hospital security to provide safe environment

Summary

Palliative care offers pain and symptom management for patients with advanced chronic illness in the hospital setting. Patients with cancer, cancer survivors, and those living with chronic medical conditions commonly experience pain and may be at higher risk for hospitalization and high utilization of healthcare services. The hospital-based palliative care team and the palliative care unit offer comprehensive care that addresses the multiple contributors of pain. The varied members of the palliative care team use the concept of total pain to simultaneously treat the biomedical, psychosocial, spiritual, and emotional mediators of chronic pain. It offers a holistic approach to patient care and pain management while supporting patients and families.

References

1. Grant M, Dy SM. *The Hospice and Palliative Care Approach to Serious Illness*, 4th ed. Chicago: American Academy of Hospice and Palliative Care, 2013.
2. Weissman DE, Meier DE. Identifying patients in need of a palliative care assessment in the hospital setting: a consensus report from the Center to Advance Palliative Care. *J Palliat Med*. 2011;14:17–23.
3. American Cancer Society. Cancer facts and figures 2013. http://www.cancer.org/research/cancerfactsfigures/cancerfactsfigures/cancer-facts-figures-2013
4. Glare PA, Davies PS, Finlay E, et al. Pain in cancer survivors. *J Clin Oncol*. 2014;32:1739–1747.
5. Lowery AE, Krebs P, Coups EJ, et al. Impact of symptom burden in post-surgical non-small cell lung cancer survivors. *Support Care Cancer*. 2014;22:173–180.
6. Go AS, Mozaffarian D, Roger VL, et al. Executive summary: heart disease and stroke statistics—2014 update: a report from the American Heart Association. *Circulation*. 2014;129:399–410.
7. Tracy B, Sean Morrison R. Pain management in older adults. *Clin Ther*. 2013;35:1659–1668.
8. Goodlin SJ, Wingate S, Albert NM, et al. Investigating pain in heart failure patients: the Pain Assessment, Incidence, and Nature in Heart Failure (PAIN-HF) study. *J Card Fail*. 2012;18:776–783.
9. O'Donnell MJ, Diener HC, Sacco RL, Panju AA, Vinisko R, Yusuf S. Chronic pain syndromes after ischemic stroke: PRoFESS trial. *Stroke*. 2013;44:1238–1243.
10. Davison SN. The prevalence and management of chronic pain in end-stage renal disease. *J Palliat Med*. 2007;10:1277–1287.
11. Ong CK, Forbes D. Embracing Cicely Saunders's concept of total pain. *BMJ*. 2005;331:576.
12. Leleszi JP, Lewandowski JG. Pain management in end-of-life care. *J Am Osteopath Assoc*. 2005;105:S6–S11.
13. Davies PS. Chronic pain management in the cancer survivor: tips for primary care providers. *Nurse Pract*. 2013;38:28–38; quiz 38–29.
14. Burton AW, Fine PG, Passik SD. Transformation of acute cancer pain to chronic cancer pain syndromes. *J Support Oncol*. 2012;10:89–95.
15. Moskowitz MC, Todd BL, Chen R, Feuerstein M. Function and friction at work: a multidimensional analysis of work outcomes in cancer survivors. *J Cancer Surviv*. 2014;8:173–182.
16. Weinstein S, Portenoy RK, Harrington SH. *UNIPAC Three: Assessing and Treating Pain*, 4th ed. Chicago: American Academy of Hospice and Palliative Medicine, 2013.
17. Chambers WA. Nerve blocks in palliative care. *Br J Anaesth*. 2008;101:95–100.

18. Soriano A, Davis MP. Malignant bowel obstruction: individualized treatment near the end of life. *Cleve Clin J Med*. 2011;78:197–206.

19. Rutter C, Weissman DE. Radiation for palliation—part 1. *J Palliat Med*. 2004;7:865–866.

20. Rutter C, Weissman DE. Radiation for palliation—part 2. *J Palliat Med*. 2004;7:866–867.

21. Yamamura S, Takehira R, Kawada K, et al. Structural equation modeling of qualification of pharmacists to improve subjected quality of life in cancer patients. *J Pharm Pharm Sci*. 2005;8:544–551.

22. Bruhn H, Bond CM, Elliott AM, et al. Pharmacist-led management of chronic pain in primary care: results from a randomised controlled exploratory trial. *BMJ Open*. 2013;3(4), pii:e002361

23. Ise Y, Morita T, Katayama S, Kizawa Y. The activity of palliative care team pharmacists in designated cancer hospitals: a nationwide survey in Japan. *J Pain Symptom Manage*. 2014;47:588–593.

24. Keefe FJ, Porter L, Somers T, Shelby R, Wren AV. Psychosocial interventions for managing pain in older adults: outcomes and clinical implications. *Br J Anaesth*. 2013;111:89–94.

25. MacDonald JE. A deconstructive turn in chronic pain treatment: a redefined role for social work. *Health Soc Work*. 2000;25:51–58.

26. Balducci L. Beyond quality of life: the meaning of death and suffering in palliative care. *Asian Pac J Cancer Prev*. 2010;11(Suppl 1):41–44.

27. Strang S, Strang P. Questions posed to hospital chaplains by palliative care patients. *J Palliat Med*. 2002;5:857–864.

28. Rabow MW, Knish SJ. Spiritual well-being among outpatients with cancer receiving concurrent oncologic and palliative care. *Support Care Cancer*. 2015;23(4):919–923.

29. Hassed C. Mind-body therapies—use in chronic pain management. *Aust Fam Physician*. 2013;42:112–117.

30. Sohl SJ, Weaver KE, Birdee G, Kent EE, Danhauer SC, Hamilton AS. Characteristics associated with the use of complementary health approaches among long-term cancer survivors. *Support Care Cancer*. 2014;22:927–936.

31. Butchart A, Kerr EA, Heisler M, Piette JD, Krein SL. Experience and management of chronic pain among patients with other complex chronic conditions. *Clin J Pain*. 2009;25:293–298.

32. Vandergrift A. Use of complementary therapies in hospice and palliative care. *Omega (Westport)*. 2013;67:227–232.

33. Engelman SR. Palliative care and use of animal-assisted therapy. *Omega (Westport)*. 2013;67:63–67.

14

Management of Chronic Pain in Nursing Homes, Rehabilitation Facilities, Long-Term Care Facilities, Prisons and on the Psychiatric Unit

MICHAEL LUBRANO, YURY KHELEMSKY, TODD IVAN, AND KARINA

GRITSENKO

KEY POINTS

- Nearly half of all U.S. citizens will receive nursing home care prior to their deaths, with one in four ultimately dying in a nursing home. For these patients chronic pain is a recurrent component of life, as nearly 80% of all institutionalized elderly suffer from some form of pain.
- Chronic pain is typically undertreated in these settings. This problem becomes further complicated because patients in these institutions can be very sick and are not always capable of speaking for themselves. Several barriers to appropriate management of chronic pain for these patients exist. They include transfer miscommunications, poor medication reconciliation, cognitive deficits and other patient comorbidities, and issues with polypharmacy and adverse drug interactions.
- We generally recommend only short-term use of opioids for patients with chronic non-cancer pain with psychiatric comorbidities. Opioids can be utilized temporarily to facilitate rehabilitation, but then should be weaned. When a patient is admitted to the psychiatric floor on high-dose opioid therapy, chronic pain management services should be consulted, and plan to wean from opioids should be discussed with the patient.

Introduction

As patients age they invariably become sicker, requiring medical care in a variety of settings both within and outside hospitals. Prior studies estimated that 43% of U.S citizens turning 65 years old in 1990 would eventually receive nursing home care before their deaths.[1] Today, individuals who are 85 and older are part of a growing cohort of the U.S. population; this number is expected to reach 31 million by the year 2050.[2] These shifting demographics suggest that prior studies underestimate the future patient populations that will require stays in healthcare institutions, many of which exist outside of the inpatient hospital domain. Pain (especially chronic pain) is not a normal part of aging, but nearly 80% of the institutionalized elderly suffer from some form of it.[3] The goal of this chapter is to explore obstacles pertaining to managing chronic pain in a number of institutional settings (nursing homes, rehabilitation centers, psychiatric centers, and prisons) in order to provide cogent and achievable recommendations for pain management and future improvement in these areas.

Institutional Healthcare Settings

Institutionalized patients are, by definition, dependent on the center within which they permanently or temporarily reside for medical care and other services. While inpatient hospital stays may fit this categorical criterion, for the purposes of this chapter we will discuss extraneous settings where patients may also dwell. Managing chronic pain in institutionalized patients of nursing homes, rehabilitation facilities, psychiatric facilities, and prisons presents a set of obstacles that is unique to each; however, data and recommendations relevant to these populations are sparse or not available. One Dutch study found less frequency of pain reported on psychogeriatric wards. These patients subsequently received less pain medication when compared to somatic wards after controlling for cognitive status, age, gender, and a number of other variables.[4] In this section, we briefly review each setting in order to frame some treatment concerns.

NURSING HOMES

The nursing home (NH), as a term, references a class of institutionalized settings ranging from long-term care facilities where residents receive assistance with activities of daily life (ADL) to skilled nursing facilities where staff may provide dressing changes for wounds. We will use NH to reference all of these settings as a group. Chronic pain is the most common form of pain experienced by 40%–80% of NH residents, with a prevalence of 75% found in those with advanced cancer.[5] Intermittent, acute illnesses and pain episodes may also occur and complicate pain management in these settings. Frequent culprits of acute pain precipitation include dehydration, renal failure, urinary tract infections, and pneumonia with each requiring separate management in an inpatient hospital.[5] This increases the number of transfers that residents experience, which only serves to create opportunities for chronic pain mismanagement within a context of exacerbating and remitting pain. Well-known long-term effects of chronic pain include depression, appetite changes, fatigue, and insomnia, which result in adverse clinical outcomes in this already frail patient population.

REHABILITATION FACILITIES

Rehabilitation facilities (RF) receive classification by the U.S. Federal Government based on specified criteria. In order to obtain reimbursement for services, RFs must always receive their transfers directly from an inpatient hospital. At least 60% of RF patients should be capable of tolerating at least 3 hours of therapy per day.[6] An RF will subsequently place individualized treatment regimens within the RF, with access to more comprehensive therapies including physical therapy, occupational therapy, and speech therapy. Many patients found in these settings recently underwent surgery, a neurological complication such as stroke, or any number of other medical ailments that were initially stabilized in the hospital. Chronic pain management in these patients is incredibly important, especially during postoperative periods. The severity of pain both at rest and with activity has been shown to be associated with decreased quality of recovery after operations.

HOSPITAL PSYCHIATRIC FLOOR AND RESIDENTIAL PSYCHIATRIC FACILITIES

The high frequency of psychiatric comorbidities among patients with chronic pain is well known.[7] Patients with both chronic pain and some common mental health conditions will likely have higher pain intensity, wider pain distribution, and a longer history of chronic pain than patients without psychiatric comorbidities.[7] However, the cause-and-effect relationship of pain and psychiatric conditions is not well understood. Nearly two-thirds of patients with depression report symptoms of pain during diagnosis and have an elevated risk for developing chronic pain problems over the subsequent decade.[8] These patients also experience greater pain intensity, pain persistence, and functional interference as a result of their symptoms.[9] In general, 1-year prevalence of major depression is around 7%.[7] As the presence of a chronic pain condition increases, the rate of depression increases two- to fivefold. Worsening pain intensity is directly associated with worsening depression severity, and improved pain intensity is associated with improved depression severity. Similar associations were observed for anxiety disorders and PTSD. For example, approximately half of those with chronic pain have anxiety symptoms, with nearly one-third exhibiting suffi-cient signs for a diagnosis of anxiety disorder.[10] There are reports pointing to a tight relationship between mental health disease and opioid abuse or misuse in patients receiving chronic opioid therapy or, unrelated to opioid therapy, having substance use disorders, including alcohol abuse, tobacco use, and other. These patients are also more likely to have complications and negative outcomes such as overdose, opioid misuse and abuse, and emergency department and hospital admissions,[7] including psychiatric unit admission.

On the other hand, studies have shown that patients with psychiatric and substance use disorders are more likely to receive chronic opioid medications at higher doses and for longer periods than their mentally healthy counterparts, and also are more likely to have worse outcomes.[7]

Despite the fact that psychiatric disorders increase the chance of patients being on chronic opioid therapy, there is good evidence that psychiatric comor-bidity decreases the analgesic effect of opioids. Long-term opioid treatment side effects extend beyond conventional medication adverse effects.[7] In addition to hyperalgesia, endocrine, and immunosuppressive effects, they include a wide range of psychosocial derangements, opioid dependence, and concerns related to compulsive opioid-consumption behavior. In fact, opiate medications' common side effects include severe depression, insomnia, anxiety, and hallucinations, among other psychiatric symptoms, which, in turn, may trigger admission to the psychiatric floor.

Based on these findings we generally do not recommend long-term use of opi-oids for patients with chronic non-cancer pain with psychiatric comorbidities. Opioids can be used temporarily to facilitate rehabilitation, but then patients should be weaned off them. When a patient is admitted to the psychiatric floor on high-dose opioid therapy, chronic pain management services should be con-sulted, and a plan to wean from opioids should be discussed with the patient.

PSYCHIATRIC FACILITIES

Psychiatric facilities include long-term residential centers as well acute, short-term management settings. As such, the diagnoses that patients maintain range from severely debilitating psychosis or depression to more mild symptoms that allow patients to function well in community settings after discharge. Chronic pain management in the psychiatric population in the setting of a psychiatric facility is exceedingly difficult given primary psychiatric conditions themselves as well as the psychiatric medications these patients tend to be on. Patients with cognitive deficits may present with long-term resistance to care, inappro-priate behavior, abnormal thought processes, and a 50% increase in delusions.[11] In general, working with a multidisciplinary care team that includes both psy-chiatrists and pain management specialists is of utmost importance in these settings.

Correctional Facilities

Chronic pain in the prison population, like most medical conditions in this cohort, is estimated to be significantly more prevalent than in the general population.[12] The U.S. Supreme Court ruled in 1976 that the 8th amendment ensures prison inmates adequate medical care. Since this decision, three major tenets have emerged as basic rights: access to care, care that is ordered, and professional medical judgment.[13] The goals of these protections are to ensure that inmates receive care that is deemed necessary and that medical professionals make these decisions, not legislative bodies. This includes guaranteed access to pain management despite limited data related to the prevalence and treatment options for chronic pain in these populations. States such as Oregon have a quick timeline between acute pain complaint and treatment. There, as in many other states, use of narcotics is typically avoided because of concerns related to abuse potential, diversion, and extortion.[14] Pain management in prisons is thus primarily restricted to dealing with acute pain complaints rather than long-term, chronic pain issues.

One survey of incarcerated women found that reporting pain was strongly predicted by cognitive and emotional responses. These women experienced catastrophizing symptoms more frequently; one hypothesis suggests that those with chronic pain do not receive appropriate care for symptoms. There is also a paucity of reports describing behavioral pain treatment in the U.S. prison system despite its efficacy in curbing pain medication reliance and subduing emotional pain responses.[14] Much more work remains to be done to characterize the deficits in as well as opportunities for chronic pain management within the prison system.

Obstacles to Managing Chronic Pain in Institutional Settings

We have outlined a number of different institutions for short- and long-term care where patients may require chronic pain management outside of inpatient hospital settings. While each of these locations varies in staffing, overall structure, and healthcare niche, there are a myriad of overlapping themes that pertain to some or all of them. Obstacles to managing chronic pain in these settings originate from transfer of care, use of physician extenders, knowledge deficits, comorbidity challenges, and patient population concerns. For example, the prison system itself frequently has inmates with co-occurring psychiatric, substance abuse, and chronic medical conditions. As the prison population ages, geriatric and palliative care issues begin to intersect.[15] Much of the sparse literature related to chronic pain management in institutions pertains to the NH, thus we will present information predominantly related to NH settings as a model for obstacles and recommendations for extrapolation when appropriate.

ORGANIZATIONAL BARRIERS AND MISCOMMUNICATION

Patients who no longer require the acute, continuous treatment that inpatient hospitals provide will be transferred to institutional settings for further management of their care when deemed appropriate. This transition implies differences and segmentation across sites in staffing, delivery of care, and overall communication. Increased number of transfers has been shown to directly lead to miscommunication between providers. Approximately half of all adverse drug effects (ADEs) occur due to prescribing discrepancies as a result of patient transfers, with mistakes in opiate prescribing being most frequent.[16] One study found that of nearly 2000 patients entering NHs, nearly three-quarters had at least one prescription problem. Discrepancies included dosing route or frequency inaccuracies as well omission of essential drugs from the medication list altogether.[17] For patients with chronic pain, excluding a necessary analgesic can lead to provider confusion, pain precipitation, and delay of treatment.

Careful medication reconciliation upon patient transfer to institutions is thus extremely important for appropriate management of chronic pain. This requires several interventions. The first involves staffing someone to reconcile medications uniformly, with careful attention to detail in order to avoid clerical errors. The second intervention consists of informing prescribing decision-makers that there is a medication discrepancy. It is important to report the discrepancy to someone with enough influence to ultimately alter the prescribing pattern for that patient. These are areas where miscommunication or lack of influence in decision-making leads to a perpetuation of medication omissions and dosing errors.[16]

PROVIDER AND PATIENT KNOWLEDGE DEFICITS AS EDUCATIONAL OPPORTUNITIES

Physician extenders are frequently the primary deliverers of care in most institutions. In many cases, physicians are present a few days a week, with some only returning once a week. An ideal scenario would allow nurses and other professionals to know their residents extremely well in order to provide high-quality care. Unfortunately, these models are fraught with organizational problems. Low nursing salaries in many areas lead to high staff turnover and disjointed staffing patterns. Part-time and hired agency staff thus provide much of the care. This creates even more care fragmentation and miscommunication.[18] Deficits in knowledge or assessment skills may also contribute to under-detection of pain or inappropriate pain management.

Healthcare Providers and Analgesic Prescribing

NH managers admit to poor adherence to chronic pain treatment guidelines. An aversion to opiate prescribing and concerns regarding cognitive deficits in patients are the most frequent excuses for this.[19] Gaps in knowledge among providers—both physicians and other health professionals alike—lead to negative attitudes toward analgesic prescribing as well as poor pain assessment skills. One survey of oncologists found that three-quarters of providers felt that low competence in pain assessment was their largest barrier to providing appropriate management for pain. Nearly 60% felt that a reluctance toward opiate prescribing was another significant barrier.[5]

Poor competence and an aversion to opiate prescribing have significant effects on appropriate treatment for institutionalized patients. In some settings, less than half of NH residents with recurrent, chronic pain are prescribed scheduled pain medications.[20] Surgically treated hip fracture patients in one study were found to receive, on average, significantly less medications during their first 24 hours in the NH after transfer there than in the last 24 hours of inpatient hospitalization.[18] One-third did not receive an opioid analgesic, with nearly 20% receiving no analgesic at all during their initial NH day. With such reluctance to prescribe appropriate analgesics for acute pain in the immediate postoperative period, it is no surprise that analgesic prescription for chronic pain is even poorer among institutionalized patients with chronic pain.

Effective educational campaigns for healthcare providers within institutions are frequently necessary to address these many concerns. It is important to emphasize that opioids rarely cause addiction or rapid tolerance in these settings. Studies have shown that using opiates in chronic, nonmalignant pain results in very low risk for addiction in patients who have no substance abuse history.[5] They also have a wide effective dosage range, contrary to the belief of many health professionals. The effects of chronic pain management education campaigns within NHs and similar institutions have begun to be studied, with promising data to date. One institution implemented a 6-month educational and formal quality improvement plan. Topics for provider education included vital signs and pain, tolerance and addiction, sleep and pain, non-drug interventions, and side-effect management. All of these knowledge areas exhibited significant improvement among staff after program implementation.[21] One educational program lasting only 8 weeks was still able to show significant improvement in staff knowledge of pain management, with lower resident pain scores and increased use of alternative therapies.[22]

Resident Aversion to Analgesics: Underreporting

While much emphasis has been placed on improving chronic pain management on the provider end, increased attention must also be paid to appropriately educating patients. Many residents in healthcare institutions have a serious fear of analgesics, especially opiates, and associate them with addiction, tolerance,

---

Box 14.1 **Provider and Patient Barriers to Chronic Pain Management**

- Resident chooses to not report pain
  - Cultural or age difference
  - Fear of opiate addiction/tolerance
- Resident inability to report pain
  - Cognitive deficit
  - Physically unable
- Provider aversion to use of analgesics
  - Physician does not prescribe
  - Nurse does not administer
- Resident elects to not take analgesic

Box modified from Frampton.[23]

---

and side effects. Others view requiring scheduled medications for coping with recurrent symptoms as a personal weakness or even as a sign of advanced disease progression.[5] Perception of control, expectations, and social conditioning are also factors that contribute to these misperceptions.[23] These concerns lead patients to underreport symptoms or refuse scheduled analgesics for their pain. The importance of appropriate patient education in these settings cannot be understated. Educational initiatives similar to those constructed for enhancing provider knowledge may be instituted to dispel analgesic myths within these patient populations. Residents who rate providers as providing adequate education for their conditions subsequently have much higher provider satisfaction scores (Box 14.1).[24]

MENTAL STATUS AND CHRONIC PAIN ASSESSMENT

Chronic pain symptoms for institutionalized patients may be complicated, or even masked, by a myriad of emotional or psychiatric problems, including anger, depression, anxiety, and dementia.[5] Cognitive deficits are especially capable of presenting obstacles to determining whether or not a resident of an institution is in pain or not. Diseases such as dementia, stroke, and developmental or genetic disorders may cause a patient to be unable to comprehend assessment questions or even render them physically incapable of speaking altogether.

For years there has been debate in the literature regarding the relationship between cognitive abilities and the physical sensation of pain that is experienced. In a recent study, only a weak association was observed between cognition and pain.[25] This suggests that a patient with deteriorating mental status cannot be expected to experience decreased, or even increased, pain compared to normally functioning counterparts. In Alzheimer's disease, for example, the somatic sensory cortical areas are preserved despite limbic pathway deterioration.[23] With this neurological area intact, patients are reportedly able to experience acute pain more frequently than chronic pain, although both forms of pain are reported.[26]

Treating institutionalized patients, especially those with cognitive deficits, involves a highly individualized approach as well as patience on the providers' end. Elderly or mentally impaired residents tend to be depressed, tired, and potentially very sick. Adequate time for communication is therefore one of the most important components for pain assessment in this population. Those with mild to moderate cognitive impairment require this additional time in order to formulate questions in their mind. They exhibit shorter attention spans with a lower threshold for distraction. Improving the assessment of chronic pain requires attention to a number of details. It is important to face the patient directly while speaking slowly and clearly. Excellent lighting, hearing devices, and visual cues in large print are also considerations. It is not uncommon to repeat or reword phrasing, as well as frequently reaffirm the patient's understanding of the evaluator's questions.[5]

Numeric rating scales are often used within the NH setting, although some existing data suggest only modest accuracy for identifying chronic pain of clinical significance.[27] In patients with cognitive impairment, individual self-reports are more frequently used to assess pain in lieu of rating scales, as some providers feel they are more accurate.[28] One expert consensus statement for assessing pain in older persons describes how to approach patients with varied mental status. A Colored Analog Scale (CAS) for severe impairment may be useful, while most other patients may be assessed with a Verbal Descriptor Scale (VDS).[29] Experts encourage that baseline scores be acquired using a highly individualized approach, with solicitation of assistance from family or other care providers who know the patient well. Any form of assessment tool must be used under consistent circumstances if it is to be applied over time. This means that if a patient is assessed in the morning, all pain assessments should be conducted at this time.

In patients with impaired ability to communicate it is the duty of the healthcare provider to conduct a thorough patient assessment. Nonverbal cues for expressing pain become extremely important and may be the only mechanism for evaluating pain, as outlined in Table 14.1.[23] Another tool, the Non-communicative Patient's Pain Assessment Instrument (NOPPAIN) has been shown to have high inter- and intrarater reliability with significant correlation to self-reported pain and detailed behavioral coding.[30] It also has convergent validity when using a VDS in cognitively intact elders. The tool itself incorporates a number of nonverbal cues and therefore is useful in patients with serious cognitive deficits. Facial expressions, vocalizations, body movements, and alterations in behavior are all components considered by its algorithm.

Table 14.1 **Assessing Pain in Cognitively Impaired Patients**

General Assessment Recommendations	Nonverbal Indicators of Pain
• Well-lit environments	• Physical
• Appropriate hearing Devices	• Diaphoresis
• Interpreter if patient is ESL	• Tachycardia
• Face patient directly	• Hypertension
• Clear, slow pronunciation	• Behavioral
• Adequate time for thinking	• Increased agitation
• Repeat and/or reword questions	• Repetitive verbalizing
• As focused and brief as possible	• Fluctuating mental status
	• Reduced mental and physical function
	• Withdrawal

Table modified from Glajchen[5] and Frampton.[23]

MEDICAL CHALLENGES

The residents of institutional healthcare facilities are at much higher risk for having complicated medical comorbidities than the general population, by nature of their need for assisted living. In settings discussed thus far, patients are more likely to be elderly and have cognitive deficits; in the penile system they also often have comorbid substance abuse disorders. While chronic pain management in patients with substance abuse is discussed elsewhere in this book (see Chapter 22), there are many polypharmacy and drug interaction concerns among elderly and psychiatric patients worthy of discussing here. Residents with respiratory disease, cardiovascular disease, or cerebrovascular disease are much more likely to experience negative side effects from opioid pain management, including bradycardia, respiratory depression, and hypotension.[31] These additional medical challenges require providers to carefully select agents and seriously consider patient comorbid conditions prior to generating final treatment plans.

Comorbid Medical Conditions and Agent Function: Renal and Liver Failure

Organ failure can affect any age group dwelling in healthcare institutions; however, it is much more prevalent in elderly NH populations. The absorption, metabolism, and excretion of medications may be seriously affected by disease status. Dosing routes must be carefully determined on this basis. For example, if a patient has irritable bowel disease with impaired intestinal absorption, the bioavailability of any agent absorbed by the intestines could be significantly altered. Transdermal, intramuscular, or intravenous administration rather than oral dosing may be considered in these patients.

Hepatic impairment is another major consideration before selecting and dosing analgesic agents for chronic pain. A number of opiates are prodrugs that require activation by the cytochrome P450 system. For example, codeine, hydrocodone, and dihydrocodeine cannot function without CYP2D6 metabolism to their active forms: morphine, hydromorphine, and dihydromorphine, respectively.[32] Without activation, doses that initially seem appropriate will have decreased efficacy in ameliorating symptoms. The inverse problem exists for analgesics that require liver metabolism prior to bodily excretion, which may have dangerous central nervous system side effects if unrecognized. The most significant comorbid factor to consider with analgesic management for chronic pain in long-term care facilities is renal impairment (creatinine clearance <60 mL/min).[33] Opioid medications, especially renally excreted classes, may inadvertently reach plasma concentrations that are 50% higher in residents with renal failure than in those with appropriate kidney function.[31] This is one reason why slow-dose titration is important for these patients. In general, one must also consider that genetic variance may play a role in alteration of the metabolism of medications; thus, individualized care within large-scale systems continues to be important in the management of patients. Lack of attention to patient variance may affect the analgesic quality as well as the side-effect profile.

Drug–Drug Interactions

Opioids are excellent options for moderate to severe pain. Unfortunately, use of this drug has been poorly studied in long-term care facility populations. While the majority of studies focus on gastrointestinal or central nervous system side effects, polypharmacy in these patients presents legitimate concerns for cytochrome P450 disruption.[34] The average elderly patient may take an average of seven daily medications, with up to a 50% risk for drug–drug interactions (DDI).[35] Given the co-occurrence of psychiatric diagnoses and chronic pain, one of the most concerning DDIs is opiates and antipsychotics. One study found that nearly one-third of newly admitted NH residents were prescribed an antipsychotic. Of these patients, 32% had no clinical indication that could be identified upon chart review.[36] While this speaks to previously discussed issues regarding communication and pain-induced behavioral changes, it also serves to highlight how frequently a DDI with antipsychotics may require consideration. For example, medications that are metabolized by the CYP2D6 system (tramadol, codeine, etc.) should not be prescribed in conjunction with those that inhibit the same system (antidepressants such as paroxetine). This not only risks the precipitation of serotonin syndrome but also decreases the efficacy of the opiate.[34] Inversely, cytochrome P450 inducers can increase opiate metabolism and decrease opiate effects. Knowledge of medications, their effectiveness, and their interactions in various diseases as well as in the elderly is essential for appropriate chronic pain management with analgesics in long-term care facilities.

PALLIATIVE CARE AND DO NO HARM

Approximately one in four Americans dies in an NH.[37] The AARP Policy Institute reported that symptoms, needs, and illness trajectories of dying people are not sufficiently recognized by professional caregivers in these settings.[38] Many of these institutions are considered home by patients for extended periods of time. The NH is the best example of a setting where palliative care and, ultimately, hospice may take place.[33] Sources of pain for these patients include physical, emotional, social, and spiritual. Please refer to Chapter 13 for specifics on palliative care management in a chronic pain setting. Once a patient exhibits disease states, such as advanced cancer or dementia, for which palliative care would beneficial, it is incredibly important to begin these discussions with staff and family as soon as possible. Part of providing adequate treatment for these patients includes avoiding excess or unnecessary interventions. Do Not Hospitalize and Do Not Resuscitate orders should therefore be discussed with patients and their families during end-of-life care so that adverse medical outcomes do not result in transfers of patients out of their long-term care facilities for inpatient hospital treatment. One large, national study of 91,000 NH residences over the age of 65 with advance dementia found wide variability in Do Not Hospitalize orders. The prevalence was as high as 26% in Rhode Island and as low as 1% in Oklahoma.[39] Corporate chains with less overall staff including less advanced practice nurses were less likely to have Do Not Hospitalize orders signed for these patients. This identifies a need for more patient-centered approaches to end-of-life care, including avoiding unnecessary treatment or harm to patients, in long-term care institutions.

Approach to Selection of Therapy for Chronic Pain in Institutionalized Patients

Therapeutic considerations for chronic pain in healthcare institutions include analgesics (both opioid and non-opioid), adjuvant analgesics such as antidepressants, and nonpharmacological and behavioral modalities. Important steps to follow while selecting chronic pain medications may be found in Box 14.2. When choosing appropriate analgesics, the World Health Organization (WHO) pain relief ladder should be used for titrating oral medications.[40] The WHO ladder is available online and will not be reviewed here in detail. The WHO ladder is a sequential escalation guide for analgesic management, beginning from non-opioid agents and progressing first to weak opioids and then to stronger and long-acting opioids. Popular acute pain opiate medications used in NHs include Vicodin, oxycodone, Percocet, and hydromorphone. For long-acting relief, oxycodone (OxyContin) and MS Contin are may be selected.[5]

Box 14.2 **Steps for Analgesic Selection and Dosing**

1. Assess patient status, chart, and medication record
   a. Absorption and dosing route concerns
2. Explore potential for significant pharmacokinetic drug–drug interaction
   a. Metabolism: cytochrome P450 inhibitors and inducers
   b. Clearance interactions: renal function
3. Select agent, "start low and go slow"
   a. Slow titration of dose
   b. Total doses should be lower than usual
   c. Longer duration of actions are anticipated
4. Frequent assessment for efficacy and monitoring for adverse effects

_____

Box modified from Pergolizzi et al.[49]

Chronic pain has a strong connection to emotional responses in the elderly. These responses result from pain symptoms that include anxiety, migraine, nausea, incontinence, constipation, and dizziness. These physiological symptoms are associated with pain 90% of the time. Given the strong emotional tie to pain-associated symptoms, nearly two-thirds of elderly patients experiencing these effects also feel that there are no potential treatments for their pain.[41] This strong psychological component of chronic pain calls for a multidisciplinary team approach for assessing and managing chronic pain in these residents. Antidepressants may be considered "adjuvant analgesics" and are used in patients with comorbid emotional or psychiatric disorders (especially neuropathic pain and fibromyalgia). By carefully coadministering antidepressants, providers may effectively reduce the necessary opioid doses for patients. Many antidepressants function by blocking serotonin and norepinephrine reuptake, subsequently enhancing descending inhibitory neurons.[42] Tricyclic antidepressants (TCA) have been shown to be effective adjuvant analgesics for reducing chronic pain, with outcomes even greater than those with selective serotonin reuptake inhibitors (SSRIs).[43] A norepinephrine-serotonin reuptake inhibitor (SNRI), duloxetine, has received FDA approval for use in chronic diabetes and musculoskeletal pain.[44]

Nonpharmacological and behavioral therapies are also essential for managing chronic pain in long-term settings, if patients are physically and mentally able to carry them out. For emotional concerns, pain diaries and a thorough evaluation of disease experiences and behaviors are helpful in conjunction with sessions with a mental health professional. Additional helpful interventions include music therapy, cold/heat therapy, and massage therapy. There is no replacement for exercise and movement for most patients with chronic pain. This should be encouraged or ordered through physical therapy services for any resident who is healthy enough to tolerate exercise.

Addressing Adverse Drug Effects

Nausea, vomiting, confusion, and somnolence are common side effects of many therapeutic agents. These often improve after 7 to 10 days. If not, opioid rotation, dose titration, or adjuvant therapies may be considered.[5] A prophylactic bowel regimen in anticipation of constipation is also encouraged. A thorough knowledge of a patient's medical history and current prescriptions is essential for avoiding adverse drug effects and drug interactions.

ROLE OF QUALITY IMPROVEMENT IN HEALTHCARE INSTITUTIONS

Treatment guidelines are essential to assuring a higher standard of quality in care for pain management. One study found that patients receiving intravenous analgesics as needed (PRN) have worse Visual Analog Scale (VAS) scores for pain than those receiving pain medication through actual pain protocols.[24] Despite evidence-based guidelines for assessing and treating chronic pain, it is frequently not assessed and remains undertreated in institutional, especially NH, settings. A survey of NH managers found that only 60% used pain treatment guidelines in their facilities.[19] This is perplexing, considering existing data extolling their benefit, yet many of the concerns laid out in this chapter have led to an aversion to these guidelines.

Quality improvement initiatives for managing chronic pain in healthcare institutions such as NHs have been successful at improving verbal and nonverbal pain scale assessment as well as provider knowledge. They have also been shown to be instrumental in identifying potentially toxic drug interactions.[45] According to diffusion of innovation theory, an *innovation* is an idea or process that a group may consider new, while *diffusion* of the idea involves the process by which it is communicated and adopted by this group over time.[46] In order to implement quality improvement practices in healthcare institutions, one must have a comprehensive strategy. Clinician education alone has proven ineffective for changing actual clinical practice. Multifaceted interventions that incorporate aspects of education must be therefore implemented in order to see successful practice alterations.[47] Clinical education for all providers, enhanced nursing roles, implementation of algorithm guidelines, and collaborative management are all components that should be considered for inclusion when implementing quality improvement initiatives for chronic pain management in healthcare institutions.

The Advancing Excellence in America's Nursing Homes Campaign is one example of a national quality initiative that assists stakeholders of long-term care supports and services to improve the quality of care by providing educational materials and support. By 2010, at least 19 states had seen more than 50% of their NHs join. Pain complaints in long-term facilities have subsequently decreased, from 14% in 2011 to 10.5% in 2012.[48] More information and materials for this initiative can be found at www.nhqualitycampaign.org.

Summary

Chronic pain is a recurrent component of daily life for patients in these varied settings. Residents of these institutions can be very sick, are not always capable of speaking for themselves, and often have chronic pain that is undertreated. The goal of this chapter was to highlight a number of obstacles to managing chronic pain in institutionalized patients as well as provide recommended solutions for each of the obstacles. Careful medication reconciliation can decrease drug omission and dosing errors resulting from patient transfers and increased staff turnover. Educational campaigns are effective means for combating provider and patient misinformation regarding opiate addiction, tolerance, and side effects. Chronic pain assessment should be highly individualized (especially in patients with cognitive defects), and use of a number of assessment algorithms may also help standardize this process and improve its quality. Adverse drug events may be avoided through careful drug selection with attention to current medication lists, diseases affecting metabolism and clearance, and slow and low dosing titration. In addition, there is a role for quality improvement measures to be implemented at any point along this chronic pain assessment and therapeutic selection process, to avoid missed opportunities for better patient pain management. Chronic pain is an undertreated symptom in institutionalized settings, especially nursing homes. With appropriate provider education and attention to details outlined in this chapter, this problem can begin to be addressed, to improve the quality of life among this vulnerable patient population.

References

1. Kemper P, Murlaugh CM. Lifetime use of nursing home care. *N Engl J Med.* 1991;324:595–600.
2. Reinhard SC, Young HM. The nursing workforce in long-term care. *Nurs Clin N Am.* 2009;44:161–168.
3. Epps CD. Recognizing pain in the institutionalized elder with dementia. *Geriatr Nurs (Minneap).* 2001;22(2):71–78.
4. Achterberg WP, Pot AM, Scherder EJ, Ribbe MW. Pain in the nursing home: assessment and treatment on different types of care wards. *J. Pain Symptom Manage.* 2007;34(5):480–487.
5. Glajchen M. Chronic pain: treatment barriers and strategies for clinical practice. *J Am Board Fam Med.* 2001;14(3):211–218.
6. InpatientRehab. 2012. http://www.cms.gov/Medicare/Provider-Enrollment-and-Certification/CertificationandComplianc/InpatientRehab.html

7. Howe CQ, Sullivan MD. The missing 'P' in pain management: how the current opioid epidemic highlights the need for psychiatric services in chronic pain care. *Gen Hosp Psychiatry.* 2014;36(1):99–104.

8. Larson SL, Clark MR, Eaton WW. Depressive disorder as a long-term antecedent risk factor for incident back pain: a 13-year follow-up study from the Baltimore Epidemiological Catchment Area sample. *Psychol Med.* 2004;34(2):211–219.

9. Rahman A, Reed E, Underwood M, Shipley ME, Omar RZ. Factors affecting self-efficacy and pain intensity in patients with chronic musculoskeletal pain seen in a specialist rheumatology pain clinic. *Rheumatology (Oxford).* 2008;47(12):1803–1808.

10. McWilliams LA, Cox BJ, Enns MW. Mood and anxiety disorders associated with chronic pain: an examination in a nationally representative sample. *Pain.* 2003;106(1-2):127–133.

11. Tosato M, Lukas A, van der Roest HG, et al. Association of pain with behavioral and psychiatric symptoms among nursing home residents with cognitive impairment: results from the SHELTER study. *Pain.* 2012;153(2):305–310.

12. Baillargeon J, Black SA, Pulvino J, Dunn K. The disease profile of Texas prison inmates. *Ann. Epidemiol.* 2000;10(2):74–80.

13. Rold WJ. Legal considerations in the delivery of health care services in prisons and jails. In: Anno B, ed. *Correctional Health Care: Guidelines for the Management of an Adequate Delivery System.* Chicago: National Commission on Correctional Health Care; 2001:43–66.

14. Darnall BD, Sazie E. Pain characteristics and pain catastrophizing in incarcerated women with chronic pain. *J. Health Care Poor Underserved.* 2012;23(2):543–556.

15. Swartz JA. Chronic medical conditions among jail detainees in residential psychiatric treatment: a latent class analysis. *J. Urban Health.* 2011;88(4):700–717.

16. Boockvar KS, Liu S, Goldstein N, Nebeker J, Siu A, Fried T. Prescribing discrepancies likely to cause adverse drug events after patient transfer. *Qual Saf Health Care.* 2009;18(1):32–36.

17. Tjia J, Bonner A, Briesacher BA, McGee S, Terrill E, Miller K. Medication discrepancies upon hospital to skilled nursing facility transitions. *J Gen Intern Med.* 2009;24(5):630–635.

18. Feldt KS, Gunderson J. Treatment of pain for older hip fracture patients across settings. *Orthop Nurs.* 21(5):63–64, 66–71.

19. Barry HE, Parsons C, Peter Passmore A, Hughes CM. An exploration of nursing home managers' knowledge of and attitudes towards the management of pain in residents with dementia. *Int J Geriatr Psychiatry.* 2012;27(12):1258–1266.

20. Hutt E, Buffum MD, Fink R, Jones KR, Pepper GA. Optimizing pain management in long-term care residents. *Geriatr Aging.* 2007;10(8):523–527.

21. Long CO. Pain management education in long-term care: it can make a difference. *Pain Manag Nurs.* 2013;14(4):220–227.

22. Tse MMY, Ho SSK. Pain management for older persons living in nursing homes: a pilot study. *Pain Manag Nurs.* 2013;14(2):e10–21.

23. Frampton M. Experience assessment and management of pain in people with dementia. *Age Ageing.* 2003;32(3):248–251.

24. Bozimowski G. Patient perceptions of pain management therapy: a comparison of real-time assessment of patient education and satisfaction and registered nurse perceptions. *Pain Manag Nurs.* 2012;13(4):186–193.

25. Burfield AH, Wan TT, Sole M Lou, Cooper JW. A study of longitudinal data examining concomitance of pain and cognition in an elderly long-term care population. *J. Pain Res.* 2012;5:61–70.

26. Scherder EJ, Bouma A. Acute versus chronic pain experience in Alzheimer's disease. a new questionnaire. *Dement Geriatr Cogn Disord.* 11(1):11–16.

27. Krebs EE, Carey TS, Weinberger M. Accuracy of the pain numeric rating scale as a screening test in primary care. *J Gen Intern Med.* 2007;22(10):1453–1458.

28. Bruckenthal P, D'Arcy Y. Assessment and management of pain in older adults: a reveiw of the basics. *Top Adv Pract Nurs eJournal.* 2007;7(1).

29. Hadjistavropoulos T, Herr K, Turk DC, et al. An interdisciplinary expert consensus statement on assessment of pain in older persons. *Clin J Pain.* 2007;23(1 Suppl):S1–43.

30. Horgas AL, Nichols AL, Schapson CA, Vietes K. Assessing pain in persons with dementia: relationships among the non-communicative patient's pain assessment instrument, self-report, and behavioral observations. *Pain Manag Nurs.* 2007;8(2):77–85.

31. Smith H, Bruckenthal P. Implications of opioid analgesia for medically complicated patients. *Drugs Aging.* 2010;27(5):417–433.

32. Smith HS. Opioid metabolism. *Mayo Clin Proc.* 2009;84(7):613–624.

33. Dumas LG, Ramadurai M. Pain management in the nursing home. *Nurs Clin North Am.* 2009;44(2):197–208.

34. Lynch T. Management of drug-drug interactions: considerations for special populations—focus on opioid use in the elderly and long-term care. *Am J Manag Care.* 2011;17(Suppl 1):S293–298.

35. Björkman IK, Fastbom J, Schmidt IK, Bernsten CB. Drug-drug interactions in the elderly. *Ann Pharmacother.* 2002;36(11):1675–1681.

36. Chen Y, Briesacher BA, Field TS, Tjia J, Lau DT, Gurwitz JH. Unexplained variation across US nursing homes in antipsychotic prescribing rates. *Arch Intern Med.* 2010;170(1):89–95.

37. Casarett D, Karlawish J, Morales K, Crowley R, Mirsch T, Asch DA. Improving the use of hospice services in nursing homes: a randomized controlled trial. *JAMA.* 2005;294(2):211–217.

38. Wetle T, Teno J, Shield R, Welch L, Miller SC. End of life in nursing homes: experiences and policy recommendations. 2004: http://www.aarp.org/home-garden/livable-communities/info-2004/end_of_life_in_nursing_homes_experiences_and_polic.html.

39. Mitchell SL, Teno JM, Intrator O, Feng Z, Mor V. Decisions to forgo hospitalization in advanced dementia: a nationwide study. *J Am Geriatr Soc.* 2007;55(3):432–438.

40. World Health Organization. WHO's cancer pain ladder for adults. http://www.who.int/cancer/palliative/painladder/en/.

41. Zanocchi M, Maero B, Nicola E, et al. Chronic pain in a sample of nursing home residents: prevalence, characteristics, influence on quality of life (QoL). *Arch Gerontol Geriatr.* 47(1):121–128.

42. Leo RJ, Barkin RL. Antidepressant use in chronic pain management: is there evidence of a role for duloxetine? *Prim Care Companion J Clin Psychiatry.* 2003;5(3):118–123.

43. Bras M, Dordević V, Gregurek R, Bulajić M. Neurobiological and clinical relationship between psychiatric disorders and chronic pain. *Psychiatr Danub.* 2010;22(2):221–226.

44. Skljarevski V1, Zhang S, Iyengar S, D'Souza D, Alaka K, Chappell A, Wernicke J. Efficacy of duloxetine in patients with chronic pain conditions. *Curr Drug Ther.* 2011;6(4):296–303.

45. Leone AF, Standoli F, Hirth V. Implementing a pain management program in a long-term care facility using a quality improvement approach. *J Am Med Dir Assoc.* 2009;10(1):67–73.

46. Rogers EM. *Diffusion of Innovations,* 5th ed. New York: Free Press; 2003.

47. Gilbody S, Whitty P, Grimshaw J, Thomas R. Educational and organizational interventions to improve the management of depression in primary care: a systematic review. *JAMA.* 2003;289(23):3145–3151.

48. Bakerjian D, Zisberg A. Applying the advancing excellence in America's nursing homes: circle of success to improving and sustaining quality. *Geriatr Nurs.* 2013;34(5):402–411.

49. Pergolizzi J, Böger RH, Budd K, et al. Opioids and the management of chronic severe pain in the elderly: consensus statement of an International Expert Panel with focus on the six clinically most often used World Health Organization Step III opioids (buprenorphine, fentanyl, hydromorphone, met. *Pain Pract.* 2008;8(4):287–313.

Part III

ROLE OF NURSING, PHARMACY SPECIALIST, AND OTHER HOSPITAL SERVICES IN MANAGEMENT OF CHRONIC PAIN PATIENTS

15

Nursing Considerations

KIMBERLY BERGER AND CHRISTINE WIERZBOWSKI

KEY POINTS

- Chronic pain is a common condition that has a significant impact on individuals' inpatient experience. Too often it is disregarded as nurses and physicians focus instead on acute and underlying conditions.
- Persistent pain affects inpatient experience of both those who have the pain and their loved ones, visiting family and friends.
- The bedside nurse must be knowledgeable in treating chronic pain in order to provide accurate and appropriate information.
- A patient is much more likely to adhere to a pain management program when he or she has a thorough and valid understanding of why it has been prescribed and how it will help.

Introduction

Chronic pain is a common condition that can have a significant impact on individuals' inpatient experience. Too often it is disregarded as nurses and physicians focus instead on acute and underlying conditions. For example, in hospitals, approximately 67% of geriatric patients experience pain, yet less than half of these patients are treated effectively.[1]

Persistent pain, in and of itself, is a chronic disease and continues to increase across almost all demographics within the United States,[2] with approximately one-third of American adults reporting chronic pain.[3] Inadequate treatment of chronic pain is widespread, with females, minorities, and the elderly being among those at greatest risk for undertreatment of pain.[2] Ineffective pain management has been identified as a contributor to several adverse hospital outcomes.

Adult patients with chronic pain report a litany of negative effects, including less enjoyment of life, depression, reduced concentration, decreased energy, poor sleep, and decreased physical, social, and role functioning.[2] It can also lead to the contrasting effects of dependence on other people and a tendency toward isolation.[4] Patient barriers to effective pain management abound. Patients commonly suffer from multiple comorbidities that can exacerbate pain and complicate treatment.[5] Obstacles to self-management include inadequate access to services, limiting psychological attributes (fears, thoughts, beliefs, and biases), and programs that do not address the needs of the patient.[6]

Persistent pain affects inpatient experience of both those who suffer with the pain and their loved ones, visiting family and friends. Additionally, nurses and physicians are negatively affected by the increased need for support and by the stress and emotional burden associated with caring for someone in persistent chronic pain, which is typically exacerbated during a hospital stay. Given their continuous presence within the hospital unit, bedside nurses have a unique opportunity to attend to a patient's chronic pain, promote effective pain management, and improve patient experience. The substantial social impacts related to chronic pain present significant clinical implications for nursing staff. It is time for nurses to recognize the societal burden, both within the healthcare system and in the community, of chronic pain. There is growing evidence to support the critical nature of acute pain management in patients with chronic pain. Nurses must become adept at its assessment and inpatient treatment.

Nursing Staff Knowledge and Attitudes

Nursing staff experience their own challenges in caring for the inpatient chronic pain population. Abundant research has been conducted regarding nurses' knowledge of and attitudes about pain management.[7-12] The most significant modifiable nurse barrier to managing chronic pain is lack of knowledge, which can engender unwarranted bias and fears. Prejudice against chronic pain and opioid-dependent patients and a sense of powerlessness in treating them can discourage a nurse from being proactive and tenacious in resolving their concerns. Just as some regular patients tend to underreport their pain, some patients with chronic pain may exaggerate their pain, provoking potentially unsafe pain management with escalated doses of opioids. However, it is not uncommon for nurses and physicians to discount a chronic pain patient's self-report or the significance of persistent pain.[5] The most beneficial thing nurses can do for patients with chronic pain is to educate themselves, their colleagues, and their patients so that appropriate and safe care is provided that minimizes suffering and promotes good inpatient experience.

In order to treat persistent chronic pain effectively in a hospital setting, the nurse must both possess an understanding of the mechanisms and treatment of acute and chronic pain and maintain a positive attitude toward these patients and their inpatient care. A proverb familiar to every bedside nurse is, "Pain is whatever the experiencing person says it is, existing whenever he/she says it does."[13]. Patient self-report is the most valid and reliable indicator of pain—that is, of course, as long as the patient is heard and believed.[14] Unfortunately, mistaken knowledge and beliefs, borne of misinformation and a lack of evidence, can lead nursing staff to distrust their patients.

Because nurses' knowledge and attitudes toward pain impact the care they provide,[7,8] they must educate themselves in order to ensure that they provide the best patient care. Given the importance of knowledge and attitudes to the treatment of acute on chronic pain, evidence-based continuing education, along with regular reinforcement, is essential. Education is necessary to dispel the common misperceptions surrounding chronic pain that lead to biases against these patients and their treatment. An educated nurse is essential for correcting and preventing misconceptions on the part of the patient. The bedside nurse must be knowledgeable in treating pain so that he or she can provide accurate and appropriate information. A patient is much more likely to adhere to a pain management program when he or she has a thorough and valid understanding of why it has been prescribed and how it will help.

Hospital systems can serve both nurses and patients by establishing chronic pain teams. A pain resource nurse program, provided by nurses for nurses, is another option that can promote confidence in pain management knowledge and enhance practice.[15] There are many reputable sources of evidence-based guidelines that everyone, from individual nurses to entire healthcare systems, can reference to ensure the highest quality of chronic pain management. Nursing professionals can use these evidence-based guidelines to inform their practice and provide excellent pain management for their patients.

As important as knowledge is compassion, a cornerstone of chronic pain treatment. It is through compassion that a therapeutic relationship can develop. Empathy provides the foundation from which mutual trust and cooperation arise. In the initial meeting with a patient, distrust can be mutual. It is equally likely that the nurse will have to prove her- or himself to the patient. As biased as a nurse might be, the patient might be even more leery of putting faith in a healthcare worker. Wariness of health professionals after a long history of unsuccessful attempts at obtaining pain relief is a regular attitude among patients with chronic pain.[5] The nurse may have to overcome a patient's distrust before a true therapeutic alliance can begin. Development of a supportive, trusting relationship with nursing staff is paramount for successful pain management. By attempting to understand the patient's experience and approaching him or her with a positive attitude, the nurse can minimize negative bias and prejudice and ensures an objective approach to the patient's care.

Comprehensive Nursing Care of the Patient with Chronic Pain

Nursing care for chronic pain requires a comprehensive approach that extends beyond any given hospitalization. Nursing functions within this realm can be

Table 15.1 **A Comprehensive Approach to Nursing Care for Chronic Pain**

Phase of Care	Nursing Intervention	Goals of Care
Prevent	Discourage activities that increase risk for chronic pain. Aggressively manage acute pain to prevent conversion from acute to chronic pain	Stop chronic pain before it can start
Assess	Continuous comprehensive pain assessment with history and physical; WILDA; self-report when possible	Appraisal of chronic pain condition to establish goals of care and evaluate effectiveness of treatment
Treat	Multimodal treatment • Non-opioids • Opioids • Adjuvant medications • Nonpharmacological treatments	Patient reports symptom control, increased function, improved quality of life
Educate	Self-management; behavior change; realistic expectations; causes of pain; goals of treatment	Patient and family verbalize pain management regimen; demonstrate self-management techniques; establish realistic pain goals based on functional status

broadly divided into four categories: prevention, assessment, treatment, and education (Table 15.1). By attending to each of these areas, the bedside nurse can help ensure the best outcomes for the patient with persistent pain.

PREVENTION

Like any other chronic illness, the best and most effective defense against chronic pain is prevention. The hospital nurse can help patients by aggressively treating acute pain to prevent its conversion to chronic pain.[16] Additionally, educating all patients about healthy living and avoidance of situations and activities that might increase the risk for chronic pain is a wise nursing intervention. Encouraging good ergonomics can minimize risk of chronic musculoskeletal injury. When it comes to chronic pain, an ounce of prevention is worth more than a pound of cure. Certainly, many would argue that it's worth its weight in gold!

ASSESSMENT

If the patient has persistent pain, the first step in its management is the assessment. In order to do this, the nurse must first recognize persistent pain as a legitimate problem. Pain is routinely disregarded, undertreated, and undervalued as a significant health issue. It is crucial that the nurse not dismiss chronic pain as "beside the point" during a patient's hospital stay or assume that management of the pain is outside the scope of the hospitalization. Once it is recognized as a problem, thorough interdisciplinary assessment can be used to identify underlying causes, and potentially treatable contributors can be recognized and definitively addressed.[17]

On the initial patient encounter, the nurse should conduct a comprehensive pain assessment to include history, physical exam, pain assessment, psychological assessment, social support, cognitive function, and patient self-report, if possible. When self-report is not possible, direct observation and patient history are reasonable secondary options.[18] It makes sense to use a variety of terms when discussing chronic pain with a patient. It is not uncommon for a patient to deny pain and yet agree that he or she experiences symptoms of pain when asked about "discomfort" or "achiness," for example.

Once painful conditions have been identified, regular reassessments are necessary and critical to ensure that an optimal treatment regimen is in place. Assessment of physical functioning is at least as important as a pain score for chronic pain patients. Knowing that the patient will persistently experience a baseline amount of pain as well as its impact on activities of daily living and social functioning is paramount.

Patient communication about preferences related to assessment and treatment should be an important consideration in planning care of the patient with persistent pain. A thorough understanding of a patient's home pain management regimen is essential to continuing successful pain management during the hospital stay.

TREATMENT

There is much that a nurse can do to provide chronic pain management for a hospitalized patient. With their focus on holistic care, nurses are particularly well suited to providing comprehensive chronic pain management care that incorporates both pharmacological and nonpharmacological approaches.

While the nurse is not authorized to prescribe medications, in having the primary responsibility for their administration it makes sense for the nurse to have a strong grasp of pharmacological therapy. Pharmacological management can be a safe and effective method of pain control when the risks and benefits are fully considered. There are several general principles of pharmacological treatment of chronic pain. Certainly, as with any patient, the least invasive route of medication administration should be used. The oral route is, most generally, the preferred route unless swallowing difficulties preclude the option. Scheduling of medication administration should take the pain experience into account: continuous pain should be treated with long-acting medications that maintain a steady concentration in the body, and episodic pain with immediate-release short-acting medications.

Given the different physiological causes of chronic pain, the mechanism of action of a medication must suit the type of pain. For instance, a medication regimen for mild inflammatory nociceptive pain will differ from the regimen for severe neuropathic pain. A combination of medications should be considered to treat various aspects of the pain experience, as they can work synergistically and provide greater relief while also decreasing risks from higher doses of a single drug. A patient with chronic pain who is admitted to the hospital is likely to experience the same amount of pain or more during hospitalization rather than less and will, likewise, require as much or more medication than before hospitalization.

Non-opioid analgesics are the recommended first-line therapy for the treatment of many forms of mild chronic pain. Acetaminophen's relatively low risk-profile can make it an excellent first choice when reasonable safety precautions are taken, including observing safe dosing guidelines to avoid hepatic and renal complications. NSAIDs can be an appropriate choice for treatment of inflammatory conditions but are contraindicated in patients with renal, gastrointestinal (GI), or cardiovascular risks. For patients receiving chronic NSAID therapy, proton pump inhibitors should be used for GI protection.[19] Topical preparations can be effective for localized pain.

Available research and clinical evidence provide ample support for the use of opioid medications as an effective and often indispensable part of a successful pain management regimen for moderate to severe pain in adults.[20] Many clinical trials have demonstrated the short-term efficacy of opioid therapy for a wide range of chronic pain conditions, but there remains little evidence related to its efficacy in long-term use. Initial use of opioid therapy should be explored on a trial basis with clearly defined therapeutic goals. It is important that the patient understand that the trial will be discontinued if these goals are not met. If the trial is successful, the therapy can continue with vigilant monitoring and patient counseling.

While the risks of opioid therapy cannot be ignored, they should also not be given undue weight when measured against the benefits. The most consistent adverse effect of opioid therapy is constipation and should be addressed proactively. The other common side effects dissipate with long-term use. While an uncommon occurrence, respiratory depression deserves attention because of its potentially devastating effects. Respiratory depression occurs most commonly with rapid and excessive increases in dose. The adage "start low and go slow" can be particularly helpful to minimize this risk. Another very low but real risk of opioid therapy is that of addiction. However, it is equally important that nurses be cognizant of pseudo-addictive behaviors in patients seeking pain relief to avoid misinterpretation as addiction.[21] It is certainly appropriate to screen for addiction prior to initiation of opioid therapy.

Adjuvant medications are those drugs that were originally formulated to treat other conditions but have been found to be beneficial for the treatment of pain. Common adjuvant medications include antidepressants, anticonvulsants, corticosteroids, muscle relaxants, benzodiazepines, and cannabinoids. Adjuvants can be used alone but are often more effective in conjunction with other pharmacological and nonpharmacological therapies. Just as with opioid therapy, it is important to "start low and go slow" and to allow an adequate analgesic trial before a medication is discontinued for failure to provide relief.[19]

Nonpharmacological nursing interventions are an excellent option for the treatment of chronic pain and should be considered both alone and in combination with medication therapy. An individualized moderate physical activity plan should be developed and maintained for the patient during the hospital stay, taking into account the patient's needs and preferences and ensuring proper monitoring and supervision. The exercise regimen should maintain or improve flexibility, strength, and endurance. While the physical aspects of pain management are more vigorously addressed, the psychosocial aspects of living with chronic pain cannot be discounted. There is evidence to support the use of cognitive behavioral therapy (CBT) techniques by trained nursing staff to address these less tangible concerns.[22,23] While CBT is generally a longer-term, regularly scheduled therapy, there are many quick and easy techniques that can be used within the limited duration of a hospital visit. The RN should seek out other appropriate disciplines and take advantage of both established treatment modalities and newer, less common interventions.[22,24]

PATIENT EDUCATION

Despite the vast array of treatment options, the majority of chronic pain patients will continue to experience symptoms. It is thus vitally important to empower them to take control of their pain. While the patient is, by default, the expert on his or her pain, this expertise does not necessarily equate to expertise in pain management.

Medication education is of primary importance for the hospitalized patient with chronic pain. Because of the wide variety of treatment options, there are a great many medications that may or may not be familiar to the patient. In particular, the bedside nurse must be able to recognize the selection of adjuvant medications and explain their use for the specified condition. Because these medications are being used for chronic pain instead of a more usual diagnosis, the nurse must be able to clearly explain this use to ensure adherence.

Another important aspect of patient education is establishment of realistic expectations. There is no quick fix for chronic pain. The patient cannot expect a miracle to occur in the limited time span of a hospitalization. At the same time, pain management is the right of every patient admitted to the hospital, even the challenging ones. But pain management does not mean zero pain; it means controlling pain to a reasonable and acceptable level safely while maximizing functional status.

Dealing with a "Difficult" Patient

When about to deal with a patient who is upset about any aspect of chronic pain control, the first thing a nurse must, do regardless of the circumstances, is to let the patient know that he or she understands that the patient is in pain. This will open up a productive channel, as most opioid-dependent patients have to constantly convince everyone that they are in pain. Next, the nurse should verify the patient's concern with the current regimen. At this time, the nurse should stress the importance of the patient's willingness to help themselves. This is exemplified by the so-called 49/51 rule, which states that "we will do up to 49% of the work, but the patient must do at least 51%"; the patient cannot be a passive participant when he or she has chronic pain.

It is important to have a discussion on medication safety as a priority for both the patient and the healthcare team. A discussion about medication used as an adjunct to opioids, regional blocks, physical and occupational therapy, psychology, chaplain services, and integrative medicine, if available, is important to have with the patient. The patient should be helped to understand that physical therapy is not necessarily ordered to "fix" the patient's pain but to make the rest of the body stronger. It is important to explain that the hospital's psychological services do not interpret the pain as "imaginary," rather, they are about helping the patient deal with the nature of chronic pain: it affects so many areas of the patient's life that coping mechanisms are vital to successful treatment. They work mainly by separating anxiety and/or depression from pain, which, along with other psychological problems, are tightly associated with pain but cannot be effectively treated with opioids. Many patients have trouble understanding this concept, especially when they experience acute chronic pain in the hospital. They have to be ready to comprehend this information, and the nurse has to be able to gently, but persistently and nonjudgmentally, deliver these educational concepts to the patient. Patient education, including reinforcing self-help techniques and explaining known causes of pain, goals of treatment, and pain management expectations, is critical to treatment success.

Patients should also be encouraged to pursue support within the community after being discharged from the hospital. Patient and family education is crucial for any chronic pain management program, because long-term pain control requires continuous and sustained self-management (Figure 15.1). Prior to hospital discharge, the nurse can provide resources for follow-up programs to support relapse prevention and maintenance of self-management skills.[4,25]

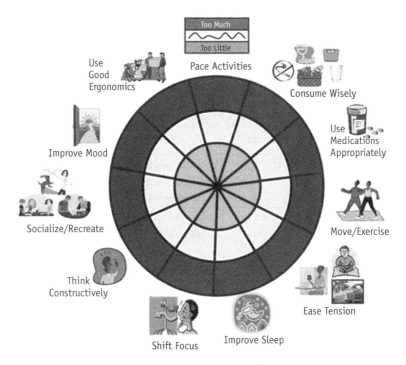

Figure 15.1 Pain self-management strategies wheel.[27] Reprinted with permission from Richard Wanlass, Ph.D., and Debra Fishman, Psy.D., University of California, Davis.

Promoting Pain Management Nursing Throughout the Hospital

The staff nurse has an excellent opportunity to have an impact on chronic pain management practices within the hospital and to provide excellent care (Table 15.2). She or he can be an expert clinician in matters of chronic pain and act as a mentor and role model in the implementation of evidence-based pain management practice. Considering the nearly universal tendency to discount the pain experience of patients with chronic pain, nurses will serve their colleagues well by being educated in the area of pain management and then providing and supporting education for their peers. Establishment of a pain resource nurse program can promote nurse involvement and highlight the important role of nurses in successful pain management.[15]

Nurses can benefit from hospital-specific clinical pathways for management of chronic pain with a focus on providing care across the continuum. The establishment of quality assurance and improvement programs can allow for assessment and feedback regarding chronic pain care. Chronic pain management must receive adequate funding within healthcare financial systems.

Table 15.2 **Nursing Activities and Associated Chronic Pain Outcomes**

Activity	*Outcomes of Practice*
Incorporate both pharmacological and nonpharmacological approaches to chronic pain management, including complementary and alternative medicine	Patients will receive a multimodal approach to chronic pain management; pain will be well controlled.
Address psychosocial aspects of chronic pain	Patients and families will develop effective coping skills and address psychosocial contributors to chronic pain.
Patient/family self-management education	Long-term pain control, realistic expectations, relapse prevention, and maintenance of self-management skills
Act as a practitioner, mentor, and role model in the implementation of evidence-based chronic pain management practice	Evidence-based practice skills are demonstrated and nurses practice on the basis of evidence with resulting positive patient outcomes.
Staff is educated in chronic pain management	Pain management education programs are developed, implemented, and evaluated with a focus on evidence-based practice and patient outcomes.
Establishment of a pain resource nurse program	Nurse involvement in pain management is promoted, and the important role of nursing in successful pain management is highlighted.
Comprehensive policies and procedures to address acute and chronic pain management	Evidence-based pain management practices are implemented throughout the organization; references are available for staff to ensure effective pain management.
Quality assurance/improvement practices	Pain management practices are continuously attended to within the organization to ensure treatment of the highest quality.

Education is needed—not just for nurses, but for all healthcare clinicians and for patients.

Knowing that integrative approaches to pain control can be particularly effective, at even the smallest scale within a healthcare organization, the RN can promote multidisciplinary collaboration in pain management.[25,26] As the conduit between the patient and the rest of the medical team, the bedside nurse is the linchpin that ensures successful treatment. The importance of communication with physicians, patients, interdisciplinary team members, and among nurses themselves cannot be stressed enough.

The need for attention throughout the hospital to management of chronic pain provides the staff nurse with abundant opportunities to effect change on an even larger scale. The universal need for chronic pain treatment presents an occasion for the nurse to advocate for improved pain management practices at the system level. Comprehensive policies and procedures to address chronic pain can be an effective means of promoting evidence-based practice.

Quality assurance and improvement practices can reinforce organizational commitment to serve this undertreated population. Effective pain management results in improved patient outcomes. Expected measureable results include improved functional capacity, increased ability to perform ADLs, reduced pain, occupational readiness, reduced disability, improved health-related quality of life, decreased healthcare usage, decreased depression and anxiety, and improved coping.[4,25,26] Tools and scales for the measurement of these outcomes are abundant. Monitoring and assessing these outcomes can support implementation of a robust chronic pain program.

Summary

While chronic pain is currently appreciated as a chronic illness, the prevalence of uncontrolled acute on chronic pain, the systemic undertreatment of this condition, and the major complications related to inpatient opioid overdose make it clear that acute on chronic pain deserves immediate and thorough attention. Pain management is a universal human right, and it is time to ensure that this right is safeguarded for the most vulnerable among us. The bedside nurse plays an important role in guaranteeing excellent pain management for the hospitalized patient with chronic pain.

References

1. Gianni W, Madaio RA, Di Cioccio L, et al. Prevalence of pain in elderly hospitalized patients. *Arch Gerontol Geriatr.* 2010;51(3):273–276.
2. Institute of Medicine Committee on Advancing Pain Research, Care, and Education. *Relieving Pain in America: A Blueprint for Transforming Prevention, Care, Education, and Research.* Washington DC: National Academies Press; 2011. http://iom.nationalacademies.org/reports/2011/relieving-pain-in-america-a-blueprint-for-transforming-prevention-care-education-research.aspx.
3. Johannes CB, Le TK, Zhou X, Johnston JA, Dworkin RH. The prevalence of chronic pain in United States adults: results of an Internet-based survey. *J Pain.* 2010;11(11):1230–1239.
4. Frich LMH, Sorensen J, Jacobsen S, Fohlmann B, Hojsted J. Outcomes of follow-up visits to chronic nonmalignant pain patients. *Pain Manage Nurs.* 2012;13(4):223–235.

5. Denny DL, Guido GW. Undertreatment of pain in older adults: an application of beneficence. *Nurs Ethics*. 2012;19(6):800–809.

6. Bruckenthal P. Integrating nonpharmacologic and alternative strategies into a comprehensive management approach for older adults with pain. *Pain Manag Nurs*.
2010;11(2):S23–S31.

7. Al-Shaer D, Hill PD, Anderson MA. Nurses' knowledge and attitudes regarding pain
assessment and intervention. *Medsurg Nurs*. 2011;20(1):7–11.

8. McNamara MC, Harmon D, Saunders J. Effect of education on knowledge, skills and attitudes around pain. *Br J Nurs*. 2012;21(16):958–964.

9. Prem V, Karvannan H, Chakravarthy RD, Binukumar B, Jaykumar S, Kumar SP. Attitudes
and beliefs about chronic pain among nurses- biomedical or behavioral? A cross-sectional
survey. *Indian J Palliat Care*. 2011;17(3):227–234.

10. Schreiber JA, Cantrell D, Moe KA, et al. Improving knowledge, assessment, and attitudes related to pain management: evaluation of an intervention. *Pain Manage Nurs*.
2014;15(2):474–481.

11. McKenna L, Boyle M, Brown T, et al. Levels of empathy in undergraduate nursing students. *Int J Nurs Pract*. 2012;18(3):246–251.

12. Desai G, Chaturvedi SK. Pain with no cause! nurses' perception. *Indian J Palliat Care*.
2012;18(3):162–164.

13. McCaffery M. *Nursing Practice Theories Related to Cognition, Bodily Pain, and Man–Environment
Interactions*. Los Angeles: University of California at Los Angeles Bookstore; 1968.

14. Gregory J, Richardson C. The use of pain assessment tools in clinical practice: A pilot survey. *J Pain Relief*. 2014;3(2):140–146 .

15. Grant M, Ferrell B, Hanson J, Sun V, Uman G. The enduring need for the pain resource
nurse (PRN) training program. *J Cancer Educ*. 2011;26(4):598–603.

16. Voscopoulos C, Lema M. When does acute pain become chronic? *Br J Anaesth*.
2010;105:i69–85.

17. American Geriatrics Society Panel on Persistent Pain in Older Persons. The management
of persistent pain in older persons. *J Am Geriatr Soc*. 2002;50(6):S205–S224.

18. Herr K, Coyne PJ, Key T, et al. Pain assessment in the nonverbal patient: position statement with clinical practice recommendations. *Pain Manage Nurs*. 2006;7(2):44–52.

19. American Geriatrics Society Panel on the Pharmacological Management of Persistent
Pain in Older Persons. Pharmacological management of persistent pain in older persons.
Pain Med. 2009;10(6):1062–1083.

20. American Academy of Pain Medicine. *APS/AAPM Clinical Guideline for the Use of Chronic
Opioid Therapy in Chronic Noncancer Pain*. Chicago: AAPM; 2013.

21. Arnstein P. Balancing analgesic efficacy with safety concerns in the older patient. *Pain
Manage Nurs*. 2010;11(2):S11–S22.

22. Jelin E, Granum V, Eide H. Experiences of a Web-based nursing intervention—interviews
with women with chronic musculoskeletal pain. *Pain Manage Nurs*. 2012;13(1):2–10.

23. Nash VR, Ponto J, Townsend C, Nelson P, Bretz MN. Cognitive behavioral therapy, self-efficacy, and depression in persons with chronic pain. *Pain Manag Nurs*.
2013;14(4):e236–e243

24. Teixeira ME. Meditation as an intervention for chronic pain: an integrative review.
Holistic Nurs Pract. 2008;22(4):225–234.

25. Dysvik E, Kvaloy JT, Natvig GK. The effectiveness of an improved multidisciplinary
pain management programme: a 6- and 12-month follow-up study. *J Adv Nurs*.
2012;68(5):1061–1072.

26. Ravenek MJ, Hughes ID, Ivanovich N, et al. A systematic review of multidisciplinary outcomes in the management of chronic low back pain. *Work*. 2010;35(3):349–367.

27. Wanlass R, Fishman D. *Pain Self-Management Strategies*. Davis, CA: UC Davis Medical Center;
2008:3. http://www.ucdmc.ucdavis.edu/nursing/Research/INQRI_Grant/Long-Term%20Non-
Surgery%20Pain%20Management%20Strategies%20Booklet%20WebFINAL082311.pdf.

16

Role of the Pharmacist in Management of Patients' Chronic Pain in the Hospital Setting

GLENN R. RECH AND PAMELA S. MOORE

KEY POINTS

- The hospital pharmacist is an essential member of the healthcare team caring for a patient with chronic pain while in the hospital. Pharmacists are medication therapy management experts with in-depth knowledge of the pharmacokinetics and pharmacodynamics of the medications used in the treatment of pain.
- A patient may experience changes in physiological processes during hospitalization that may dramatically alter the body's normal processing and response to the patient's chronic medications.
- The pharmacist can assist with the medication adjustments that will be necessary to keep the patient safe and to maintain effective pain control throughout the hospital stay. The pharmacist should also participate in education to staff members and patients in setting realistic expectations and goals for pain management.
- As medication experts, pharmacists are uniquely suited to conducting medication histories, interpreting prescription monitoring reports, performing medication reconciliations, and recommending alternative options and equianalgesic dosing should the patient's chronic pain medication not be available on formulary.
- The pharmacist can also act as a liaison between the prescriber and the governing bodies of the hospital in the creation of order sets and policies and in ensuring compliance with the recommendations and standards of safety and regulatory agencies. For the hospital pharmacist who is not a pain management expert, there are many resources and training programs available to learn more and improve skills in managing pain.

Introduction

Healthcare has evolved over the last several decades into an integrated team approach. As medication experts, pharmacists work as members of interdisciplinary teams in an effort to improve patient care outcomes. Giberson and colleagues outlined the numerous examples of how pharmacists have assisted in improving patient care in a 2011 report to the U.S. Surgeon General.[1] Examples specific to pain management may include pharmacists working in ambulatory care clinics, inpatient services to manage patient controlled analgesia, medical teaching services focusing on oncology pain management services,[2] and treating hospitalized patients with pain and substance abuse history or those with chronic pain.

Transitions of Care: The Tipping Points

In the area of chronic pain management, the medication history should be complete. Include all the prescribed and over-the-counter medication or supplement names, dosage strengths, and frequency. Pain medications consumption must be noted. Complete histories include the name of the prescribing physician, the average number of as-needed doses taken on a typical day, the number of as-needed doses taken on a day when pain is well controlled and on a day when the pain is at its worst, as well as the effectiveness of the as-needed doses and any regularly scheduled pain medications. Many patients forget to mention topical agents, patches, and implanted pumps, so these should be specifically asked for. The medication history is an opportune time to ask about typical adverse effects, such as constipation, and what medications are being used to treat them. Conversely, some patients exaggerate their opioid dosing, hoping to increase the opioid dose and its euphoric effect.

In the United States, legislation has allowed prescription record reporting for Drug Enforcement Agency (DEA)-categorized controlled medications, including opioids, sedatives, and stimulants. In states where prescription monitoring programs (PMP) are available, all practitioners, including pharmacists, should apply for and utilize the programs as allowed within the boundaries of the law. This information is useful when determining the patient's "opioid load" with a hospital admission, as the reports that are generated are essential tools in obtaining and evaluating medication histories. The information included in the PMP reports varies by state, and the practitioner must be knowledgeable about the structure, format, potential for errors and omissions, and method of interpretation and use the report as one piece of the puzzle, not relying on the document as the only piece of information. For example, the Ohio Automated Rx Reporting System (OARRS) reports do not reflect information regarding prescriptions filled at Veterans Administration pharmacies, prescriptions dispensed to extended care facilities, or medications directly administered to a patient, such as those administered under direct observation at an opioid addiction maintenance clinic.

CASE STUDY

"Hello, my name is Glenn; I am a pharmacist here at the Center for Pain Medicine." This is my introduction to the patients, staff, and prior authorization (PA) medication insurance specialist. (Only the prior authorization specialist seemed confused with a pharmacist in a setting outside of a pharmacy.)

A pharmacist, as a member of the healthcare provider team, is a collaborator for the medication management of a patient with pain. Patients suffering from pain deserve a multidisciplinary approach to treatment. Medications have been the cornerstone of treatment, although a more diversified approach may be appropriate. Understanding the pharmacokinetics, pharmacodynamics, drug interactions, and adverse effects (pain patients seldom tolerates gabapentin) of medications and focusing on the patient's expectations are aspects that pharmacists can provide as team members. The following case is a situation in which a pharmacist would be helpful. If you find yourself on-call without a supporting network, please talk to a   pharmacist.

You receive a call from the ER informing you of a new admission to the hospital. A patient, MK, is being admitted to a medical-surgical floor with the chief complaints of headaches, neck pain, and numbness in the left arm. A recent radiographic workup demonstrated a C5-6 disk bulge. ER medications administered included oxycodone/acetaminophen 5/325 mg orally at 17:29, morphine 2 mg IV at 19:44, 20:02, 22:24, and meperidine (case was from December 2006) 25 mg IV at 23:16. You have been following this patient in the hospital. Medications on the floor during the following two days included meperidine 25–50 mg IV, oxycodone/acetaminophen 10/325 mg every 4 hours as needed, sustained-release oxycodone 20 mg twice daily, and diazepam 10 mg three times daily. Patient-controlled analgesia (PCA) with hydromorphone was ordered and discontinued within 45 minutes. Hydromorphone 2–3 mg IV every 2 hours as needed for severe pain replaced the PCA order. On the morning of day 3 at 05:30, a lab tech called the nurse, stating that the patient wouldn't wake up. Noted was a bloody discharge from the nasal orifices, respirations were minimal, and pulse thready. A Code Blue was called. Initial respirations were 4–6 per minute, pulse oximetry was recorded as 34%. Naloxone was administered at 0.1 mg times 4 doses over 1 hour. The patient was transferred to the ICU and a naloxone infusion was started.

Clearly this patient incurred an opioid-induced respiratory arrest. The patient had fallen getting out of bed, hitting her head, causing a nose bleed. The Code Blue could have been prevented. Most opioid-induced respiratory arrests can also be prevented. Patients with chronic pain are often managed with an opioid in the ambulatory setting, in this case, oxycodone/acetaminophen. Tolerance to the analgesic and euphoric effects can develop. A myriad of opioids was offered to this patient, including oral, parenteral. Additionally, for spasms of the neck, diazepam was prescribed. The added risk of opioids induced respiratory depression with the combination of other sedating agents was not obvious for medical team until the major complication has occured. The point to make here is that one needs a reference value to aggregate the opioid load, as well as awareness of which medications may contribute, in combination, to respiratory depression. This is important in a hospital setting, where opioid combinations and different routes of administration are provided. For example, MK's morphine equivalency was 22 on day one, 128 on day two, and 193 on day 3.

Challenges with Opioid Conversions

For patients taking more than one opioid, the morphine equivalent dose of the different opioids must be added together to determine the cumulative dose. A multitude of different equianalgesic tables and electronic opioid dose calculators can be found on the Internet and in print resources. The following are just a few examples.

> www.nhms.org/sites/default/files/Pdfs/Opioid-Comparison-Chart-Prescriber-Letter-2012.pdf
> www.ohiopaininitiative.org/resources/42_OPI%20Anaglesic%20Table%20 2011.pdf
> www.agencymeddirectors.wa.gov/guidelines.asp
> www.clincalc.com
> www.globalrph.com
> www.hopweb.org
> www.medcalc.com
> http://opioidcalculator.practicalpainmanagement.com

It is important to recognize the limitations inherent in such tools,[3] read the disclaimers, and understand that the equivalent dose calculations are just one part of the opioid conversion process.[4] Practitioners should familiarize themselves with a particular table or tool, determine whether it is a conservative or aggressive approach, and adjust the prescription accordingly. A specific limitation is that not all tables or calculators are appropriate to use in a bidirectional manner, meaning that they might be intended to aid in conversion from product A to product B, but not from product B to product A. [due to significant risk of dose error]

Tools to Assess Risks

In addition to assessing and treating pain, it is equally necessary for healthcare providers to evaluate the risks for administering medications, especially for the opioids. There are a number of tools designed to assist in assessing a patient's appropriateness to be treated with opioids as it pertains to the risk of misuse or abuse. The following are a few examples:

Screener and Opioid Assessment for Patients with Pain (SOAPP®)
Current Opioid Misuse Measure (COMM™)
Opioid Risk Tool (ORT)
Diagnosis, Intractability, Risk, Efficacy (DIRE)
Screening Instrument for Substance Abuse Potential (SISAP)

Assessment tools such as the Pasero Opioid Sedation Scale[5] may be used to assist in determining if it is safe to give the next dose of an opioid to a patient who is awake enough to report pain but may be exhibiting other signs that indicate otherwise. Screening for identifying patients at risk for sleep apnea such as the STOP-Bang[6] or questionnaires evaluating sleep hygiene may also be helpful in identifying patients at higher risk for opioid-induced respiratory depression.

Discussion of Expectations

The expectations of patients experiencing chronic pain must be addressed. Patients should be taught that the management of chronic pain is different than the treatment of acute pain. Managing the patient from a multidisciplinary approach reinforces for the patient that nothing will completely eliminate this unpleasant feeling. Medications may be just one part of the treatment plan containing other treatment modalities.

The expectations of prescribers must also be considered. Although standardization of the comprehensive approach to pain management should be viewed as a positive, hospital policies, protocols, and order sets should not be designed as "one-size-fits-all". Rather in a manner that allows for a standardized process of individualization of the medications, routes, doses, regimens, as-needed indications, and monitoring parameters. Patient A reporting a pain score of 5 on a visual analog scale of 0–10 may desire a dose of pain medication, whereas patient B with a pain score of 7 may request no additional pain medication.[7] Because of this, one may have to adjust preprogrammed orders where for any patient with a pain score of 1–3 a particular medication and dose is given, a score of 4–7 receives a different medication/dose, and a pain score greater than 8 would receive yet a different medication/dose. Such ordering strategies can be

---

Box 16.1 **Medications to Avoid in Patients with Renal System Failures**

Renal: (CrCL <30 mL/min)
- Meperidine
- Codeine
- Morphine
- Nonsteroidal anti-inflammatory agents

---

used, but the pain scores in the as-needed indication as well as the medications and doses should be individualized for the needs of the given patient.

Medications cause adverse effects. Boxes 16.1, 16.2, and 16.3, provide guidelines for the use of drugs in patients with system failures, information on medications with active metabolites and common drug interactions. A question common to all pain providers is, Why are some patients always allergic to all the adjuvant medications? Patients report pedal edema or drowsiness from gabapentin or pregabalin, nausea or dizziness from duloxetine or venlafaxine. Patients are experts at funneling their therapy to the medications they desire. If the patient reports an allergy to a medication, then the physician won't prescribe it. Certain patients refuse any opioid therapy for fear of addiction. Still others have a history of addiction to a medication and are concerned with a repeating problem.

Formulary Management, Safety, and Regulatory Issues

Unless you work in an institution with an open formulary, which is very rare, you are most likely aware of the challenges of working within the confines of a formulary [list of medications available at an institution]. Formularies are designed to promote safety, efficacy, and cost containment. Chronic pain management needs can vary greatly from one patient to the next, but that doesn't mean that all pain medications available on the market can or should be available on formulary. A sufficient number and variety of medications, including

---

Box 16.2 **Medications with an Active Metabolite**

- Codeine (prodrug-activation required)
- Tramadol
- Hydrocodone
- Oxycodone

Box 16.3 **Common Drug Interactions within Chronic Pain Medications**

- Tramadol, tapentadol—SSRI (increase risk of seizures and serotonin syndrome)
- Tramadol, tapentadol—TCA (increase risk of seizures and serotonin syndrome)
- Tizanidine—ciprofloxacin, fluvoxamine (increase risk of sedation)
- Methadone—too many to list, consult your pharmacist

---

opioids, non-opioid pain medications, and adjuvant medications, should be available on formulary in order to meet the needs of most patients through the process of opioids conversion discussed earlier.

Ensuring that all pharmacists are capable of performing basic equianalgesic conversions is important in order to assist prescribers in identifying alternative agents and dosages to be substituted while the patient is in the hospital. Regularly reviewing safety information such as that from the Institute of Safe Medication Practices (ISMP) and regulatory recommendations such as the Sentinel Event Alerts from The Joint Commission[8] will assist the pharmacy department in evaluating formulary options and developing policies and procedures regarding pain medications. Pharmacists should be essential members of interdisciplinary committees committed to the safe and effective management of patients' pain.

A newer concept is that of pain medication stewardship.[9] Similar to antimicrobial or anticoagulant stewardship programs, which also manage high-risk medications, a pharmacist may work in conjunction with a prescriber to screen patients and ensure that opioids and other medications used to treat pain are being utilized in a safe and cost-effective manner. Depending on how the program is set up and the governing laws and regulations, the pharmacist may need to be credentialed[10] and privileged to conduct stewardship activities. Please see Box 16.4 for more details.

Additional Resources and Training

There are many options available for hospital-based pharmacists wanting to improve their knowledge and skills regarding pain management. Ranging from resources such as textbooks, journal articles, continuing education programs, and webinars to traineeships and postgraduate year-two residency programs for pain management and palliative care, the various programs offer different levels of education, practice-based involvement, and time commitment to fit the needs of the learner. Please refer to Box 16.5 for more details.

Box 16.4 Role of Pharmacist as Pain Medication Expert

- Understanding acute with chronic pain
- Pharmacokinetics and pharmacodynamics
- Opioid tolerance and dangers when it wears off
- When to increase and when to decrease medications
- Pharmacists as hospital generalist
- Pharmacists as hospital specialist
- Working with a pain management specialist/interdisciplinary team—membership on interdisciplinary team and committees—knowing your role
- Working without a pain management team—stewardship, credentialing, and privileging
- Setting expectations—key phrases ("manage" not "eliminate")
- Support for nursing and generalist staff members by providing formal and informal education
- Evaluating polypharmacy and triggers to trim the list

ESSENTIAL TASKS

- Ability to take a medication history—pitfalls
- Ability to perform medication reconciliations
- Access and interpret prescription monitoring reports
- Assist with formulary management to support the needs of the patient population with chronic pain, including development and review of order sets and protocols
  - Intrathecal pumps
  - Adjuvants
  - Mitigate risks (Pasero Opioid Sedation Scale, capnography)
  - Support conversion between non-formulary medications on the home medication list and formulary alternatives
  - Examples, scenarios/cases, references, and resources, understanding the limitations of conversion tables and online calculators
  - Ensure adherence to regulatory and safety recommendations—The Joint Commission sentinel event alert, ISMP reports
  - Pharmacist as pain management specialist—opportunity for pain and palliative care residency training, certified pain educator, ASHP traineeship

```
┌─────────────────────────────────────────────────────────────────┐
│                  Box 16.5 Additional Resources                    │
│                                                                   │
│ Lipman AG. Pain Management for Primary Care Clinicians. 2004       │
│ American Pain Society www.americanpainsociety.org Principles of    │
│     Analgesic Use in the Treatment of Acute and Cancer Pain Management, │
│     educational conferences                                       │
│ American Society of Pain Educators www.paineducators.org educational │
│     conferences, Certified Pain Educator (CPE) credentialing exam │
│ PainEDU www.painedu.org online continuing education, resources for │
│     practice and education                                        │
│ American Society of Health-System Pharmacists pain and palliative care │
│     traineeship www.ashpfoundation.org/painmanagement             │
│ American Society of Health-System Pharmacists postgraduate year two │
│     residencies in pain management and palliative care http://accred. │
│     ashp.org/aps/pages/directory/residencyProgramSearch.aspx      │
└─────────────────────────────────────────────────────────────────┘
```

Summary

The hospital pharmacist is an essential member of the healthcare team caring for a patient with chronic pain while in the hospital. Pharmacists are medication therapy management experts with in-depth knowledge of the pharmacokinetics and pharmacodynamics of the medications used in the treatment of pain. A patient may experience changes in physiological processes during the hospitalization that may dramatically alter the body's normal processing and response to his or her chronic medications. The pharmacist can assist with the medication adjustments that will be necessary to keep the patient safe and to maintain effective pain control throughout the hospital stay. The pharmacist should also participate in education to staff members and patients in setting realistic expectations and goals for pain management. As medication experts, pharmacists are uniquely suited to conducting medication histories, interpreting prescription monitoring reports, performing medication reconciliation, and recommending alternative options and equianalgesic dosing should the patient's chronic pain medication not be available on formulary. The pharmacist can also act as a liaison between the prescriber and the governing bodies of the hospital in the creation of order sets and policies and in ensuring compliance with the recommendations and standards of safety and regulatory agencies. For the hospital pharmacist who is not a pain management expert, there are many resources and training programs available to learn more and improve skills in managing pain.

References

1. Giberson S, Yoder S, Lee MP. Improving Patient and Health System Outcomes through Advanced Pharmacy Practice. A Report to the U.S. Surgeon General. Office of the Chief Pharmacist. U.S. Public Health Service. December 2011.
2. Lothian ST, Fotis MA, Von Gunten CF, Lyons J, Von Roenn JH, Weitzman SA. Cancer pain management through a pharmacist-based analgesic dosing service. *Am J Health-Syst Pharm.* 1999;56:1119–1125.
3. Shaheen PE, Walsh D, Lasheen W, Davis MP, Lagman RL. Opioid equianalgesic tables: are they all equally dangerous? *J Pain Symptom Manage.* 2009;38(3):409–417.
4. McPherson ML. *Demystifying Opioid Conversion Calculations.* Bethesda, MD: American Society of Health-System Pharmacists; 2010.
5. Pasero C, McCaffery M. Monitoring sedation: it's the key to preventing opioid-induced respiratory depression. *Am J Nurs.* 2002;102:67–69
6. STOP-Bang Questionnaire. http://www.stopbang.ca.
7. Blumstein HA, Moore DS. Visual analog pain scores do not define desire for analgesia in patients with acute pain. *Acad Emerg Med.* 2003;10:211–214.
8. Joint Comission. Safe use of opioids in hospitals. www.jointcommission.org/assets/1/18/SEA_49_opioids_8_2_12_final.pdf
9. Ghafoor VL, Phelps P, Pastor J. Implementation of a pain medication stewardship program. *Am J Health-Syst Pharm.* 2013;70:2070–2075.
10. Juba KM. Pharmacist credentialing in pain management and palliative care. *J Pharm Pract.* 2012;25(5):517–520.

17

Role of the Clinical Psychologist

KEY POINTS

- The psychological consultation of a chronic pain patient in an acute care inpatient setting is different in essential ways from the outpatient psychological assessment. Its underlying assumptions, goals, and the method for gathering information are directed at a different outcome.
- The inpatient consultation is also limited by the time available to the clinician to gather information and make an intervention as well as the psychological availability of a patient in the midst of an acute medical or pain crisis.
- The manner in which the attending or consulting pain specialist introduces the assessment and its purpose to the patient will have a direct impact on the quality of the psychologist's evaluation and intervention as well as the manner in which it will be conducted.
- The naïve patient may meet the clinician with openness, if not also a little surprise, curiosity, and a cooperative attitude. On the other hand, many patients see the very presence of a psychologist as an explicit declaration that their pain does not have a basis in physical injury or dysfunction but rather is a consequence of their emotional or mental life.
- Some patients chronically violate customary doctor–patient or office–patient boundaries. When this occurs, the consultant will be able to provide explicit direction to the team about how to interact with the patient so that treatment objectives may be advanced.
- Box 17.1 and Box 17.2 present important tips for referring physicians and consultants.

Introduction

The psychological consultation of a chronic pain patient in an acute care inpatient setting is different in essential ways from the outpatient psychological assessment. Its underlying assumptions, goals, and the method for gathering information are directed at a different outcome. The inpatient consultation is also limited by the time available to the clinician to gather information and make an intervention as well as the psychological availability of a patient in the midst of an acute medical or pain crisis.

In the current healthcare climate there is great pressure placed on physicians to minimize the number of days a patient remains in the hospital. For this reason, the patient is discharged to a less intense medical setting as soon as possible—and often this effectively ends the clinician's opportunity to contribute to the patient's care. Although this creates challenges for the clinician, there are still opportunities to provide useful assessments and interventions.

The following comments are meant to serve as suggestions for clinicians working in an acute inpatient medical setting. The conditions of this particular setting call for a kind of hybrid assessment of the patient suffering with pain that cannot be as in-depth as a multisession outpatient assessment complete with psychological testing. Nonetheless, it can be a very useful tool to assist the attending physician in his or her treatment of a patient.

The Evaluation

The psychological evaluation and assessment begins before the patient and the psychologist ever meet. That is to say, the manner in which the attending or consulting pain specialist introduces the assessment and its purpose to the patient will have a direct impact on the quality of the psychologist's evaluation and intervention as well as the manner in which it will be conducted. For instance, sometimes a patient is not told that a psychologist is being consulted. When this occurs, the psychologist walking into a naïve patient's room to begin the consultation has particular rapport-building tasks that the forewarned patient does not require. The naïve patient may meet the clinician with openness, if not also a little surprise, curiosity, and a cooperative attitude. On the other hand, many patients see the very presence of a psychologist as an explicit declaration that their pain does not have a basis in physical injury or dysfunction but rather is a consequence of their emotional or mental life. When this is the case, patients are sometimes offended and often meet the psychologist with a defensive posture that can preclude disclosure of whatever the patient thinks the interviewer will perceive as an emotional vulnerability or weakness. Spontaneous revelations of factors that might have a bearing on the felt experience or exacerbation of their pain, or even that may offer an avenue for a later beneficial intervention, become less likely in this scenario. In more extreme cases, the failure to discuss a psychological intervention with the patient prior to the arrival of the psychologist sets the stage for covert and sometimes overt hostility directed at the physician who placed the consultation or at the psychologist trying to conduct the consultation.

Of course, when the referring physician has taken the time to discuss his or her assessment and treatment strategy with the patient and has explained the rationale for consulting a psychologist, the arrival of the psychologist in the patient's room is expected and does not catch the patient off-guard. However, there are better and worse ways of introducing the role of the psychologist in the treatment of the patient. The referring physician should never imply that the psychologist is going to eliminate the patient's pain. If the physician is able to explain, in a succinct and clear manner, the biopsychosocial model of treatment[1] and describe how psychological factors can play an important role in the pain experience, this could prepare the patient well for the later assessment and intervention. If the physician does not have the time or the ability to do this it may be better not to try. Rather, the physician could simply acknowledge that the pain itself can be an overwhelming and stressful experience and would like the help of the psychologist to guide him or her in the development of a treatment plan and to help the patient manage the burden of chronic pain. Needless to say, the referring physician should never implicitly or explicitly communicate the belief that the patient is inventing the pain, or malingering, is mentally unbalanced, or that the pain is "all in his head."

Regardless of how the referring physician introduces the psychological consultation, the psychologist still has to accomplish a great deal in a short amount of time. Indeed, as just noted, there is great pressure to shorten the length of stay of patients, and because of this the psychologist may only have one session to contribute to the patient's treatment. In this short amount of time the psychologist must build rapport, justify his or her presence, gather information, develop a treatment plan, and, if possible, actually begin treatment.

With regard to building rapport it is advised that the consultant present him- or herself in a friendly, relaxed manner and to do all that is possible to put the patient at ease. Casual conversation about immediate events (e.g., the quality of the patient's meal if the meal tray is evident) can create an atmosphere that is nonthreatening and can ease the transition into the actual consultation. Permission should also be asked for and granted before proceeding with formal questioning, as well as overt consent to ask personal questions. As an illustration, I introduce myself to patients as follows: "Your physician is aware that you have been going through a lot lately and he thought that maybe I would be able to contribute something to your care. I told him that I wouldn't know that until I met you and we had a chance to talk. Would it be alright with you if I asked you a few questions to get to know you as well as some questions about your illness and treatment? Is this an ok time to do that?" In this example, the rationale for the interview has been established, permission to interview has been requested, and emphasis has been placed on the patient's suffering and the search for relief. The perceptive consultant will be alert to the patient's manner of greeting and receiving him or her as a possible indication of receptivity to later psychological questions or interventions or an indication of where work may need to be done.

As an aside, the setting in which the consult is conducted is very often less than ideal. It is likely that the patient will not be in a private room and that the roommate may be able to hear the questions and answers of the interview. Or the patient's roommate may have visitors, or be loud, or be in the midst of an interview by another medical specialist. It is common for there to be many interruptions during the course of the interview. Nurses may come and go providing the patient with scheduled medications, aides may arrive to collect vitals, other consultants may enter the room to do their consultations, a hospital chaplain or the patient's pastor may arrive for a visit, or the patient's family and friends could appear just as the psychologist is in the midst of the interview. All of these interruptions must be managed in a way that is respectful of the patient and visitors, preserves the patient's privacy, and advances the purpose and effectiveness of the consultation. In some cases, the business and commotion in the patient's room which, at first glance, might seem to be a hindrance to good assessment may just as easily serve as an in vivo demonstration of the patient's response to routine challenges and stressors.

The initial portion of the interview is usually focused on gathering general demographic data. Starting here allows for a smooth and natural transition into the particulars of the patient's illness and experience of pain. During this exchange the patient's manner of answering questions is likely to provide strong hints to later receptivity to a referral to a psychologist and overtly psychological interventions in the management of the pain.

Knowing the end goal of the consultation enables the psychologist to guide the interview in an effective and efficient manner. When the consultation is complete the psychologist should have a reasonably clear understanding of the patient's experience of his or her illness and pain, the history of both medical and psychological interventions as well as their outcome, and opportunities for further intervention. The psychologist should be able to comment on the presence of overt mental illness in the patient, his or her expectations, the patient's own understanding of his or her condition and treatment options, social or psychological factors contributing to the patient's pain experience, patient assets and strengths relative to capacity to endure the pain and to participate in treatment, personal traits that could complicate treatment, and the patient's acute attitude toward, and interest in, psychological interventions.

Obstacles to Psychological Treatment

At times there are hidden, intentional, or unintentional secondary reinforcers of pain behaviors. An effective consultation will be able to identify these when present and to discern their contribution to the patient's experience. Patients often enter into an illness with assumptions, often unexamined, about health-care and human suffering. For instance, many patients believe that there is a cure for all medical conditions—as in, "Don't tell me that we can put a man on the moon but we don't know how to fix this pain. I don't believe it. Somebody needs to try harder." Some patients believe that their physician is ineffective because he or she lacks compassion— as in, "If he had this pain himself he sure as hell would find some way to fix it." Implicit in both of these expectations is an essential lack of trust that all is being done that can be done. Unfortunately, this lack of trust makes any psychological intervention that requires the patient to pursue a treatment strategy that is not immediately face valid, easily under-stood, or worse, appears paradoxical or counterproductive all the more difficult.

Culturally, we are bombarded with pharmaceutical advertisements that, when taken collectively, imply that there is a pill for anything that ails us. Many patients carry the expectation that, if there is not a pill to fix them, then surely there is surgery. Curiously, this belief can be maintained by patients who have undergone numerous surgeries with minimal improvement and some-times worsening of their chronic pain. Alternatively, the idea, for instance, that physical activity could play an essential (and sometimes even curative) role in a patient's chronic pain is often received with great skepticism if not outright rejection. This is so even in the face of much research demonstrating the value of functional restoration programs in recovery from chronic pain.

Fear and catastrophic beliefs play hugely complicating roles in the patient's experience of chronic pain and the clinician's treatment of it must attend to these if they are present.[1] The characteristic arousal profile of overt fear and the stress response worsen one's response to the prospect of pain and can serve to trap the patient in a cycle of catastrophic fear, avoidance of movement, debility, and persistent pain.[2,3] Fear often serves as a hindrance to the pursuit of anything that may alter the patient's current treatment regimen—especially when the new treatment strategy may involve the loss of a treasured medication. Finally, the suggestion that there may be no cure for their pain and that acceptance of it and learning to live their life around it may be the goals of treatment can be very difficult for a patient to accept. There should be nothing surprising in this as it is almost a modern heresy to suggest that some of life's physical discomforts cannot be avoided.

Of course, it is highly unlikely that any clinician is going to be able to assess and successfully challenge all of these personal and cultural expectations in one or two inpatient encounters. Rather, the successful inpatient consultation will proceed in such a way that the patient's curiosity is piqued and interest is generated in alternatives to the current treatment regimen. Ideally, the patient's encounter with the psychologist will have been instructive and therapeutic. When the interaction during the consultation is marked by respect for the patient, genuine curiosity of the clinician for the patient's experience, compassion, and authentic interest in working to better the patient's condition, the patient is likely to be motivated to pursue more of the same. After all, if you are a patient in pain, what's not to like about a pain professional expressing an avid interest in your welfare and by example modeling hope for improvement?

Preparation for the Future

The consulting psychologist is, either explicitly or implicitly, a member of a treatment team. As such he or she has a particular role to play with regard to that team. In addition to the tasks mentioned previously, the psychologist should be preparing the patient for work with another psychologist or similar clinician—if the consulting psychologist does not have an outpatient practice. If the patient's encounter with the inpatient consultant was positive and inspired hope for improvement together with the dawning realization that he or she will improve fastest when taking an active role in his or her own care, the treatment team's work is made easier and the outpatient psychologist will receive a patient ready to work. If the pain specialist would like to engage the patient in a conversation about altering the medication regimen it is likely to proceed more productively when the patient perceives the specialist and the rest of his or her team as supportive and genuinely trying hard to improve control of the patient's pain. The time and the quality of the interaction that the consultant has with the patient set the stage for future problem-solving dialogues by modeling, in the behavior and manner of the consultant during the interview, an open, nonjudgmental, nonthreatening investigation into the patient's pain dilemma.

It is almost always the case that a request for a psychological consultation signals that the conventional forms of treatment already applied to the patient's pain have been unsatisfactory to the patient or to the treatment team. Side effects from medications, ineffective medications, complaints by family members that their loved one is too sedated or has had negative changes in personality, and debilitation by surgery or medication are all commonly reported. It is hoped that the psychological consultation will provide the treatment team such insight into the patient that alternative and more effective treatment strategies tailored to this particular patient with this specific constellation of physical and psychological dynamics will become possible. To this end, the consultant's findings should give some new direction to the current ineffective interventions being used.

In order for this to be possible it becomes the task of the consultant, although an admittedly difficult one, to prepare the patient for alternatives to the usual forms of intervention (e.g., surgery, opiates, benzodiazepines) that characterized treatment prior to this consultation. In a peculiar twist, the consultant must instigate a kind of rebellious attitude in the patient toward standard treatment as he or she has known it so that the patient begins to inquire about alternatives to the usual fare. No treatment comes without costs and side effects. Medications, surgical interventions, implantable devices, herbs, potions, physical therapy, and psychological interventions all have their intended and unintended effects. Even no treatment will have overt and covert consequences for the patient. If the consultant is able to trigger thoughtful reflection by the patient on the total cost to him or her of his treatment strategy and to compare this to its actual outcome, the treatment will now have an engaged and, hopefully, a motivated patient interested in trying alternative therapies. It is not likely that the psychologist will be able to identify an exact, perfectly tailored alternative treatment in one or two encounters with the patient. Nonetheless, the consultant's role is to till the earth and plant a few seeds that will bear fruit in future encounters with the rest of the treatment team. To facilitate such an attitudinal shift in a patient is no small task, but, when accomplished, new opportunities for treatment and an improvement in quality of life become possible.

In addition to the work that the consultant does with the patient directly, his or her interview can provide new direction to the treatment team. No chronic pain patient requiring a psychological consultation has an easy-to-treat condition. The usual common methods have been tried and have been found wanting. Sometimes, this is because of psychological factors unique to the patient. When this is the case, the consultant's report can provide the team with a better understanding of possible obstacles to the current regimen's effectiveness. For instance, some patients present with fully realized personality disorders or just features of personality disorders. When this is the case, the consultant can advise the team with regard to their behavior with the patient. Some patients chronically violate customary doctor–patient or office–patient boundaries. When this occurs, the consultant can provide explicit direction to the team about how to interact with the patient so that treatment objectives may be advanced.

Limitations of Psychological Consultation

As already noted, the inpatient consultation is limited by time and setting. Furthermore, the very nature of the presenting problem poses challenges for the consultant. As noted by Bouckoms and Hackett (1991) years ago:

Trying to separate functional from organic factors in long-standing pain is both vexing and unprofitable. Nevertheless, it is a task all too frequently requested.[4]

Pain is not simple. For the observer it is always a subjective phenomenon. When my neighbor hits his thumb with his hammer, I cannot feel his pain. But for my neighbor the pain is as objective and real a phenomenon as he has ever known. This murky region of assessment and treatment, combining both objective and subjective characteristics into a condition causing such great suffering, requires a humble attitude on the part of the consultant. Whereas there are many clinically meaningful contributions that the consultant may make to the patient's care, the consultant should always be wary of assuming that he or she fully "understands" the nature of the patient's pain or knows "what the patient needs." Any recommendations that the consultant offers should be made with the full realization that things are not always as they seem and that however clear the problem and its solution may seem, the treatment plan proposed is always subject to change.

Summary

It is almost always the case that a request for a psychological consultation signals that the conventional forms of treatment already applied to the patient's pain have been unsatisfactory to the patient or the treatment team. Box 17.1 and Box 17.2 present important tips for referring physicians and hospital psychology consultants.

Box 17.1 **Tips for Referring Physicians**

- Do tell the patient that a psychological consultation is being requested.
- Do tell the patient why the consultation is expected and how it is likely to benefit the patient.
- Emphasize that the consultant is a valued member of your treatment team but not the last word.
- Do not communicate to the patient in word, deed, attitude, or tone of voice that the consultation is being requested because "nothing more can be done."
- Tell the consultant why a consultation is being requested now.
- Articulate an answerable question. Ask yourself what should be in the completed consultation that will convince you that asking for a psychological consultation was a good idea. Being able to do this will help clarify the referring question.

Box 17.2 **Tips for Consultants**

- Take the time necessary to establish rapport.
- Identify the purpose of the consultation and what you hope to accomplish during your time with the patient.
- Know the question that the completed consultation is expected to answer.
- Remember that the consultant is, ultimately, an advocate for the patient's welfare. The presence of this attitude is likely to increase the patient's trust of the clinician and therefore improve the quality and quantity of the patient's disclosure.
- Demonstrate genuine interest in the patient and authentic concern for the patient's suffering.
- Remember that the consultation itself is a brief intervention as well as an introduction to future psychological treatment.
- Avoid psychological jargon in the written report and speak clearly and directly to the referring question.
- Provide concrete recommendations for treatment and, if necessary, specify who will follow through with the next phase of treatment or further assessment.

References

1. Turk DC, Monarch ES. Biopsychosocial perspective on chronic pain. In Turk DC, Gatchel RJ, eds., *Psychological Approaches to Pain Management*, 2nd ed. New York: Guilford Press; 2002:3–29.
2. Vlaeyen JW, Linton SJ. Fear-avoidance and its consequences in chronic musculoskeletal pain: a state of the art. *Pain*. 2000;85:317–332.
3. Vlaeyen JW, Linton SJ. Fear-avoidance model of chronic musculoskeletal pain: 12 years on. *Pain*. 2012;153(6):1144–1147.
4. Bouckoms A, Hackett TP. The pain patient: evaluation and treatment. In Cassem NH, ed., *Handbook of General Psychiatry*, 3rd ed. St. Louis: Mosby Year Book; 1991:39–68.

18

Physical Medicine and Rehabilitation Consultation of the Inpatient with Chronic Pain

DANIELLE SARNO, STEFAN C. MUZIN, JOSEPH WALKER III,

AND SUSAN M. LUDWIG

KEY POINTS

- Early inpatient rehabilitation consultation and therapy for patients with chronic pain are associated with improved patient outcomes and satisfaction as well as overall cost savings.
- Physiatrists specialize in nonsurgical treatment of nerve, muscle, and bone disorders for decreasing pain and restoring function. Physiatric consultation is instrumental for assessment of patients with chronic pain in the acute care setting and for coordination of the multidisciplinary rehabilitation team.
- Understanding of specific factors associated with physical impairment, disability, and handicap is helpful in determining the level of required rehabilitation services, the barriers to providing these services, and strategies for reducing these barriers.

Introduction

With advances in medicine and technology, people are living longer with chronic and complex medical issues and are utilizing more healthcare resources. Every day, 10,000 individuals turn 65[1]—by 2030, there will be an estimated 80 million people over the age of 65. In this age group, there is a 50% prevalence of multimorbidity (greater or equal to two chronic conditions), which is associated with decreased functional status, greater symptom burden, and increased healthcare costs.

Physical medicine and rehabilitation physicians, or physiatrists, specialize in nonsurgical treatment of nerve, muscle, and bone disorders for decreasing pain and restoring function. The unique physiatric approach to patient care is a multidisciplinary one, treating the whole person and not just one symptom or condition. The physiatrist takes a lead role in implementing a plan of care to facilitate the patient's medical and functional recovery. Very often, this involves collaboration with a team of medical professionals, which can include neurologists, orthopedic surgeons, nurses, physical therapists, occupational therapists, speech and language pathologists, and case managers.

By providing pain management and a plan of care for the individual as a whole, rehabilitation medicine is a valuable resource in the inpatient setting. Potential benefits of consulting physiatry in acute care service include earlier access to treatment by physical and occupational therapists, early screening/ diagnosis of other medical comorbidities, appropriate patient disposition, decreased length of stay, fewer medical complications, decreased readmission rates, greater patient satisfaction, decreased long-term insurance costs, and development of a long-term plan to maximize function and improve quality of life.

The physiatrist's role is very important in acute care settings. In addition to the variety of medical comorbidities managed throughout the rehabilitation process, pain is a significant factor to be addressed. Pain is associated with many injuries and diseases and is sometimes the disease itself. Pain may arise from a particular etiology, such as postoperative pain or pain associated with a malignancy, or pain may be the primary problem or diagnosis.

Millions of people suffer from acute or chronic pain, resulting in increased healthcare costs for treatment and decreased worker productivity. In addition, patients and their families experience significant emotional and financial burdens due to pain.[2] Suboptimal pain management can result in longer hospital stays, increased rates of rehospitalization, increased outpatient visits, and decreased ability to function. According to the Institute of Medicine report, "Relieving Pain in America: A Blueprint for Transforming Prevention, Care, Education, and Research," pain is a significant public health problem that costs society at least $560–$635 billion annually.[3] This includes the total incremental cost of healthcare due to pain, ranging from $261 to $300 billion, and lost productivity (based on days of work missed, hours of work lost, and lower wages), estimated at $297 to $336 billion.[3]

It is important to understand the difference between acute and chronic pain. According to the American Academy of Pain Medicine, *acute pain* is a normal sensation triggered in the nervous system to alert a person to possible injury and the need to take care of oneself.[2] *Chronic pain* is persistent, with pain signals firing in the nervous system for weeks, months, or even years. Although there usually is an initial inciting event, some people suffer from chronic pain in the absence of any past injury or evidence of body damage.[2]

Chronic pain itself can become the main diagnosis as well as the impairment. The pain typically persists despite medical and surgical treatment. Chronic pain can interfere with physical, vocational, and/or psychological functioning.[4] As chronic pain often leads to decreased sleep, appetite, and decreased physical and social activities, there is a strong association with frailty, negatively affecting functional status and quality of life.[5] Furthermore, chronic pain has been shown to be a cause of poor self-rated health[6] and associated with impairment of activities of daily living (ADL).[7]

Chronic pain often involves headache, low back pain, cancer pain, arthritis, or neurogenic pain (resulting from damage to the peripheral nerves or to the central nervous system itself). More than 1.5 billion people worldwide suffer from chronic pain, and approximately 3%–4.5% of the global population suffers from neuropathic pain, with incidence rate increasing with age.[2] Chronic pain affects more Americans than diabetes, heart disease, and cancer combined. At least 100 million Americans are affected by chronic pain alone.[2] Table 18.1 depicts the number of chronic pain sufferers compared to other major health conditions.[2]

Impairment and Disability

The terms *impairment, disability*, and *handicap* often are used interchangeably. However, the differences in meaning are important for understanding the rehabilitation plan and goals in the treatment of chronic pain. The most commonly cited definitions are those provided by the World Health Organization in The International Classification of Impairments, Disabilities, and Handicaps.[8]

Impairment is defined as any loss or abnormality of psychological, physiological, or anatomical structure or function that is due to an underlying diagnosis.[8] *Disability* is defined as any restriction of ability to perform an activity in the manner or within the range considered normal for a human being that results from impairment.[8] *Handicap* refers to a disadvantage, due to a disability, for a given individual that limits or prevents fulfillment of a role in society.[8]

Disability is an umbrella term, covering impairments, activity limitations, and participation restrictions.[9] An activity limitation is a difficulty encountered by an individual in executing a task or action, while a participation restriction is a problem experienced by an individual that is related to involvement in life situations.[9] In this way, disability reflects the interaction between features of a person's body and features of the society in which he or she lives.[9] Overcoming the difficulties faced by people with disabilities requires interventions to adjust environmental and social barriers.

Table 18.1 **Number of Americans with Chronic Pain Compared to Other Major Health Conditions**

Condition	Number of Sufferers	Source
Chronic pain	100 million Americans	Institute of Medicine of the National Academies*
Diabetes	25.8 million Americans (diagnosed and estimated undiagnosed)	American Diabetes Association†
Coronary heart disease	16.3 million Americans	American Heart Association‡
Stroke	7 million Americans	
Cancer	11.9 million Americans	American Cancer Society**

*Institute of Medicine Report from the Committee on Advancing Pain Research, Care, and Education. *Relieving Pain in America, A Blueprint for Transforming Prevention, Care, Education and Research*. Washington, DC: National Academies Press; 2011.

http://books.nap.edu/openbook.php?record_id=13172&page=1.

†American Diabetes Association.

http://www.diabetes.org/diabetes-basics/diabetes-statistics/

‡Heart Disease and Stroke Statistics—2011 Update: A Report From the American Heart Association. *Circulation*. 2011;123:e18–e209, p. 20.

http://circ.ahajournals.org/content/123/4/e18.full.pdf

**American Cancer Society. Prevalence of Cancer.

http://www.cancer.org/docroot/CRI/content/CRI_2_6x_Cancer_Prevalence_How_Many_People_Have_Cancer.asp

Determining Level of Services

For patients with chronic pain on an inpatient service, these concepts are factored into determining goals of treatment for physical/occupational therapy and can guide post–acute care discharge planning. The physiatrist evaluates patients for appropriate discharge planning from the acute care setting, taking the following four options into consideration: (1) admission to an acute inpatient rehabilitation facility (IRF); (2) admission to a skilled nursing facility (SNF) or subacute rehabilitation facility; (3) discharge to home with home services; or 4) discharge to home without home services, with or without outpatient rehabilitation.

The more functionally independent the patient, the fewer services that are needed. Admission to an acute IRF may be considered appropriate when a patient is expected to achieve significant functional improvement in a reasonable amount of time, measured against his or her condition at the start of the rehabilitation program. In general, the following criteria are usually required for IRF admission:

1. The patient must need active therapeutic intervention of multiple therapy disciplines, including physical therapy and occupational therapy. Speech-language pathology and/or prosthetics/orthotics therapy may be needed.
2. The patient must be able to tolerate at least 3 hours of therapy per day, at least 5 days per week.
3. The patient must be medically able and psychologically willing to actively participate in the intensive rehabilitation therapy program at the time of admission to the IRF. Functional gains are measured and should be attained within a prescribed period of time.

The differences between an acute inpatient rehabilitation facility and a skilled nursing facility are outlined in Table 18.2.

Barriers to Providing Services

As previously described, early implementation of rehabilitation therapy in the acute care setting is beneficial for patients with chronic pain. Unfortunately, several barriers to quality care exist, including increasing cost and limited rehabilitation staff resources.

The cost of care is an enormous obstacle in the management of patients with chronic pain given the financial burden for and emotional toll on patients and their families. One analysis revealed that in 2008, the annual economic cost for management of chronic pain in the United States was $635 billion.[3] Medicare covered one-fourth of this cost, comprising 14% of medical expenditures in that year. Combined state and federal programs, including Medicaid, Medicare, the Department of Veterans Affairs, and other government programs, spent $99 billion in 2008 for expenditures related to treating chronic pain.[3] This does not include loss of tax revenue related to decreased productivity, further adding to the expense.[10] Lost productive time from common painful conditions was estimated to be $61.2 billion per year, while 76.6% of lost productive time was due to reduced work performance, not absenteeism.[2]

Another potential barrier to early initiation of rehabilitation therapy in the acute care setting is the patient's perception and/or fear that early physical mobilization will increase pain. This fear may be validated if the patient experiences moderate to severe pain during rehabilitation therapy, which could be a result of inadequate pain medication prior to treatment. This experience may negatively impact the patient's motivation to continue with the rehabilitation treatment regimen. Furthermore, a healthcare provider may underestimate the amount of pain expected during therapy and fear prescribing opioid analgesics due to regulatory constraints or concerns about development of dependence, tolerance, and/or adverse effects.[11] When healthcare providers underassess and

Table 18.2 **Differences between an Acute Inpatient Rehabilitation Facility and a Skilled Nursing Facility**

Services	Typical IRF	Typical SNF
Physician visits	Daily	1 to 3 times per week
Type of physician	Physiatrist—24-hour availability	Geriatrician, internist, family practitioner—limited availability
Consultants	All specialties readily available	Limited specialist availability
Nursing hours of care	5.5 and higher hours per day primarily RNs; 24-hour availability	2–3 hours daily, primarily CNAs
Function	Complex level of care Patient and family education	Basic level of care
Integration of care	Coordinated multidisciplinary team directed by physician	Several individual disciplines
Typical length of stay	10–35 days, depending on diagnosis	24–60 days
Therapy intensity	3–5 hours daily	1–2 hours daily
Team meetings	A coordinated multidisciplinary team meeting led by physician and includes family	Several individual disciplines
Neuropsychologists	Full-time	Limited
Physical therapy and occupational therapy	Registered physical (PT) and occupational (OT) therapists	Certified PT and OT assistants and aides deliver much of the care
Audiologist, therapeutic recreation, social worker	Full-time	Limited
Speech language therapist	Full-time	Limited
Accreditation	JCAHO and CARF	None

CAN, certified nursing assistant; IRF, inpatient rehabilitation facility; SNF, skilled nursing facility.

undertreat pain, severe pain may prevent a patient from leaving his or her bed, leading to further deconditioning.

In addition, a patient may have medical comorbidities and/or physical or mental limitations precluding full participation in a standard rehabilitation therapy program. For example, a patient may have advanced heart or lung disease, or obesity, along with an associated decrease in exercise tolerance. Rehabilitation therapy needs to be modified in these circumstances for patient safety. Patients may also be depressed, lack interest or motivation, or be unaware of the advantages associated with early physical mobilization. Other possible barriers include family refusal, short hospital stays, and the inability of providers to identify patients who would benefit from rehabilitation therapy.

Strategies for Reducing Barriers

For effective rehabilitation involving patients with chronic pain, adequate control of incident and breakthrough pain is important. *Incident pain* is pain occurring as a direct and immediate consequence of a movement or activity. Understanding the barriers to managing incident pain can help the physician provide appropriate pain management prior to rehabilitation therapy. For example, the opioid dosage needed for incident pain may far exceed the dosage needed for background pain control and effective premedication before activity may be time consuming. An ideal analgesic to treat incident pain is one that is easily administered, has a rapid onset, and has a short duration of action. Therefore, a short-acting analgesic may be administered prior to rehabilitation therapy to obtain maximum benefit.

Breakthrough pain (BTP) is severe pain of rapid onset that can be disabling or even immobilizing.[12] Patients with BTP should be assessed after baseline persistent pain has been stabilized with around-the-clock (ATC) analgesics. A patient's history, including a pain diary, may provide clues about the cause and pattern of BTP. Effective treatment can greatly improve the patient's quality of life and should be tailored for each patient, taking into consideration the cause and type of BTP episodes.[12] Short-acting opioid analgesics are the primary treatment for BTP. The dose and/or dosing frequency of the ATC analgesic should be adjusted for patients with end-of-dose BTP. Short-acting oral opioids are useful when given prophylactically in patients with predictable incident BTP, while rapid-onset transmucosal lipophilic opioids are most effective for patients with unpredictable incident or idiopathic BTP. Use of non-opioid adjuvant pain medications should be considered, as they can decrease the need for opioids and help manage pain. For example, NSAIDs, anxiolytics, tricyclic antidepressants, and neuropathic medications are indicated for various diagnoses.

In addition, nonpharmacological strategies often are helpful in alleviating pain and anxiety and should be used to supplement pharmacological intervention for BTP.[12] Nonpharmacological options to consider for pain control include transcutaneous electrical nerve stimulation (TENS), heat, ice, ultrasound, acupuncture, therapeutic exercise, soft tissue mobilization, as well as other modalities and manual therapies.[12]

As common side effects of opioid medications include nausea and constipation, it is important to keep nausea and bowel management in mind for effective rehabilitation therapy. For nausea management, one should consider prophylactic intervention and choose appropriate medication based on the cause (e.g., gastric stasis or chemoreceptor trigger zone mediated).[13] For bowel management, a peristaltic laxative is useful whenever opioids are ordered and should be initiated at the same time as the opioid.

Other strategies used to minimize barriers to effective rehabilitation include recognizing coexisting medical issues, consulting other services as needed, providing a support system, tailoring rehabilitation therapy specific to the individual's needs, and discussing available post-discharge resources for continued rehabilitation.

As the patient is preparing for discharge from the hospital, it is important to provide information about available community resources for further rehabilitation. For example, the patient may be referred to outpatient exercise programs, depending on the diagnosis. Self-management programs (e.g., arthritis self-help program) are evidence based, although few older adults take these courses. Cognitive-behavioral therapy (CBT) is also evidence based, but there is a lack of providers skilled in delivering CBT.[14,15] An example of translating effective interventions into practice and reaching more individuals with pain is an adapted exercise program for seniors with back pain, implemented in 10 New York City senior centers.[16] This intervention was associated with clinically significant reductions in pain and pain-related disability and improved self-efficacy to manage pain.[16] The program has continued at most of the centers and could be translated to the inpatient setting for patients with chronic back pain.

Benefits of Early Physiatric Intervention

Earlier involvement of rehabilitation services for patients with chronic pain may lead to cost savings within our healthcare system. Back pain is a huge burden on society, as the direct costs may be as high as $90 billion per year in the United States; the personal suffering and indirect impact on the patient, family, and society are even greater.[17] Therefore, development of efficient and effective systems of care around the primary care–physiatrist–surgeon axis could be an important strategy for reducing costs and suffering. In a prospective study, Fox et al. sought to determine whether an insurer rule requiring physiatrist consultation before non-urgent surgical consultation would affect surgery referrals and surgery rates.[17] Priority Health, a major health plan in Western Michigan, created a Spine Centers of Excellence program to reduce surgical costs and the total number of spine surgical procedures in its patient population.[17] The development of the program was based on previous studies demonstrating the following: for many types of back and neck pain, outcomes for nonoperative care are comparable to those with surgery; implementation of multidisciplinary spine centers has been shown to reduce surgery rates; and patients fully informed of all their treatment options tend to choose more conservative treatment than when surgeons are the decision-makers.[17] In another study, Deyo and Diehl demonstrated a 22% reduction in surgery rates when patients used shared decision-making tools that explored all treatment options available for the condition being treated.[18] Priority Health's Spine Centers of Excellence program also supported the Triple Aim goals of the Institute for Healthcare Improvement to (1) improve the health of the population, (2) enhance the patient experience of care (including quality, access, and reliability), and (3) reduce, or at least control, the per capita cost of care.[17]

Physiatrists were chosen to lead the Spine Centers of Excellence because of their broad-based experience and expertise. During their training, physiatrists gain experience in management of spinal disorders and obtain pertinent core competencies and skills that are not part of either surgical or primary care training.[17] These skills may include electrodiagnostic testing, manual medicine diagnostics and treatment, and spinal injections. Physiatrists are also trained in leading multidisciplinary evaluation and treatment teams and in management of patients' return to work and activity despite impairment. Given their unique training and perspectives and the evidence supporting physiatric intervention, it was thought that a physiatrist-led approach would provide an evidence-based alternative to the surgeon-first approach prevalent in the region of Western Michigan.[17] In the 12 months after implementation, total spine care costs decreased by 12.1% and surgical costs decreased 25.1%, representing a net decrease of more than $14 million in 1 year.[17]

Thus, Priority Health's policy, which required a physiatrist consultation before surgery, significantly reduced surgery rates and costs.[17] The authors concluded that results from changes across multiple hospital service areas in a wide region of a state are not due to some individual clinician or group but instead can be generalized across communities, hospitals, and practices. This particular study demonstrated that a required physiatrist consultation for elective spine surgery radically decreased the operative rate while maintaining patient satisfaction across a large region.[17] Although experiences might be different in other settings, policies such as this one have the potential to improve spine care and decrease cost.

Physiatrists offer an expert intermediate step that provides alternative choices and highlights the importance of shared decision-making.[17] Physiatric consultation may give patients a more balanced understanding of their diagnosis, prognosis, and treatment options. The physiatrist may spend more time counseling patients about these issues and may uncover an alternative diagnosis, find treatable secondary musculoskeletal pain generators, and detect psychosocial factors that would make surgery inappropriate.[17] Finally, treatments resulting from the visit might be more successful than those provided initially by the primary care physician. The Fox et al. study looked only at actions and costs that could be measured from an insurance database. Potentially, the total cost savings related to less time off work, less litigation, and other factors likely were higher.[17] The authors theorized that this type of policy would have a similar or even greater positive effect on the workers' compensation and Medicare populations. Although this study took place in the outpatient setting, similar benefits of physiatric care in the inpatient setting are likely.

Another study indicated that use of endurance exercises was the most consistent predictor of better outcome in patients with spinal impairments.[19] This effect appeared in both the physical and emotional health dimensions. These results are consistent with the findings of Lindstrom et al., who found that a group of workers with low back pain who participated in an individualized exercise program that included some form of endurance exercise returned to work more quickly and had less long-term sick leave than a control group who did not have exercise instruction.[19] The findings also provide support for the Agency for Health Care Policy and Research's guideline for acute low back pain, which recommends endurance programs and low-stress aerobics. Inclusion of endurance exercises in a physical therapy regimen may convince patients to try physical activities they have avoided and may improve their aerobic capacity, allowing them to perform activities with less perceived exertion.[19] Endurance exercise also may reduce sensitivity to pain, increase blood flow to painful muscles, and increase endorphin levels. In addition to endurance exercise, other treatments, including manipulation or mobilization, strengthening exercises, and flexibility exercises, are related to better outcomes for patients with cervical impairments. These findings suggest use of a multimodal approach to physical therapy care for patients with cervical impairments.[19]

Deyo and Diehl studied similar disabilities as measured by the Sickness Impact Profile.[18] In all cases, patients with back pain demonstrated the greatest disability in role functioning. The physical functioning and pain scales for the SF-36 and SF-20 in these studies were also considerably lower than for the general population.[18] The authors concluded that individuals with vertebral impairments have decrements in both the physical and emotional dimensions of health, with pain being a major problem. Over a course of physical therapy, improvements in health occurred in nearly all areas for those with spinal pathology.[18]

The Physical Medicine and Rehabilitation Prescription

Rehabilitation prescriptions are based on physiatric medical and functional evaluations, noting the patient's diagnosis, relevant medical comorbidities, functional impairments, functional goals, frequency of treatment, and precautions. A physiatrist should perform the initial rehabilitation consultation in order to determine the appropriate therapeutic intervention with respect to the patient's medical condition. All rehabilitation therapy prescriptions must include the following components: (a) the patient's diagnosis (including relevant medical history); (b) precautions/parameters; (c) goals; (d) estimated length of therapy; (e) which disciplines are treating the patient; and (f) the prescriber's signature. In order to enhance physician supervision throughout the rehabilitation process and encourage physician–therapist communication, the prescription for rehabilitation therapy should be more detailed than "evaluation and treat." Examples of precautions include bleeding risk (e.g., if a patient is on Coumadin), orthostasis, cardiac (usually with parameters for heart rate and blood pressure), respiratory, skin conditions/wounds, deep vein thrombosis, safety/falls, and seizures. The physician-led team decides on therapeutic goals, which are objectives related to functional abilities. Rehabilitation therapy disciplines include physical therapy, occupational therapy, speech and language pathology, psychology, social services, recreational therapy, respiratory therapy, and case management.

Rehabilitation modalities are prescribed based upon the patient's initial physical status and are adjusted as functional gains and losses occur. In general, passive modalities are utilized initially as they are easier for a patient to tolerate. Active, self-powered therapy against gravity is more difficult and thus accomplishing active tasks is the goal of many rehabilitation mobility/pain programs. The gradation of therapeutic difficulty in both physical therapy (PT) and occupational therapy (OT) is noted in Figure 18.1. A sample of PT/OT prescription is presented in Appendix 18.1.

Summary

Early diagnosis and intervention among patients with chronic pain are critical to optimize patient outcomes. There are multiple benefits associated with early inpatient rehabilitation therapy, including improved patient outcomes and satisfaction and overall cost savings. Future directions in this area may include inpatient physiatry consultation on all chronic pain patients within 24 hours of admission. There also should be consideration of tele-rehabiliation medicine in areas with limited accessibility.

According to the World Health Organization, rehabilitation is an excellent investment because it builds human capacity.[9] It should be incorporated into

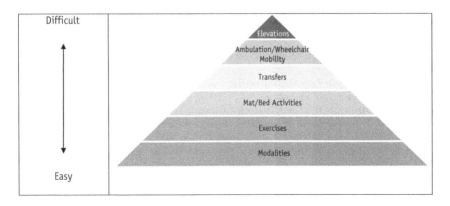

	PT	OT
Modalities	Ultrasound, Heat/Ice, Whirlpool, TENS	Paraffin, Hydrotherapy, Fluidotherapy, Heat/Ice
Exercises (isometric, isotonic, isokinetic)	Lower Extremity	Upper Extremity
Mat/Bed	Hi Level/Low Level	Bed Mobility
Transfers	Wheelchair to Mat, Sit to Stand	Functional Transfers (bed, tub, toilet)
Ambulation/Wheelchair Mobility		Equipment
Elevations/Advanced Wheelchair Skills		ADL evaluation and training

Figure 18.1 Gradation of therapeutic difficulty in both physical therapy (PT) and occupational therapy (OT).

general legislation on health, employment, education, and social services and into specific legislation for people with disabilities. Early intervention is important to carry out, as rehabilitation promotes functioning in people with a broad range of health conditions, including chronic pain. For established services, the focus should be on improving efficiency and effectiveness, by expanding coverage and improving quality and affordability.[9] Integrating rehabilitation into primary and secondary healthcare settings can improve availability of services. Referral systems between different modes of service delivery (inpatient, outpatient, home-based care) and levels of health service provision (primary, secondary, and tertiary care facilities) can improve access. Rehabilitation interventions delivered in communities are an important part of the continuum of care.

By shifting the focus from health condition to functioning, the International Classification of Functioning (ICF) places all health conditions on an equal footing, allowing them to be compared via a common framework.[8] Overall, patients and society will benefit when the focus of healthcare shifts to value function.[21]

References

1. Facts & Figures: Health in Aging Foundation. http://www.healthinagingfoundation.org/who-we-are/facts-figures/
2. American Academy of Pain Medicine—Get the Facts on Pain. http://www.painmed.org/PatientCenter/Facts_on_Pain.aspx
3. Institute of Medicine (US) Committee on Advancing Pain Research, Care, and Education. *Relieving Pain in America: A Blueprint for Transforming Prevention, Care, Education, and Research*. Washington, DC: National Academies Press; 2011.
4. Reid MC, Williams CS, Gill TM. Back pain and decline in lower extremity physical function among community-dwelling older persons. *J Gerontol A Biol Sci Med Sci.* 2005;60:793–797.
5. Blyth FM, Rochat S, Cumming RG, et al. Pain, frailty and comorbidity on older men: the CHAMP study. *Pain.* 2008;140:224–230.
6. Mäntyselkä PT, Turunen JHO, Ahonen RS, Kumpusalo EA. Chronic pain and poor self-rated health. *JAMA.* 2003;290:2435–2442.
7. Leveille SG, Fried L, Guralnik JM. Disabling symptoms: what do older women report? *J Gen Intern Med.* 2002;17:766–773.
8. Svestková O. International classification of functioning, disability and health of World Health Organization (ICF). *Prague Med Rep.* 2008;109:268–274.
9. World Health Organization. Disabilities. http://www.who.int/topics/disabilities/en/
10. Gatchel RJ, McGeary DD, McGeary CA, Lippe, B. Interdisciplinary chronic pain management: past, present, and future. *Am Psychol.* 69:119–130.
11. Rich BA. An ethical analysis of the barriers to effective pain management. *Camb Q Healthc Ethics.* 2000;9:54–70.
12. McCarberg BH. The treatment of breakthrough pain. *Pain Med.* 8(Suppl 1):S8–S13.
13. Carver AC, Foley KM, Management of cancer pain. In: Bast RC Jr, Kufe DW, Pollock RE, et al., eds., *Holland-Frei Cancer Medicine*, 5th ed. Hamilton, Ontario: BC Decker; 2000: Chapter 14.
14. Morley S, Eccleston C, Williams A. Systematic review and meta-analysis of randomized controlled trials of cognitive behaviour therapy and behaviour therapy for chronic pain in adults, excluding headache. *Pain.* 1999;80:1–13.
15. Lunde L-H, Nordhus IH, Pallesen S. The effectiveness of cognitive and behavioural treatment of chronic pain in the elderly: a quantitative review. *J Clin Psychol Med Settings.* 2009;16:254–262.
16. Beissner K, Parker SJ, Henderson CR Jr, et al. A cognitive-behavioral plus exercise intervention for older adults with chronic back pain: race/ethnicity effect? *J Aging Phys Act.* 2012;20:246–265.
17. Fox J, Haig AJ, Todey B, Challa S. The effect of required physiatrist consultation on surgery rates for back pain. *Spine (Phila. Pa. 1976).* 2013;38:E178–184.
18. Deyo RA, Diehl AK. Measuring physical and psychosocial function in patients with low-back pain. *Spine (Phila. Pa. 1976).* 1983;8:635–642.
19. Jette DU, Jette AM. Physical therapy and health outcomes in patients with spinal impairments. *Phys Ther.* 1996;76:930–941; discussion 942–945.
20. Bottemiller KL, Bieber PL, Basford JR, Harris M. FIM score, FIM efficiency, and discharge disposition following inpatient stroke rehabilitation. *Rehabil Nurs.* 2006;31:22–25.
21. AAPM&R—American Academy of Physical Medicine and Rehabilitation. http://www.aapmr.org/Pages/default.aspx.
22. Rehab Measures—Functional Independence Measure. http://www.rehabmeasures.org/Lists/RehabMeasures/DispForm.aspx?ID=889.

Appendix 18.1 Inpatient Rehabilitation Prescription Outline

Diagnosis/Impairment (including relevant medical history):	Psychological:
	Industrial Rehab:
Precautions:	Education:
Physical Therapy:	Social Services:
Occupational Therapy:	Recreational Therapy:
Speech Language Pathology (speech and/or swallow):	Signature:
Prevocational:	

Sample Prescriptions
A

Admitting Diagnosis/Impairment: Severe bilateral knee osteoarthritis status post bilateral total knee replacements on 6/11/14; history of hypertension.

Currently: FIM score 3.*

Discharge Goal: Independent with bed mobility and transfers, independent with ambulation ~100 feet, active range of motion 5–90 degrees.

Estimated length of stay (LOS): 2 weeks.

Precautions: bilateral knee surgical wounds; fall precautions; weight bear as tolerated (WBAT).**

Positioning: Elevation of legs when in bed; place pillow under the ankle, not the knee.

Occupational Therapy: 1 hour daily × 6 days per week

AROM/AAROM to bilateral upper extremities, general conditioning exercises for bilateral upper extremities, activities of daily living (ADL) evaluation and training, wheelchair management training, group activities, community skills outing when appropriate, family training, development of home exercise program.

Modalities: Ice as needed

Social Service: Discharge planning, family counseling, and evaluation for community resources.

(continued)

Sample Prescriptions (Continued)
A

Physical Therapy: 2.0 hours daily × 6 days per week	Recreational Therapy: Instruct in leisure education and recreation participation.

Active range of motion/active assist range of motion (AROM/AAROM) to bilateral lower extremities, mat activities, transfer training, standing/balance training, ambulation with assistive device as tolerated/gait training, endurance training, general conditioning exercises, ice as needed, group activities, wheelchair management and training, family training, development of home exercise program.

Pain: Transition to oral pain medications as tolerated; oxycodone-acetaminophen every 4 hours as needed (prn), Ice as needed.
Signature:

FIM Scoring Criteria [22]

Score	Description
7	Complete independence
6	Modified independence (patient requires use of a device, but no physical assistance)

Helper (Modified Dependence)

Score	Description
5	Supervision or setup
4	Minimal contact assistance (patient can perform 75% or more of task)
3	Moderate assistance (patient can perform 50% to 74% of task)

Helper (Complete Dependence)

Score	Description
2	Maximal assistance (patient can perform 25% to 49% of task)
1	Total assistance (patient can perform less than 25% of the task or requires more than one person to assist)
0	Activity does not occur

B

Assessment:	Right hip OA, status post right posterior total hip arthroplasty; severe pain
Impairments:	Currently, FIM score: 3
	Discharge goal is FIM score: 6. Estimated LOS is 3 weeks.
PT/OT consults for:	Strengthening, conditioning, ROM, functional mobility, balance, transfers, stairs, progressive gait training with assistive devices, posterior hip precautions reinforcement, ADL training, adaptive equipment and patient/family education.
Precautions:	Rest: Offer rest periods to optimize active participation in therapy.
Positioning:	If cemented total hip—weight bearing to tolerance (WBTT) with walker immediately after surgery, unless otherwise instructed by surgeon.
Pain:	If non-cemented total hip—limited (touch down or partial weight bearing depending on instruction of surgeon) for 6–8 weeks with walker.
	Position of instability for posterior dislocation - flexion + adduction + internal rotation (avoid)
	Position of instability for anterior dislocation - extension + adduction + external rotation (avoid)
	Abduction pillow—used while asleep or resting in bed for 5–6 weeks, up to 12 weeks. Discontinue use as per instruction by physician.
	Transition to oral pain medications, Percocet every 4–6 hours prn.

*The Functional Independence Measure (FIM) is a widely accepted scale used to measure the functional abilities of patients undergoing rehabilitation.[22]

**First-time knee replacement: weight bear as tolerated (WBAT); revision: 50% weight bearing for the first 6 weeks.

19

Integrative Medicine in Treatment
of Inpatients' Chronic Pain

JOSEPH WALKER III, ANDREE MAUREEN LEROY,

KRISTIANNE SEELYE, AND RICHARD RYNAKSI

KEY POINTS

- Integrative medicine, via mind–body practices, can introduce many adjuvant treatment benefits for chronic pain patients who are inpatients.
- Chronic pain has many disparate pathological threads, including symptomatic, sociological, and psychological ones, that the multidisciplinary nature of integrative medicine can help sew together.
- Some evidence-based integrative medicine treatment modalities, such as acupuncture, massage, and relaxation techniques, can help chronic pain patients in an inpatient environment.
- Integrative medicine may be used to address and treat aspects of pain that traditional medicine has difficulty addressing, such as stress responses to pain and the individual biopsychosocial impacts of the pain.
- Selection of a specific treatment modality within an integrative medicine approach should depend on an individual patient's needs.
- Selection of a specific treatment modality within an integrative medicine approach should be based on available validated evidence.
- There are relatively few contraindications for ordering and utilizing integrative modalities in an inpatient hospital-based setting.

Introduction

According to the National Center for Complementary and Alternative Medicine (NCCAM), 1 of the 27 institutes and centers that make up the National Institutes of Health (NIH) within the U.S. Department of Health and Human Services, in 2007, approximately 38% of U.S. adults aged 18 years and over and approximately 12% of children used some form of complementary and alternative medicine CAM.[1] In 2007, U.S. adults spent $33.9 billion out of pocket on visits to CAM practitioners and purchases of CAM products, classes, and materials.[2] Generally, CAM modalities are used in numerous subspecialties in medicine, most notably oncology and mental health. In these disciplines, optimal health delivery outcomes depend on addressing both the mental and physical components of the patient's concerns. This is also the case for optimally treating patients with chronic pain. In this context, treatment with pain medicine is also fertile ground for the incorporation of integrative medicine, especially while chronic pain patients are inpatients.

Conventional medicine is defined as the Nation Cancer Institute at the NIH as a system in which medical doctors and other healthcare professionals (such as nurses, pharmacists, and therapists) treat symptoms and diseases using drugs, radiation, or surgery. It is also called allopathic medicine, biomedicine, mainstream medicine, orthodox medicine, and Western medicine. *Complementary medicine* generally refers to using a non-mainstream approach together with conventional medicine. *Alternative medicine* refers to using a non-mainstream approach in place of conventional medicine. In general, true alternative medicine is not common. Most people use a combination of non-mainstream approaches along with conventional treatments. And the boundaries between complementary and conventional medicine overlap and change with time. Complementary approaches may become conventional approaches. For example, guided imagery and massage, once considered complementary or alternative, are used regularly in some hospitals to help with pain management. *Integrative medicine* as defined by the Consortium of Academic Health Centers for Integrative Medicine as the practice of medicine informed by evidence that focuses on the whole person by making use of all appropriate therapeutic approaches (conventional and nonconventional) to achieve optimal health and healing. In a team setting, various healthcare professionals and disciplines work together to achieve this goal (Figure 19.1).

Benefits of Integrative Medicine for Patients with Chronic Pain

Although there have been many therapeutic advances in the treatment of chronic pain, many patients with chronic pain become resistant to conventional medical treatments or suffer adverse effects from widely used prescription medications with high addictive potential, such as opiates or nonsteroidal anti-inflammatory agents. Patients may then turn to integrative medicine, which provides patient-centered care and addresses the full range of physical, emotional, mental, social, spiritual, and environmental influences that affect a person's health.[3]

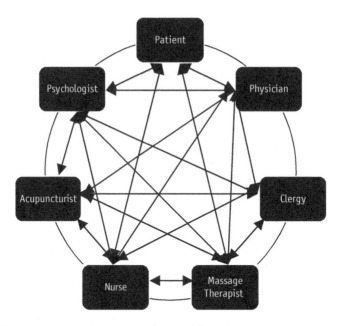

Figure 19.1 Integrative interconnectedness of disciplines.

Dusek et al., in their 2010 study, showed that inpatient integrative medicine had a significant impact on pain scores for hospitalized patients, reducing self-reported pain by more than 50%, without placing patients at increased risk for adverse effects.[4] The individual goals of a patient-focused integrative pain therapy approach vary yet may include the following[5]:

a) Empowering patients to actively participate in pain control strategies
b) Improving the ability to function physically and perform activities of daily living
c) Improving the ability to function in social and family roles
d) Improving understanding of the role of emotions, behavior, and attitudes in pain
e) Developing the skills and knowledge needed to increase the patient's sense of control over pain
f) Promoting awareness and understanding of the factors that contribute to physical and emotional distress related to pain
g) Reducing or eliminating pain
h) Using medicines that are appropriate, provide sustained benefits, have tolerable side effects, and support the functional goals of the patient
i) Reducing distress and enhancing comfort, peace of mind, and quality of life
j) Educating patients in ways to maintain rehabilitation gains and avoid re-injury
k) Supporting the patient's ability to return to work and function on the job

Dusek et al. also noted in their study that although most patients (66%) had never previously received integrative services, provision of integrative services had immediate and beneficial effects on pain scores.[4] Utilizing an individualized strategy that considers the patient's unique needs, circumstances, and situation, integrative medicine employs the most appropriate interventions from an array of scientific disciplines to heal illness and help people regain and maintain optimum health. When the patients are inpatients, complete change is unlikely to occur during the short inpatient time, but the seeds of change toward a whole health-positive outlook for the patient can begin with introduction of some complementary approaches in a team setting.

The NCCAM generally uses the term *complementary health approaches* when discussing the practices and products and divides the approaches as generally falling into one of two subgroups—natural products or mind–body practices. This chapter will use those terms as well, mainly focusing on mind–body practices. The goal of this chapter is to introduce a few of these complementary health approaches that may be conducive to integration into the inpatient treatment of chronic pain in patients.

Mind–Body Practice: Acupuncture

BACKGROUND

Acupuncture is widely known to date back thousands of years. The first records are from 100 years b.c.e. The written classic Chinese medicine handbook, *Yellow Emperor's Classic of Medicine*, also known as the "Huang Di Neijing," is the first indigenous writings to include acupuncture. The Neijing provides foundational and fundamental principles of acupuncture, whereby the human body is regarded as a microcosmic reflection of the macrocosm of the universe. These philosophies emphasize the importance for humans to understand, integrate, and abide by the laws of nature, rather than resist or alter them, in order to achieve health and wellness. It's all about harmony and balance in our environment. Another way to interpret these teachings is to view ourselves as not only *in* this universe but *of* the universe. There are 12 main meridians (plus two extra) that correlate to the energy of organ systems. *Qi* (chee or chi) translates to "life force." It is believed that when qi does not flow properly within the body this causes stagnation. When qi is not flowing properly in the body or organ systems this improper flow will cause disease that manifests in various forms of disharmony (i.e., pain, anxiety, insomnia, nausea).

Acupuncture is based on a holistic approach of not only the patient's bodily conditions but also on his or her mental, emotional, and spiritual state at the time of treatment and disease. All three play a part in where a disease or condition originates and how the disease or ailment will manifest. Traditional

Chinese medicine, or TCM, is the most common system taught and practiced in North America. The term *traditional Chinese medicine* or *TCM* was developed during installation of the People's Republic of China, in 1949. It is thought that traditional forms of medicine were brought back into circulation at that time, possibly for nationalistic motives but also as a practical means of providing basic levels of healthcare to serve China's massive population.[6,8]

Most of TCM's ancient citations are connected with the history of China, although there are other cultures that embrace this treasured meridian method of medicine as well, such as Japan, Korea, Vietnam, and France. All have validity in their healing capabilities. Their differences vary, in needle size, depth of insertion, manipulation of the needles once inserted, whether or not herbal medicines are used in conjunction with needling, and how practitioners evaluate the body for diagnostic purposes. For instance, a Japanese acupuncture intake differs from other methods in its use of abdominal palpation for diagnosis, depth of insertion, and use of moxabustion; Korean acupuncture uses primarily the microsystem of the hand to treat disease. There are also specialized systems of acupuncture, including scalp and auricular acupuncture, primarily developed in the 18th century. In TCM, herbal medicine is also used in a number of ways—to expel a pathogenic factor, as a circulatory stimulant to release the qi and/or blood stagnation, or as to tonify deficient conditions within the body.

TCM sees stagnation of qi and blood as the major cause of chronic pain. One method of approaching pain within TCM is via painful obstruction syndrome (POS), or the bi-syndrome model. The POS model is a derivative of six stages, four levels, triple burner, and pathogenic factors models (detailed later in this chapter) and is used to explain how pathogens enter and affect the body and cause qi and blood to stagnate (and cause pain).

Qi, blood, or both become stagnated due to a handful of factors, generally referred to as external (or internal) pathogenic factors. *Pathogenic factors* is a quite general term and should not be confused with Western pathogenic factors (i.e. bacteria, virus, and other microbes), although Western pathogenic factors could result in a TCM pathogenic factor— for instance, a bacteria (Western pathogen) could present as an external wind cold pathogenic factor, or a bacteria (Western pathogen) enters the body and causes aversion to cold, as well as cough and pain in the muscles and joints (TCM pathogenic factor external wind/cold). When herbal medicine is used, herbs to expel the TCM pathogenic factor are used, as are circulatory stimulants to release the qi and/or blood stagnation, and herbs to tonify deficient conditions within the body. In other words, multiple herbs are used to address multiple elements within the POS model.

In summary, when pathogenic factors enter the body, they can cause pain due to qi and blood stagnation. Chinese medicine is used to expel the pathogenic factor and to eliminate the pain by removing the qi/blood stagnation, and correct any imbalance which allowed the pathogenic factor to enter the body.

Table 19.1 **Pathogenic Causes**

Common external pathogenic factors	Wind, cold, damp
Other external pathogenic factors	Heat, summer heat, dryness, pestilential factor
Internal/emotionally derived pathogenic Factors	Anger, fear, shock, joy, pensiveness, worry, sadness
Other internally derived pathogenic factors	Irregular food intake Overindulgence in alcohol and/or greasy food Overexertion, excessive births Traumatic injuries Excessive sexual activity Parasites and poisons

When treating a patient for pain, the acupuncturist determines the (TCM) pathogenic factors involved and the underlying root cause. Pathogenic factors must be expelled and the underlying root cause corrected.

Table 19.1 and Table 19.2 provide examples of pathogenic factors that cause qi and blood stagnation and the manifesting symptoms.

APPLICATIONS

The NIH and the World Health Organization cite over 52 common problems that acupuncture can address. Acupuncture is one of the most widely used treatments for pain conditions in an acute care setting. Considering that chronic pain can manifest as a number of disruptive complaints, an inpatient provider may also order acupuncture for conditions such as insomnia, nausea, and anxiety when conventional medicine is not able to provide relief. Although many

Table 19.2 **Clinical Symptoms**

Typical symptoms from wind POS	Pain and soreness of the muscles and joints Moves from joint to joint
Typical symptoms from dampness POS	Feeling of heaviness and numbness of the limbs and joints Pain is fixed in one location Aggravated by damp weather
Typical symptoms from cold POS	Severe pain and soreness of the muscles and joints Pain usually not bilateral
Typical symptoms from chronic POS	Muscle atrophy Joint deformity

people have sought out acupuncture for pain relief, there has been controversy around whether the relief is from a placebo or therapeutic effect. Researchers from the Acupuncture Trialists' Collaboration, a group established to synthesize data from high-quality randomized trials on acupuncture for chronic pain, conducted an analysis of individual patient data from 29 high-quality randomized controlled trials, including a total of 17,922 people. These trials investigated the use of acupuncture for back and neck pain, osteoarthritis, shoulder pain, or chronic headache. For all pain types studied, the researchers found modest but statistically significant differences between acupuncture versus simulated acupuncture approaches (i.e., specific effects), and larger differences between acupuncture versus a no-acupuncture controls (i.e., nonspecific effects). (In traditional acupuncture, needles are inserted at specific points on the body. Simulated acupuncture includes a variety of approaches that mimic this procedure; some approaches do not pierce the skin or use specific points on the body.) The sizes of the effects were generally similar across all pain conditions studied.[6]

The authors noted that these findings suggest that the total effects of acupuncture, as experienced by patients in clinical practice, are clinically relevant. They also noted that their study provides the most robust evidence to date that acupuncture is more than just placebo and a reasonable referral option for patients with chronic pain.[6] Systematic reviews on use of acupuncture for postoperative as well as chemotherapy-induced nausea and vomiting have also been conducted. For postoperative nausea and vomiting, results from 26 trials showed acupuncture-point stimulation was effective for both nausea and vomiting. For chemotherapy-induced nausea and vomiting, results of 11 trials differed according to modality, with acupressure being effective for first-day nausea. Experimental studies showed effects of P6-stimulation on gastric myoelectrical activity, vagal modulation, and cerebellar vestibular activities in functional magnetic resonance imaging. There is good clinical evidence from more than 40 randomized controlled trials that acupuncture has some effect in preventing or attenuating nausea and vomiting.[7]

A number of clinical studies, mainly randomized controlled clinical trials, have shown positive effects in acupuncture treatment of insomnia. Some of the studies demonstrated that acupuncture treatment appeared to be better than conventional pharmacological drugs for reducing insomnia. These encouraging findings are nonetheless limited by quality problems of the methodology used in these clinical studies. The clinical efficacy of acupuncture appears to be supported by evidence obtained from basic neuroendocrinological studies. A number of studies have demonstrated that acupuncture may modulate a wide range of neuroendocrinological factors following stimulation of acupoints. Evidence has suggested that the clinical efficacy of acupuncture in treatment of insomnia is potentially mediated by a variety of neurotransmitters, including norepinephrine, melatonin, gamma-aminobutyric acid, and β-endorphin.[9]

A pilot study has shown that acupuncture may help people with posttraumatic stress disorder (PTSD). Hollifield and colleagues conducted a clinical trial examining the effect of acupuncture on the symptoms of PTSD. They analyzed depression, anxiety, and impairment in 73 people with a diagnosis of PTSD. The participants were assigned to receive either acupuncture or group cognitive-behavioral therapy (CBT) over 12 weeks, or were assigned to a wait-list as part of the control group. The people in the control group were offered treatment or referral for treatment at the end of their participation. The researchers found that acupuncture provided treatment effects similar to those with group CBT; both interventions were superior to no intervention. Additionally, treatment effects of both the acupuncture and the CBT group therapy were maintained for 3 months after the end of treatment.[10]

There are several randomized controlled trials that suggest positive benefits of acupuncture in treating chronic pain. Acupuncture appears to provide improvement in function and pain relief as an adjuvant therapy for osteoarthritis compared to sham acupuncture or no treatment. In an individual-patient meta-analysis of 31 randomized controlled trials, acupuncture provided more pain relief than sham acupuncture or no acupuncture for chronic back and neck pain, osteoarthritis, and chronic headache.[11,12] In a review of patients with chronic low back pain, several studies demonstrated improvement in pain symptoms at 8 weeks and 12 weeks in comparison to routine care but no significant difference in pain relief after 6 to 12 months.[13]

HERBAL COMBINATIONS USED TO TREAT CHRONIC PAIN

Herbal treatment alone is rarely administered in the hospital setting. However, moxibustion is a common acupuncture variation. As a reference, Table 19.3 lists some common herbal combinations (natural product categorization) used to for moxibustion as overall for treatment of chronic pain (called painful obstructive syndrome [POS] in TCM, organized by TCM pathogenic cause) that an inpatient physician may come across.

Table 19.4 lists common herbs used for chronic pain treatment in TCM.

Table 19.5 lists some examples of herb–drug interactions.

CONTRAINDICATIONS

There are a great many acupuncture points, some of which carry little or no risk and others having the potential of serious injury, particularly in unskilled or inexperienced hands.

Special care should be taken in needling points in proximity to vital organs or sensitive areas. Because of the characteristics of the needles used, the particular sites for needling, the depth of needle insertion, the manipulation techniques

Table 19.3 Common Herbal Combinations Used in Traditional Chinese Medicine for Treating Pain

TCM Herbal Formula	Expels Pathogen
Fang Feng Tang (Ledebouriella decoction)	Wind
Juan Bi Tang (remove painful obstruction decoction)	Wind
Da Qin Jiao Tang—major large gentian decoction	Wind
Ma Huang Tang (Ephedra decoction)	Cold
Ge Gen Tang (Kudzu decoction)	Cold
Gui Zhi Fu Zi Tang (Ramulus Cinnamomi-Acontium decoction)	Cold
Yi Yi Ren Tang (Coix decoction)	Damp
Chuan Bi Tang (eliminating painful obstruction syndrome decoction)	Damp
Ma Huang Lian Qiao Chi Xiao Dou (Ephedra-Forsythia-Phaseolus decoction)	Damp
Bai Hu Jia Gui Zhi Tang (white tiger Ramulus Cinnamomi decoction)	Heat
Xuan Bi Tang (clearing painful obstructino syndrome decoction)	Heat
Xi Jiao San (Cornu Bisontis decoction)	Heat
Du Huo Ji Sheng Tang (Angelica pubescens-Loranthus decoction)	Chronic/bone
Qin Jiao Si Wu Tang (Gentiana macrophylla four substances decoction)	Chronic/bone
Shen Tong Zhu Yu Tang (Cnidium and Notopterygium decoction)	Chronic/bone

Table 19.4 Common Herbs Used in Traditional Chinese Medicine for Chronic Pain Treatment

Botanical Name	PinYin Name
Herba Ephedrae	Ma Huang
Ramulus Cinnamomi	Gui Zhi
Radix Glycyrrhizae	Zhi Gan Cao
Radix Puerariae	Ge Gen
Radix Paeoniae Alba	Bai Shao
Rhizoma Zingiberis Recens	Sheng Jiang
Fructus JuJube	Da Zao
Radix Glycyrrhizae	Gan Cao
Semen Coicis lachrymal jobi	Yi Yi Ren
Rhizoma Atractylodis Ianceae	Cang Zhu
Radix Aconti Lateralis Preparata	Zhi Fu Zi
Fructus Forsythiae suspensae	Lian Qiao
Radix Angelicae pubescentis	Du Huo

Table 19.5 **Herb–Drug Interactions**

Absorption	Bind to other substances in GI tract inhibiting transfer to bloodstream
Drugs	Questran, Colestid, Xenical
Herbs	[authors have to place herbs here]
	Buplrurum, Astragalus, Condonopsis

Bloodstream	Amplify or attenuate effects
Drugs	Beta blockers
Herbs	Ma Huang
Drugs	Anticoagulants
Herbs	Dang Gui (Radicis Angelicae Sinensis)

Metabolism	Speeds up livers rate of breakdown
Drugs	Phenobarbitals
Herbs	Milk thistle (*Silybum marianum*)

Toxicity	Some type of toxic effect on the body
Drugs	Antibiotics, chemotherapy, immunosuppressants, antihyperlipidemics, chronic stimulant laxatives, ACE inhibitors, NSAIDs, aspirin, mesalamine
Herbs	Fu Zhi (Radix Aconiti)
	Datura Metel (devil's trumpet)
	TCM formulas containing aristolochic acid (Guang Fang Ji (Radix Aristolochiae) and Guan Mu Tong (Caulis Aristolochiae Manshuriensis)

used, and the stimulation given, accidents may occur during treatment. In most instances they can be avoided if adequate precautions are taken. If they do occur, the acupuncturist should know how to manage them effectively and avoid any additional harm.[14]

Points on the chest, back, and abdomen should be needled cautiously, preferably obliquely or horizontally, so as to avoid injury to vital organs. Attention should be paid to the direction and depth of insertion of needles.

Injury to the lung and pleura caused by too deep insertion of a needle into points on the chest, back, or supraclavicular fossa may cause traumatic pneumothorax. Cough, chest pain, and dyspnea are the usual symptoms and occur abruptly during the manipulation, especially if there is severe laceration of the lung by the needle. Alternatively, symptoms may develop gradually over several hours after the acupuncture treatment.

As a precaution, we recommend not needling patients with an INR greater than 4 or platelet levels lower than 50. Patients with bleeding and clotting disorders should be identified prior to treatment and before consent. Patients who are on anticoagulant therapy or taking drugs with an anticoagulant effect should be treated with great caution.[15]

Acupuncture and moxibustion are contraindicated for puncture points on the lower abdomen and lumbosacral region during the first trimester of pregnancy. After the third month, points on the upper abdomen and lumbosacral region and points causing strong sensations should be avoided, as well as ear acupuncture points that may induce labor.

Care should be taken in needling areas of poor circulation (e.g., varicose veins) and where there is a risk of infection. Practitioners need to avoid accidental puncture of arteries (sometimes aberrant), which may cause bleeding, hematoma, arterial spasm, or more serious complications when pathological change is present (e.g., aneurysm, atherosclerosis).[15]

HOW TO ORDER

Acupuncture should be ordered as adjuvant treatment to any conventional medicine regimen of treatment. Most commonly, acupuncture is used in cases when patients are not able to obtain relief from conventional medicine treatments alone. An order for acupuncture is recommended when any of the following diagnoses have been determined (please check your ICD diagnoses codes): chronic pain, fibromyalgia, back pain, neck pain, insomnia, anxiety disorders, neuropathies, pain due to chemotherapy, nausea, vomiting, headaches, migraines, vertigo, depression, pain from stroke, spinal cord injuries, traumatic brain injuries, gastrointestinal disorders, PTSD, and smoking cessation.

Treatment protocols will vary depending on the many factors of a patient's intake. Each acupuncturist will have their own means of determining how long a treatment series is expected to last. A series of 12 treatments is a starting point for most practitioners. Evaluation of efficacy of treatment can be better determined at that point—that is, whether or not a patient is finding relief from treatment.

Mind–Body Practice: Chaplain Services

Spiritual care is vital to the well-being of a person. Spiritual connection is where some people find their purpose and direction in life, as well as their values, self-worth, and morality. For many individuals who find themselves facing the realities of suffering and pain, it is their connectedness to God that comforts and sustains them. One's physical, emotional, and spiritual care are all connected to one's health.[16]

BACKGROUND

The word *chaplain* is derived from the Latin word for "cloak." In the fourth century, St. Martin, on his duty as a soldier to protect the emperor, came across a beggar whose clothes were so ragged that he was practically naked. If St. Martin had met the man's need by giving him his own cloak, he would have shifted the problem to himself, so instead, he tore his own cloak in two and shared it—half for the beggar and half for himself. From this the understanding, a chaplain is someone who shares support with those in the storms of life, offering spiritual help and direction during their difficult times. The chaplain also has the strength to share and offer support, but not at the detriment of his or her own health; a chaplain keeps clear boundaries and strength that does not waver.[17]

Hospital chaplains provide a wide range of services offered to many people of many different denominations. Most hospitals will locate a chaplain of a person's denomination, if requested. A qualified hospital chaplain will offer services for both patients and visitors. Their expertise is to listen and offer spiritual and emotional support for those in crisis or grief. Some may share prayer and sacraments and lead worship while others offer reflection and consultation on ethical concerns and decisions.[17] The 2002 National Health Interview Survey of Adults using Complementary and Alternative Medicine indicated that 24% of adults participated in prayer by others for one's own health, and 43% of adults used prayer specifically for one's own health.[1]

Chaplains pray with patients, regardless of the chaplain's own trained denomination; help families make difficult end-of-life decisions; or simply offer a sympathetic ear (Box 19.1). As interest has risen in the links between religion, spirituality, and health, there has been a new push to establish chaplaincy in the medical mainstream and to apply more rigorous scientific research in this area. The Association of Professional Chaplains, which certifies healthcare chaplains, issued its first standards for practice in 2009, including the requirement that chaplains document their work in patient medical records and stay abreast of new research. Medical schools are adding courses on spirituality and health and training residents to consider patients' spiritual needs. Two-thirds of U.S. hospitals provide chaplaincy services; others rely on local clergy and lay volunteers.[16]

APPLICATIONS

In general, more research support is needed to study the impact of pastoral care and spiritual counseling on patients with chronic pain. Over time, spiritual

---

Box 19.1 **An Abbreviated Spiritual History**[20]

Following are some of the screening questions that many healthcare professionals use to address spiritual issues with patients:

- *Faith, Belief, Meaning*
  What is your faith or belief?
  What things do you believe give meaning to your life?
- *Importance and Influence*
  How have your beliefs influenced your behavior during this illness?
  What role do your beliefs play in regaining your health?
- *Community*
  Are you part of a spiritual or religious community?
  Is there a person or group of people you really love or who are really important to you?
- *Address/Action in Care*
  How would you like me, your healthcare provider, to address these issues in your health care?

---

support has increasingly become more mainstream and recognized as an integral part of the holistic healthcare system. There are some studies that point to this importance.

Mandziuk et al. noted that pastoral caregivers have a unique role in bringing the expertise of their profession as well as the traditions of prayer and meditation toward easing a person's suffering from chronic pain. The pastoral attending can be a key component for relational support.[18] A separate qualitative study showed that self-examination and exploration into spirituality can enable chronic pain sufferers to rediscover life's meaning by helping them understand both the meaning of suffering and the interrelation of pain, emotions, and addiction.[19]

A $3 million grant from the John Templeton Foundation has enabled the Health Care Chaplaincy to oversee six national research projects examining the role of healthcare chaplains. Additionally, George Washington University's Institute for Spirituality and Health (GWish), which the Foundation has supported with grant funding, is overseeing the National Spiritual Care Demonstration Project. Overall, it is important that teaching doctors and nurses to be sensitive to patients' spiritual needs helps uncover "critical information required for effective diagnosis and treatment."[17]

CONTRAINDICATIONS

There are currently no known contraindications to use of a chaplain's services.

HOW TO ORDER

Anyone may request to have a chaplain visit. A chaplain is seen not only by patients but also for support of family and friends in times of need. Chaplains are sometimes called to serve when difficult decisions have to be made about patient care. A qualified hospital chaplain, with qualifications set by the Association of Professional Chaplains and the National Association of Catholic Chaplains, must have four units of Clinical Pastoral Education (CPE) from an accredited CPE facility. He or she must have a Master in Divinity or its equivalent, and a church endorsement from his or her denomination.

Mind–Body Practice: Energy Healing (Reiki)

BACKGROUND

The U.S.-based NCCAM distinguishes between healthcare involving scientifically observable energy, which it calls "veritable energy medicine," and healthcare methods that invoke physically undetectable or unverifiable "energies," which it calls "putative energy medicine."[1] Reiki is an example of putative energy medicine. Reiki is an energetic healing method developed by the Japanese Buddhist monk Mikao Usui, around the turn of the 19th century. Reiki is a method of interacting with the energy field of the patient to correct imbalances in that energy field and restore the patient to optimal health.

There are three levels in the path of becoming a Reiki practitioner. Level 1 is the initiation level; the other levels involve a deeper understanding of Reiki. In level 1, the student is introduced to the process of Reiki healing. One of the elements of this level is the initiation, during which the Reiki master welcomes the student into Reiki. This might be described as being similar to baptism in Christianity, where the intent of the student is amplified with a formal procedure. This commitment helps bind the student to the path of Reiki. In level 1, the energy model of the human body is presented (chakras), as this is the basis for Reiki healing.

In level 2, the practitioner receives three symbols and their phrases. According to Reiki, these Japanese symbols and phrases, when used during the treatment, enhance the effects of the Reiki treatment. Specifically, these symbols and phrases are power, mental, and distance.

Level 3 involves a continuation of level 2, where the practitioner is drawn deeper into the process of Reiki. The student now becomes a master and can initiate new Reiki students into the Reiki healing method. There are additional levels of Reiki beyond level 3.

Reiki, like other forms of energy work, is a model to channel the love of the universe into a point, for example, the palm of one's hand. It is the use of Gods' love to heal. We are all connected to a fabric of love, and often our connection to this fabric needs repair. The Reiki practitioner uses love and a model of how energy is distributed through the body in order to repair this connection. Reiki can be done locally, in the presence of the patient, or remotely, when the patient is not present with the practitioner. Remote Reiki healing is similar to prayer. In remote Reiki healing, practitioner directs the healing power of love, by intent, to the patient.

APPLICATIONS

Overall there is a lack of high-quality research on Reiki, and studies that have been done show conflicting results. Research on Reiki has generally focused on symptom management or well-being. An NCCAM-funded study found that in the treatment of fibromyalgia, neither Reiki nor touch had any effect on pain symptoms.[21]

CONTRAINDICATIONS

1. Overall, Reiki appears to be generally safe, and no serious side effects have been reported.
2. If the patient does not believe in Reiki, there may be an uncomfortable experience with the process of hands-on Reiki healing. Someone who has never been introduced or exposed to alternate medicine might have an obstacle to a healing process that involves unfamiliar hands on the body. A negative, uncomfortable experience could have an emotional impact on the patient.
3. Do not use Reiki to replace conventional care or to postpone seeing a health-care provider about a health problem.

HOW TO ORDER

There is no formal credential or license required for practicing or teaching most energy healing techniques. However, the techniques may be used or taught by licensed professionals, including physicians, acupuncturists, recreational therapists, and psychologists. Creating and defining the scope of the hospital consultation services will depend on hospital's needs.

Mind–Body Practice: Massage

BACKGROUND

Massage therapy dates back thousands of years, with references to massage appearing in ancient writings from China, Japan, India, and Egypt. In general, massage therapists work on mobilizing muscle, ligament, connective tissues, and other soft tissue structures. In Swedish massage, the therapist uses long strokes, kneading, deep circular movements, vibration, and tapping. Sports massage combines techniques of Swedish massage and deep tissue massage to release chronic muscle tension. It is adapted to the needs of athletes. Myofascial trigger point therapy focuses on trigger points—areas that are painful when pressed and associated with pain elsewhere in the body. Massage therapy is sometimes done using essential oils as a form of aromatherapy.

APPLICATIONS

Much of the scientific research on massage therapy is preliminary or conflicting, but much of the evidence points toward beneficial effects on pain and other symptoms associated with a number of different conditions. Much of the evidence suggests that these effects are short term and that people need to keep getting massages for the benefits to continue.[22]

A 2008 systematic review and 2011 NCCAM-funded clinical trial concluded that massage may be useful for chronic low-back pain.[23,24] Massage may help with chronic neck pain, a 2009 NCCAM-funded clinical trial reported. Massage may help with pain due to osteoarthritis of the knee, according to a 2012 NCCAM-funded study.[25] Studies suggest that for women in labor, massage provided some pain relief and increased their satisfaction with other forms of pain relief, but the evidence is not strong, a 2012 review concluded. A 2010 review concluded that massage therapy may help temporarily reduce pain, fatigue, and other symptoms associated with fibromyalgia, but the evidence is not definitive.[26] The authors noted that it is important that the massage therapist not cause pain. Clinical trials on the effects of massage for headaches are preliminary and only somewhat promising.

CONTRAINDICATIONS

Massage therapy should not be used to replace conventional care or to postpone seeing a healthcare provider about a medical problem. Forceful and deep tissue massage should be avoided by people with conditions such as bleeding disorders or low blood platelet counts, and by people taking anticoagulant medications such as warfarin (also known as blood thinners). Massage should not be done in any potentially weak area of the skin, such as wounds. Deep or intense pressure should not be used over an area where the patient has a tumor or cancer, unless approved by the patient's healthcare provider.[27,28]

HOW TO ORDER

Most states that regulate massage therapists require them to have a minimum of 500 hours of training from an accredited training program. The National

Certification Board for Therapeutic Massage and Bodywork certifies practitioners who pass a national examination and fulfill other requirements.[29] Creating and defining the scope of the hospital consultation services will depend on the hospital's needs (Box 19.2).

Box 19.2 **Sample Abbreviated Massage/Reflexology History**

1. How would you rate your state of health? Excellent ___ Good ___ Fair ___ Poor ___

2. Have you ever had any type of body work (i.e., massage) before?

   _____

3. Are you currently under a doctor's care? If so, explain

   _____

   _____

   _____

4. Do you have any allergies? If so, please list them:

   _____

   _____

5. For women—are you pregnant? If yes, for how long?

   _____

   _____

6. Are you taking any medications? If so, for what conditions?

   _____

   _____

   _____

   _____

7. List any previous major illnesses, accidents, surgeries, or broken bones:

   _____

   _____

   _____

   _____

---

8. For **reflexology**, are you experiencing any problems with your feet? For **massage**, do you have any skin conditions?

If yes, explain_____

_____

_____

9. Where is tension most evident in your body? On the diagram, please shade in the areas where you feel symptoms associated with your complaints.

Mind–Body Practice: Meditation and Relaxation Techniques

BACKGROUND

Relaxation techniques include a number of practices, such as progressive relaxation, guided imagery, mindfulness-based stress reduction (MBSR), biofeedback, self-hypnosis, and deep breathing exercises. The goal is similar in all: to consciously produce the body's natural relaxation response, characterized by slower breathing, lower blood pressure, and a feeling of calm and well-being. In addition to reducing pain, such techniques may be used by some to release tension and to counteract the ill effects of stress, induce sleep, and calm emotions. Meditation as defined by Goleman and Schwartz is the intentional self-regulation of attention from moment to moment. It is neither contemplation nor rumination. There are two major classes of meditation practice: concentration meditation, which can include forms of transcendental meditation, relaxation response, biofeedback, guided imagery, autogenic training, and self hypnosis; and mindfulness meditation, which include deep breathing, such as qi gong, and MBSR.

Types of relaxation response/meditation techniques include the following:

1. *Biofeedback*. Biofeedback-assisted relaxation is the process of gaining greater awareness of physiological function by primarily using instruments that provide information on the activity of physiological systems with the goal of being able to alter the physiological function at will. At times, electronic devices can be used to provide the feedback to relax muscles, thereby reducing pain.[30]
2. *Deep breathing or breathing exercises*. To relax using this method, one consciously slows one's breathing and focuses on taking regular and deep breaths.
3. *Guided imagery*. For this technique, one focuses on pleasant images to replace negative or stressful feelings and relax. Guided imagery may be directed by oneself or by a practitioner through storytelling or descriptions designed to suggest mental images (also called visualization).
4. *Mindfulness-based stress reduction* (MBSR) utilizes training in a form of meditation known as mindfulness or awareness meditation as the major self-regulatory activity. Three basic methods are used, including a body scan, which focuses on proprioception, or placing attention to the body; mindfulness of breath; and Hatha yoga postures. All practices used in MBSR are taught independent of the religious and cultural beliefs associated with them.[31,32]
5. *Self-hypnosis*. In self-hypnosis one produces the relaxation response with a phrase or nonverbal cue (also called a "suggestion").
6. *Autogenic training*. When using this method, one focuses on the physical sensation of one's own breathing or heartbeat and pictures one's body as warm, heavy, and/or relaxed.

In contrast to the stress response, in which the body releases hormones that produce the fight-or-flight response, the relaxation response slows the heart rate, lowers blood pressure, and decreases oxygen consumption and levels of stress hormones. Because relaxation is the opposite of stress, the theory is that voluntarily creating the relaxation response through regular use of relaxation techniques could counteract the negative effects of stress.[33]

According to the 2007 National Health Interview Survey, which included a comprehensive survey on the use of complementary health approaches by Americans, 12.7% of adults used deep-breathing exercises, 2.9% used progressive relaxation, and 2.2% used guided imagery for health purposes. Most of those people reported using a book to learn the techniques rather than seeing a practitioner.[1]

APPLICATIONS

People may use relaxation techniques as part of a comprehensive plan to treat, prevent, or reduce symptoms of a variety of conditions including stress, chronic pain, insomnia, depression, labor pain, headache, and anxiety.

Current research has examined relaxation techniques for the following:

Anxiety: Studies have suggested that relaxation may assist in the conventional treatment of phobias or panic disorder. Relaxation techniques have also been used to relieve anxiety for people in stressful situations, such as when undergoing a medical procedure.

Depression: In 2008, a major review of the evidence that looked at relaxation for depression found that relaxation techniques were more effective than no treatment for depression, but not as effective as cognitive-behavioral therapy.[34]

Fibromyalgia: Some preliminary studies report that using relaxation or guided imagery techniques may sometimes improve pain and reduce fatigue from fibromyalgia.

Headache: There is some evidence that biofeedback and other relaxation techniques may help relieve tension or migraine headaches. In some cases, these mind and body techniques were more effective than medications for reducing the frequency, intensity, and severity of headaches.

Insomnia: There is some evidence that relaxation techniques can help reduce chronic insomnia.

Irritable bowel syndrome: Some studies have indicated that relaxation techniques may prevent or relieve symptoms of irritable bowel syndrome (IBS) in some participants. One review of the research found some evidence that self-hypnosis may be useful for IBS.

Nausea: Relaxation techniques may help relieve nausea caused by chemotherapy.

Smoking cessation: Relaxation exercises may help reduce the desire to smoke.

Temporomandibular disorder (pain and loss of motion in the jaw joints): A review of the literature found that relaxation techniques and biofeedback were more effective than placebo in decreasing pain and increasing jaw function.

CONTRAINDICATIONS

1. Relaxation techniques are often used as part of a treatment plan and not as the only approach for potentially serious health conditions.
2. There have been rare reports that certain relaxation techniques might cause or worsen symptoms in people with epilepsy or certain psychiatric conditions, or in those with a history of abuse or trauma.

HOW TO ORDER

There is no formal credential or license required for practicing or teaching most relaxation techniques. However, the techniques may be used or taught by licensed professionals, including physicians, recreational therapists, and psychologists. Creating and defining the scope of the hospital consultation services will depend on hospital's needs.

Mind–Body Practices: Meditative Movement Therapies

BACKGROUND

Meditative movement therapies, or MMT, are a new category of exercise defined by (a) some form of movement or body positioning, (b) a focus on breathing, (c) and a clear or calm state of mind with the goal of (d) deep states of relaxation. The three most commonly used forms of meditative movement therapy include qi gong, tai chi, and yoga.[35]

Qi gong is an ancient Chinese practice dating back 2500 to 4000 years. It focuses on the integration of physical postures, breathing techniques, and focused intentions.[36] It can easily be adapted to accommodate people who have physical limitations, as many of the exercises can be performed in a standing, seated, or supine posture.[36]

Tai chi is an ancient martial art developed in China in the late 17th century. It involves gentle, flowing movement exercises of the upper extremities combined with constant weight shifting of the lower limbs with meditation, and breathing to move the qi (in the Chinese belief, qi is the internal energy of the body).[37]

The classical techniques of yoga date back more than 5000 years. The word *yoga* means "to yoke" or "join together" and joins together the mind, body, and spirit through practice. The system of yoga is built upon three main structures: exercise, breathing, and meditation. There over 100 different schools or types of yoga.[38] An estimated 14 million Americans practiced yoga in 2002, including more than 1 million who used it as a treatment for back pain. Approximately 1.2% of Americans practiced tai chi for health reasons, and 0.3% of Americans practiced qi gong.[39]

Applications

There is growing evidence to support the use of such therapies for chronic pain interventions; however, the number of randomized studies is small.[40] In a meta-analysis of seven studies examining the efficacy and safety of meditative movement therapies in fibromyalgia, yoga interventions resulted in statistically significant reduction in pain, fatigue, health-related quality of life, and depression at final treatment. Qi gong and tai chi yielded a reduction in fatigue, sleep disturbance, and depression but no significant differences in pain levels once interventions were completed. However, safety and acceptance of such therapies with supervised intervention remained high.[41] The American Pain Society recommends that clinicians consider offering yoga to patients with chronic low back pain. There is fair evidence for viniyoga and poor evidence for Hatha yoga for patients with chronic to subacute low back pain.[42]

HOW TO ORDER

In the various meditative movement therapies, treatment duration ranged from as few as four 20-minute sessions of qi gong to 24 weekly sessions of yoga. Most patients will not remain in the inpatient setting for longer periods of time, but these therapies can be introduced in the inpatient setting and transitioned to outpatient once a patient is discharged. It is recommended that each of these disciplines be practiced under the guidance of a well-trained instructor. However, there is significant variability in the amount of time practitioners spend in training, and there are many practices that have not been regulated by licensure.[39,41] There are many physical, occupational, and recreation therapists that have training in these disciplines and elements of them can be incorporated as a part of the therapy session. There are various styles of yoga that range in intensity, but viniyoga, chair yoga and hatha yoga are the types that have been researched.[39,41,43] Many patients may feel more comfortable observing a session prior to deciding to participate.

CONTRAINDICATIONS

Hatha yoga, viniyoga, and chair yoga are generally low impact and safe when practiced under the guidance of a well-trained instructor. However, rare side effects are possible. Yoga is contraindicated in patients with uncontrolled hypertension and with glaucoma. Yoga should be modified or certain poses should be avoided by women who are pregnant and by patients with sciatica. Patients with a history of stroke, Chiari malformation, or advanced cervical stenosis should avoid headstand or shoulder stand poses.[39] Patients who have been diagnosed with advanced spinal stenosis or severe osteoporosis should avoid extreme extension poses of the spine, such as back bends.[39,44]

Tai chi and qi gong are relatively safe; however, there are some precautions.[45] Instructors do not recommend practice right after a meal or when patients are extremely fatigued. Movements must be modified in patients with pregnancy, hernias, or severe osteoporosis. Tai chi and qi gong are contraindicated in patients with orthostatic hypotension or active infection. There have also been case reports of abnormal psychosomatic responses, or mental disorder may be induced when qi gong is practiced inappropriately or excessively, or when pre-disposed individuals practice qi gong unguided. In one study, 62% of abnormal psychological reactions to qi gong practice were in patients with pre-existing mental disorders of varying degrees, and disease onset appeared after beginning exercises. Reactions may take the form of emotional disturbances, depression, anxiety, neurosis, or schizophrenia. Qi gong–triggered disorders are usually transient and normalize after practice is terminated.[45]

How to Create an Inpatient Integrative Pain Medicine Program

As with other inpatient consultative services, optimal patient service delivery begins with developing a structure. Three ways of ordering integrative services are as follows: (1) the hospitalist or caring physician has standing orders, (2) implementation of nurse-driven protocols, or (3) the hospitalist or caring physician consults an integrative medicine practitioner so that the practitioner directs integrative care. In our opinion, having an initial inpatient consultation order directed to a physician or advanced nurse practitioner may be the more efficient structure. The specified practitioner with an integrative medicine focus can determine the appropriate mind–body service or services from which the patient would best benefit. Each culture that resides within an institutional setting has its own needs; the delivery structure will depend on this culture.

Assessing a Hospital's Complementary Care Needs

Next it is important to identify what the hospital's complementary care needs are as well as to determine how the program can fill those gaps. The following are departmental and institutional questions that should be addressed:

1. Determine what the needs are in the hospital.
2. Who supports integrative health?
3. Who has been trained in integrative medicine therapies? Many nurses have familiarity of acupressure, aromatherapy, guided imagery, and hand massage techniques.
4. Find out who is interested in learning more about integrative medicine. Provide a few courses for nursing staff to get involved when the integrative team is not on staff.
5. What are the solutions and who are the providers of care to meet that hospital's needs? Provide evidence-based medicine research that supports your integrative team.

6. Determine the needs and challenges of the solutions needed.
7. Who will provide the care? Will the spiritual care team or chaplain be willing and able to work with the team?
8. Start with a holistic approach within the system and structure you would like to build. Place each professional as part of the community; each will have a voice, concern, opinion, and their own insight as to what is needed. Listen without judgment. Honor each professional's personality and persona.
9. Do your research. Find out more about all professions proposed. What are the qualifications needed in order to provide optimum healthcare to the community who will be served?
10. Where will the funding come from? What is the primary source of healthcare services provided to the community at large? Are there other hospitals offering this service? What is lacking? What is successful?
11. Find the support systems within your system. Look within your hospital's already formed organizations. Call on a local foundations board, administrative staff, or an outside philanthropist that is willing to support your integrative clinic and its mission.
12. Is your target institution an existing accountable care organization (ACO)? Is it planning to become one? Is it a hospital gobbling up primary care practices? Does it manage patient-centered medical homes (PMCH)? The Affordable Care Act (ACA) is beginning to shift how institutions and providers are reimbursed and incentivized. ACOs are reimbursed at higher levels to reduce hospital readmissions and improve patient satisfaction rates. If a CMS (Medicare, Medicaid) patient is hospitalized longer due to preventable infections, the institution loses money through "partial" reimbursements. Those extra days of hospitalization will not be covered. This shift brings renewed focus to the precepts of health promotion, education, true prevention, and the core tenets of integrative health.
13. Evidence-based medicine research emphasizes the importance of proper nutrition, exercise, stress reduction, and overall behavioral change for creating and maintaining good health. When sharing your integrative vision and building your coalition, you must share this literature liberally. Include other literature that supports each modality through the validity of evidence-based medicine research studies.

STRUCTURING

There are over 402 integrative clinics in the United States, and the number is growing. Check out the resources online. Call and find out if you can visit these institutions. Many integrative clinics are open for a tour if planned in advance. Structuring a group of committees to provide not only a sense of community in building the core structure of the integrative clinic but also providing a direct connection to the people within the community for outreach is essential.

The following are structural questions to address:

- How many therapists are needed
- Which areas they will work in
- How many hours per week
- Supplies and equipment needed
- Supplies and equipment kept
- Space provided to chart, have meetings
- Who they will be accountable to
- Will the specific modality be credentialed or validated (credentialing refers only to licensed practitioners)
- How to educate staff, family, and patients about the program
- How will patients access the service(s)? This is usually done through nursing staff, who are usually first to find out that conventional medicine is not working to reduce their patients' pain scores. Educate, educate, educate, and build advocates.
- Where and how will orders and documents be executed? Contact your legal department when creating documentation practices for providers.

PROGRAM EXPANSION

- Quarterly data collection assessments from patients and providers can provide information on the benefits or areas of work. This information in turn can be used to decide whether to expand, retract, or hold services stable. This information is also valuable to locate areas of excess and/or areas of shortage.

FURTHER FUNDING DESIGNS

- Apply for Medical staff grants
- Seek out contributions from areas interested in becoming pilot units
- Tap into Department of Medicine funding
- Apply for hospital auxiliary grants
- Foundation grants
- Philanthropic donations
- Fund-raising events
- Research grants

PROGRAM EVALUATION

There are several ways in which program evaluations can be done. The use of multiple approaches simultaneously can be beneficial. Collecting data is essential in determining the hospital pre- and post-assessment scores. Pain, anxiety, nausea, vomiting, and ability to cope are just a few common areas for which assessment scores need to be obtained pre- and post-treatment. Staff, patients, families, and practitioners can provide valuable information for formal outcome measurements as well as informal feedback. This information can then be used to maintain, revise, and expand the program. As in most organizations, formal data collection is usually more convincing to those qualified to empower a group to move forward and/or to provide future funding.

Summary

The various components of integrative medicine can assist in the treatment of inpatients with chronic pain in a number of ways. First, the holistic nature of the treatments, such as acupuncture and massage, done in the medicalized environment, can help the patient see that some complementary treatments are evidence based, accepted by traditional medicine, and have the potential to help. Second, holistic adjuvant treatments, such as meditation or chaplain services, may address and treat aspects of pain care that traditional medicine has difficulty addressing, such as stress responses to pain and the individual biopsychosocial impacts of the pain. A large part of integrative medicine is the teaching and awareness of self-care. Third, introducing integrative components to inpatients with chronic pain may start the transfer of the responsibility of health maintenance and awareness from the provider back to the patient. This ultimately may help in treating these patients as outpatients, because they may feel empowered to seek care that allows less reliance on medications, surgeries, and procedures. While creating and introducing a hospital-based integrative medicine consultation service can be laborious, the long-term benefits in an outcomes-based, patient-centered healthcare environment can be fruitful for patients, providers, and healthcare systems.

References

1. Barnes PM, Bloom B, Nahin R. CDC National Health Statistics Report #12. Complementary and Alternative Medicine Use Among Adults and Children: United States, 2007. National Health Statistics Reports. No. 12, December 10, 2008. http://www.cdc.gov/nchs/data/nhsr/nhsr012.pdf.
2. Nahin, RL, Barnes PM, Stussman BJ, Bloom B. Costs of complementary and alternative medicine (CAM) and frequency of visits to CAM practitioners: United States, 2007. *Natl Health Stat Report*. 2009;18:1–14.

3. Abrams DI, Dolor R, Roberts R, et al. The BraveNet prospective observational study on integrative medicine treatment approaches for pain. *BMC Complement Altern Med.* 2013;13:146.

4. Dusek JA, Finch M, Plotnikoff G, Knutson L. The impact of integrative medicine on pain management in a tertiary care hospital. *J Patient Safe.* 2010;6(1):48–51.

5. Rosomoff HL. Low back pain. Evaluation and management in the primary care setting. *Med Clin North Am.* 1999;83(3):643–662.

6. Vickers AJ, Cronin AM, Maschino AC, et al. Acupuncture for chronic pain: individual patient data meta-analysis. *Arch Intern Med.* 2012;172(19):1444–1453.

7. Streitberger K, Ezzo J, Schneider A. Acupuncture for nausea and vomiting: an update of clinical and experimental studies. *Auton Neurosci.* 2006;129(1-2):107–117.

8. White A, Ernst E. A brief history of acupuncture. *Rheumatology.* 2004;43:662–663.

9. Zhao K. Acupuncture for the treatment of insomnia. *Int Rev Neurobiol.* 2013;111:217–234.

10. Hollifield M, Sinclair-Lian N, Warner TD, Hammerschlag R. Acupuncture for posttraumatic stress disorder: A randomized controlled pilot trial. *J Nerv Ment Dis.* 2007;195:504–513.

11. Ezzo J, Hadhazy V, Birch S, et al. Acupuncture for osteoarthritis of the knee: a systematic review. *Arthritis Rheum.* 2001;44:815–825.

12. Vickers A, Cronin A, Maschino AC, et al. Acupuncture for chronic pain: individual patient data meta-analysis. *Arch Intern Med.* 2012;172(19):1444–1453.

13. Hutchinson AJ. The effectiveness of acupuncture in treating chronic non-specific low back pain: a systematic review of the literature. J Orthop Surg Res. 2012 Oct 30;7:36.

14. Birch S, Felt R. *Understanding Acupuncture.* London: Churchill Livingstone, 1999.

15. World Health Organization. Guidelines on Basic Training and Safety in Acupuncture. Geneva: World Health Organization; 1999. http://apps.who.int/iris/bitstream/10665/66007/1/WHO_EDM_TRM_99.1.pdf

16. Swift C. *Hospital Chaplaincy in the Twenty-first Century: The Crisis of Spriitual Care on the NHS* (Explorations in Practical, Pastoral and Empirical Theology). Farnahm, UK: Ashgate; 2009.

17. Bay PS, Beckman D, Trippi J, Gunderman R, Terry C. The effect of pastoral care services on anxiety, depression, hope, religious coping, and religious problem solving styles: a randomized controlled study. *J Relig Health.* 2008;47(1):57–69.

18. Mandziuk PA. Easing chronic pain with spiritual resources. *J Relig Health.* 1993;32(1):47–54.

19. Sorajjakool S, Thompson KM, Aveling L, Earl A. Chronic pain, meaning, and spirituality: a qualitative study of the healing process in relation to the role of meaning and spirituality. *J Pastoral Care Counsel.* 2006;60(4):369–378.

20. Landro L. The informed patient: bigger roles for chaplains on patient medical teams. *Wall Street Journal.* December 6, 2011.

21. Assefi N, Bogart A, Goldberg J, et al. Reiki for the treatment of fibromyalgia: a randomized controlled trial. *J Altern Complement Med.* 2008;14(9):1115–1112.

22. Nahin RL, Barnes PM, Stussman BJ, Bloom B. Costs of complementary and alternative medicine (CAM) and frequency of visits to CAM practitioners: United States, 2007. *Natl Health Stat Report.* 2009;18:1–14.

23. Cherkin DC, Sherman KJ, Kahn J, et al. A comparison of the effects of 2 types of massage and usual care on chronic low back pain: a randomized, controlled trial. *Ann Intern Med.* 2011;155(1):1–9.

24. Furlan AD, Imamura M, Dryden T, et al. Massage for low-back pain. *Cochrane Database Syst Rev.* 2008;(4):CD001929.

25. Kalichman L. Massage therapy for fibromyalgia symptoms. *Rheumatol Int.* 2010;30(9):1151–1157.

26. Perlman AI, Ali A, Njike VY, et al. Massage therapy for osteoarthritis of the knee: a randomized dose-finding trial. *PLoS One.* 2012;7(2):e30248.

27. Corbin L. Safety and efficacy of massage therapy for patients with cancer. *Cancer Control.* 2005;12(3):158–164.

28. Hillier SL, Louw Q, Morris L, et al. Massage therapy for people with HIV/AIDS. *Cochrane Database Syst Rev.* 2010;(1):CD007502.

29. U.S. Department of Labor, Bureau of Labor Statistics. Occupational Outlook Handbook. Massage Therapists. www.bls.gov/ooh/Healthcare/Massage-therapists.htm

30. Giggins OM, Persson UM, Caulfield B. Biofeedback in rehabilitation. *J Neuroeng Rehabil.* 2013,10:60.

31. Kabat Zinn J. An outpatient program in behavioral medicine for chronic pain patients based on the practice of mindfulness meditation. *Gen Hosp Psychiatry.* 1982;(4):33–47.

32. Zeidan F, Martucci KT, Kraft RA, et al. Brain mechanisms supporting modulation of pain by mindfulness meditation. *J Neurosci.* 2011;31(14):5540–5548.

33. Dusek JA, Benson H. Mind-body medicine: a model of the comparative clinical impact of the acute stress and relaxation responses. *Minn Med.* 2009;92(5):47–50.

34. Jorm AF, Morgan AJ, Hetrick SE. Relaxation for depression. *Cochrane Database Syst Rev.* 2008;(4):CD007142.

35. Larkey L, Jahnke R, Etnier J, Gonzalez J. Meditative movement as a category of exercise: implications for research. *J Phys Act Health.* 2009;6(2):230–238.

36. National QiGong Association. What is qigong? http://nqa.org/resources/what-is-qigong/. Accessed May 9, 2014.

37. Peng PW. Tai chi and chronic pain. *Reg Anesth Pain Med.* 2012;37(4):372–382.

38. American Yoga Association. General yoga information. www.americanyogaassociation. org/general.html.

39. National Institutes of Health, National Center for Complementary and Integrative Health. Yoga for Health. NCCAM Pub No. D472. http://nccam.nih.gov/health/yoga/introduction. htm#status.

40. Keefe F, Porter L, Somers T, Shelby R, Wren V. Psychosocial interventions for managing pain in older adults: outcomes and clinical implications. *Br J Anaesth.* 2013;111(1):89–94.

41. Langhorst J, Klose P, Dobos G, Bernardy K, Hauser W. Efficacy and safety of meditative movement therapies in fibromyalgia syndrome: a systematic review and meta-analysis of randomized controlled trials. *Rheumatol Int.* 2013;33:193–207.

42. Chou R, Qaseem A, Snow V, et al. Diagnosis and treatment of low back pain: a joint clinical practice guideline from the American College of Physicians and the American Pain Society. *Ann Intern Med.* 2007;147: 478–491.

43. Sherman KJ, Cherkin DC, Erro J, Miglioretti DL, Deyo RA. Comparing yoga, exercise, and a self-care book for chronic low back pain: a randomized, controlled trial. *Ann Intern Med.* 2005;143:849–856.

44. Barnes P, Powell-Griner E, McFann K, Nahin RL. Complementary and alternative medicine use among adults: United States, 2002. *Adv Data.* 2004;343:1–19.

45. An evidence-based review of qi gong by the Natural Standard Research Collaboration. *Nat Med J.* 2010;2(5). http://naturalmedicinejournal.com/journal/2010-05/evidence-based-review-qi-gong-natural-standard-research-collaboration.

46. Goleman D, Schwartz G. Meditation as an intervention in stress reactivity. *Journal of Consulting and Clinical Psychology.* 1976;44(3):456–466.

MANAGEMENT OF CHRONIC PAIN IN SELECTED PATIENT CATEGORIES

20

Chronic Pain in Hospitalized Patients with Selected Medical Conditions

TIM SABLE

KEY POINTS

- Proper evaluation and treatment of acute on chronic pain in patients admitted to the hospital are critical for healthcare delivery.
- It is important to avoid inducing withdrawal due to miscommunication or errors in medicine reconciliation on admission.
- Assessment of acute on chronic painful conditions should include review of multisystem disease involvement, such as sickle cell disease, diabetes, and autoimmune disorders.
- Treatment should be geared to analgesia, improved ambulation and function, and shortened length of hospital stay.

Introduction

In the hospital setting, pain management can be complex. Often patients have coexisting acute on chronic pain syndromes, and frequently patients have complex coexisting disease processes that complicate pain control. These processes have their own unique features that require consideration when optimizing the patient's pain control and functionality, and, ultimately, shortening length of stay or expediting discharge. In this chapter, we will explore the different nuances of pain management in commonly encountered scenarios of inpatient care. We will review specific painful conditions in major systemic diseases, including the hematological, urological, vascular, cardiac, gastrointestinal, infectious, endocrine, and musculoskeletal systems. After reviewing this chapter, the reader should have a better grasp on tailoring pain management techniques in these unique patient populations and be able to improve outcomes in the inpatient setting.

General Principles

When encountering a patient with significant pain history in the hospital, it is important to gather a pertinent history and physical. Major organ systems should be covered, particularly renal and hepatic disease, as this can drastically alter metabolism and clearance of many analgesic medications. It is also useful to know the history regarding chronic pain treatment as an outpatient, including the amount of opiate used daily, as this can be useful as a starting point for inpatient dosing. Commonly, one would call the prescribing physician, do a thorough chart review, or consult the prescription monitoring program online (this is useful when trying to resolve contradictory information).

The WHO ladder, as seen in Figure 20.1, was designed by the World Health Organization to help guide practitioners in the treatment of cancer pain, but it is also a useful starting point when managing acute on chronic pain in the hospital (Figure 20.1).

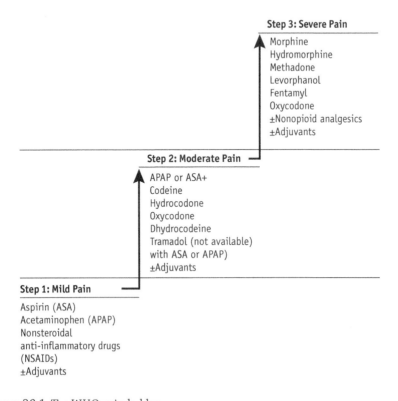

Step 3: Severe Pain

Morphine
Hydromorphine
Methadone
Levorphanol
Fentamyl
Oxycodone
±Nonopioid analgesics
±Adjuvants

Step 2: Moderate Pain

APAP or ASA+
Codeine
Hydrocodone
Oxycodone
Dhydrocodeine
Tramadol (not available)
with ASA or APAP)
±Adjuvants

Step 1: Mild Pain

Aspirin (ASA)
Acetaminophen (APAP)
Nonsteroidal
anti-inflammatory drugs
(NSAIDs)
±Adjuvants

Figure 20.1 The WHO pain ladder.

Sickle Cell Disease

Sickle-cell disease (SCD) is a hemoglobinopathy, producing severe anemia and various severe events that have been termed *crises*. It is caused by a point mutation in the β-globin chain of hemoglobin; the hydrophilic amino acid glutamic acid is replaced with the hydrophobic amino acid valine at the sixth position. This causes "sickling" of red blood cells and loss of elasticity, particularly in the setting of hypoxia, acidosis, hypothermia, and infection. This results in vaso-occclusion, the primary pathology of sickle cell crises.

Sickle cell disease results in crises of many types, including the vaso-occlusive crisis, aplastic crisis, sequestration crisis, hemolytic crisis, and others. However, acutely painful episodes of sickling are the most common reason for patients with SCD to seek medical attention.[1] While the annual incidence rate of pain episodes increases with age, reported rates for adults with SCD are relatively low because the majority of such episodes are managed at home.[1,2]

Vaso-occlusion results in tissue ischemia, and inflammation is the basis for much of SCD-related pain. Acute episodes of vaso-occlusive pain may also occur along with chronic pain due to the presence of such SCD-related complications as compression fractures, avascular necrosis, arthropathies, or leg ulcers; or they may be due to coexisting conditions not related to SCD (e.g., trauma or arthritis).[3] The main locations for acute pain in SCD are upper back (63%), left arm (61%), and, in decreasing order of frequency, legs (38%), chest (26%), and lower back (12%).[4]

When adults with SCD present to the hospital for a pain episode, the pain has been rated as a mean of 95 mm (out of 100 mm) on the visual analogue scale on admission, and 48 mm on hospital discharge (see Appendix 20.1).[5] When asked in a systematic fashion to describe the character of their pain, adults with SCD often use descriptors associated with nociceptive (secondary to tissue ischemia) and neuropathic (secondary to aberrant somatosensory input) pain. Despite the observation that ,during a pain episode, neuropathic pain symptoms have been described in adults with SCD,[5] the majority of symptoms are secondary to nociceptive pain and therapy should be directed at treatment of nociceptive pain, not neuropathic pain.

Most SCD patients do not take opioid medications for chronic pain at home. However, despite absence of indication in most cases, many of these patients will be on chronic opioid therapy between crises, and thus recognition of tolerance for acute pain crises in the hospital is expected.

Given the compromise of renal blood flow in patients with SCD and the risk of acute or chronic renal insufficiency or failure, coupled with the evidence that adjuvant NSAIDs do not decrease pain in patients concomitantly treated with morphine and acetaminophen,[6] NSAIDs should be used sparingly and based on clinical judgment, and probably should not be used beyond 5 days.

With regard to opiates, the standard WHO ladder algorithm should apply. Many patients with SCD also likely have genetic insensitivity to codeine.[7] Pain management for acute pain crises in the hospital is typically accomplished with scheduled opiates or opiate infusion. It is important to watch for pre-existing renal insufficiency and be wary of starting or maintaining doses of opiates, particularly morphine. High levels of the metabolite morphine-6-glucuronide occur in renal dysfunction and cause sedation and respiratory depression.[8]

All patients should be assessed with objective pain tools and sedation scales. Oxygen saturation monitoring is helpful in managing patients during severe painful episodes. Orders should include temporary cessation of analgesia and physician notification if oxygen desaturation or bradypnea occurs. Patient-controlled analgesia (PCA) is also a good choice for acute pain crises, and while not shown to improve pain scores or complications in this set of patients, it does result in higher patient satisfaction.[9]

Nontraumatic Acute Flank Pain

Among the diverse urological causes of nontraumatic acute flank pain are renal or ureteral stones, urinary tract infection (pyelonephritis, pyonephrosis, or renal abscess), ureteropelvic junction obstruction, renal vascular disorders (renal infarction, renal vein thrombosis), papillary necrosis, intra- or perirenal bleeding, and testicular cord torsion.

Regarding analgesia, a slow intravenous (IV) infusion of dipyrone, 1 g or 2 g, is just as effective as diclofenac (75 mg bolus). IV papaverine (120 mg) can effectively and safely relieve pain in patients not responding to conventional agents (diclofenac) and can be an alternative to diclofenac in patients with contraindications to NSAIDs. A combination of morphine and ketorolac IV can also be very effective and seems to reduce the need for rescue analgesia.[10]

Loin Pain Hematuria Syndrome

Loin pain hematuria syndrome (LPHS) is a condition sometimes encountered in pain medicine that is characterized by severe flank pain and hematuria, as the name implies. It was first described in 1967 in a report of three women who had recurrent episodes of severe unilateral or bilateral loin (flank) pain that were accompanied by gross or microscopic hematuria. The major causes of flank pain and hematuria were not present on workup. Renal arteriography suggested focally impaired cortical perfusion, while renal biopsy showed interstitial fibrosis and arterial sclerosis. Since this original report, several hundred cases have been reported in the medical literature.[11,12]

Several treatments have been described for LPHS. In general, these patients are admitted for 3–5 days in the hospital for control of severe pain and nausea. With severe nausea and vomiting, PO medications are not tolerated, so often these patients are treated with intermittent IV opiates, PCA, or transdermal routes. Sodium thiosulfate infusions, retrograde capsaicin infusion, surgical denervation, intrathecal opiates, and celiac plexus block have all been described with variable reports of success.[13–15] In general, these patients have normal renal function.

Peripheral Vascular Disease

Eight to ten million Americans suffer from arterial occlusive disease, with approximately 500 to 1000 new cases of chronic limb ischemia per million occurring per year.[16] Generally, patients are admitted when pain control is poor and/or there is evidence of significant limb ischemia.

Patients tend to be managed surgically with revascularization, particularly when critical limb ischemia is present. Often these patients have severe pain as well as coexisting renal disease, so judicious use of opiates and adjuvants is recommended. PCA again can have good utility. Neuropathic pain medications can be of good use to reduce the opiate dose needed, and often there is an element of neuropathic pain in these patients that responds well. Caution should be used with gabapentinoids when there is a high likelihood of coexisting renal disease, cardiac disease, and limb edema. Sympathetic blocks have been used as well for pain control with modest success.[17]

Spinal cord stimulation (SCS) is another modality used for pain control when medically and surgically maximized. Initial studies suggested that SCS was effective for pain relief and might improve rates of amputation and limb survival.[18,19] A recent controlled trial with 120 randomly assigned patients (SCS plus best medical therapy versus best medical therapy alone) found that rates of survival, amputation, and pain scores were the same in both groups, but the SCS group was able to reduce use of pain medications by approximately 50%.[20]

Considerations for Cardiac Disease

Patients admitted to the hospital with coexisting pain and heart disease can pose unique challenges. Depending on the etiology of their heart disease, they may have multisystem organ impairment. Caution should be used when starting membrane stabilizers that can cause edema (gabapentin, pregabalin) as these can worsen pre-existing fluid overload and congestive heart failure (CHF).[21] Topiramate is theoretically preferred in these scenarios.

Table 20.1   COX activity in selected NSAIDs.

NSAIDs should also be avoided in patients with pre-existing cardiac disease and cerebral vascular disease, particularly those with COX-2 action (Table 20.1).

Inflammatory Bowel Disease

Patients with inflammatory bowel disease (IBD), most commonly ulcerative colitis and Crohn's disease, are often frequent fliers in the hospital because of acute attacks of inflammation, bowel obstructions, and acute on chronic pain. They are often on chronic opiate therapy at home, so checking history, getting prior records, and checking state prescription monitoring programs are crucial in assessment.

NSAIDs may worsen acute exacerbations of pain and inflammation, but use of COX-2 inhibitors has shown promise in reducing pain without increasing flares. Tricyclic antidepressants and anticonvulsants have also shown promise in treatment of pain (Figure 20.2).[22]

Chronic Pain Patients with History of Bariatric Surgery

Many patients being admitted to the hospital with long-standing chronic pain may also have a history of bariatric surgery. Often absorption of long-acting

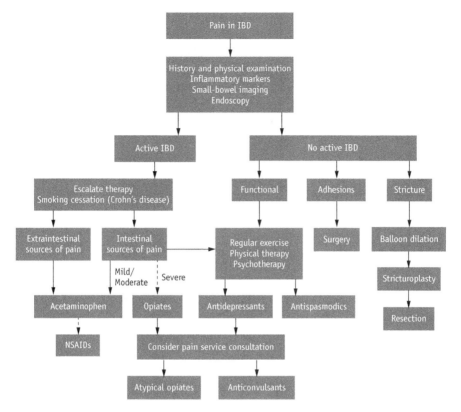

Figure 20.2 Management of acute on chronic pain in patients with ulcerative colitis and Crohn's disease.

formulations of opiates is altered in these patients. It is useful to consider rotation to transdermal opiates for these patients (fentanyl/buprenophine), or IV medication can be considered. In general, NSAIDs are to be avoided in these patients given the increased risk of gastrointestinal bleeding.

Gastroparesis

Commonly patients with severe abdominal pain have elements of gastroparesis, either disease induced (diabetes) or drug induced (opiates). Often reducing opiates in these patients improves bowel function and reduces pain. Tricyclic antidepressants can also cause decreased gut motility because of their anticholinergic effects.

HIV Neuropathy

Peripheral neuropathy is common in individuals infected with the human immunodeficiency virus (HIV). Peripheral neuropathy may arise as a complication of

HIV infection itself, drug therapy, or other host factors, such as diabetes. It can present as painful autonomic neuropathy, radiculopathy, or mononeuropathy. The incidence of herpes zoster virus is also higher in this population.

Patients with autonomic neuropathy have a high incidence of orthostatic hypotension, and many neuropathic pain medications can worsen this. Nortriptyline and desipramine are tricyclic agents with a relatively low incidence of postural hypotension and their use may minimize this problem.[23] For mononeuropathies a short oral steroid burst can be used successfully.

Care should also be taken in this population regarding use of a combination of many antiretroviral medications which are CYP3A4 inducers, as these may cause methadone or buprenorphine withdrawal through increased metabolism.[24]

Herpes Zoster

Herpes zoster, also known as shingles, results from reactivation of endogenous latent varicella zoster virus infection within the sensory ganglia, resulting in a painful, unilateral vesicular eruption. This commonly occurs in a restricted dermatomal distribution. It is typically present in older patients.

Antiviral treatment with drugs such as Acyclovir is first-line treatment.[25] Otherwise, one can follow the WHO ladder algorithm. Anticonvulsants such as pregabalin can be tried, as well as topical lidocaine and capsaicin. Interventional options depending on location of pain can include epidural steroid injections or sympathetic blocks.

Diabetes Mellitus

Chronic pain is common in the diabetic population, largely through disease-induced neuropathic pain. These patients also have a high incidence of comorbidities, including cardiac and renal impairment.

Treatments that may be beneficial for painful diabetic neuropathy include a number of antidepressants (e.g., amitriptyline, duloxetine, venlafaxine) and anticonvulsants (e.g., pregabalin, sodium valproate) as well as capsaicin cream, lidocaine patch, alpha-lipoic acid, isosorbide dinitrate topical spray, and transcutaneous electrical nerve stimulation (TENS).

A management algorithm outlined by a statement published in 2005 from the American Diabetes Association (ADA) recommended treatment in sequential steps[26]:

- Stabilize glycemic control (insulin not always required in type 2 diabetes)
- Tricyclic drugs (e.g., amitriptyline 25–150 mg before bed)

- Anticonvulsants (e.g., gabapentin, typical dose 1.8 g/day)
- Opioid or opioid-like drugs (e.g., tramadol or controlled-release oxycodone)
- Consider pain clinic referral (possible interventions including sympathetic blocks/spinal cord stimulation)

Inflammatory Arthropathy

Severe arthritic pain due to inflammation includes conditions such as rheumatoid arthritis and psoriatic arthritis, among others. These conditions cause severe pain and inflammation in the joints and are a source of severe disability as well. Commonly, these patients are managed on DMARD (disease-modifying antirheumatic drugs) therapy and often on chronic steroid therapy as well.

The WHO criteria apply in initial pain treatment. Opiates should be limited to treatment of severe exacerbation of pain and inflammation on a short-term basis only, or in cases of severe joint destruction that have not responded to corticosteroid/NSAID/DMARD treatment.

Fibromyalgia

Fibromyalgia (FM) is characterized by widespread musculoskeletal pain and fatigue, often accompanied by cognitive and mood disturbances. It is considered a functional somatic disorder. Patient often have severe pain coupled with sleep disturbances. Fibromyalgia is considered to be the most common cause of generalized, musculoskeletal pain in women between ages of 20 and 55 years. In the United States and in other countries, the prevalence is approximately 2%.[27] As such, it is commonly seen on inpatient units.

Medication therapy includes amitriptyline, duloxetine, pregabalin, or milnacipran. Patients often respond best to multimodal therapy including behavioral health, counseling, sleep hygiene, and physical therapy and exercise.[28]

Opiates are not indicated for the primary treatment of fibromyalgia, as there is no proven benefit and they may worsen generalized pain through mechanisms such as opiate-induced hyperalgesia. They should be used judiciously for acute pain syndromes and postsurgical pain in patients with pre-existing fibromyalgia. Education and expectations of pain control should be discussed with the patient. Mobilization and sleep hygiene should be stressed.

Summary

Chronic pain is increasingly prevalent in the inpatient setting. Knowing how to properly evaluate and treat acute on chronic pain is more and more vital when seeing patients admitted to the hospital. It is important to review the patient's medical history, paying particular attention to history of analgesics use, adjuvant use, and disease progression. It is essential to avoid inducing withdrawal due to miscommunication or errors in medicine reconciliation on admission. This can be facilitated through careful chart review, history, and review of state prescription monitoring programs. Assessment of acute on chronic painful conditions should include a review of multisystem disease involvement, such as sickle cell disease, diabetes, and autoimmune disorders. Treatment should be tailored to avoid worsening of organ dysfunction and build-up of drugs and metabolites, which can cause adverse outcomes. Treatment should be geared toward analgesia, improved ambulation and function, and shortened length of hospital stay.

References

1. Telfer P, Bahal N, Lo A, Challands J.Management of the acute painful crisis in sickle cell disease—a re-evaluation of the use of opioids in adult patients. *Br J Haematol.* 2014;166(2):157–164.
2. Smith WR, Penberthy LT, Bovbjerg VE, et al. Daily assessment of pain in adults with sickle cell disease. *Ann Intern Med.* 2008;148:94.
3. Ballas SK. Pain management of sickle cell disease. *Hematol Oncol Clin North Am.* 2005;19:785.
4. Wilkie DJ, Molokie R, Boyd-Seal D, et al. Patient-reported outcomes: descriptors of nociceptive and neuropathic pain and barriers to effective pain management in adult outpatients with sickle cell disease. *J Natl Med Assoc.* 2010;102:18.
5. Ballas SK, Reyes PE. Peripheral neuropathy in adults with sickle cell disease. *Am J Pain Med.* 1997;71:53.
6. Schaller S, Kaplan BS. Acute nonoliguric renal failure in children associated with nonsteroidal antiinflammatory agents. *Pediatr Emerg Care.* 1998;14:416.
7. Brousseau DC, McCarver DG, Drendel AL, et al. The effect of CYP2D6 polymorphisms on the response to pain treatment for pediatric sickle cell pain crisis. *J Pediatr.* 2007;150:623.
8. Sear JW, Hand CW, Moore RA, McQuay HJ. Studies on morphine disposition: influence of renal failure on the kinetics of morphine andmia: a randomised trial. ESES Study Group. *Lancet.* 1999;353:1040.
9. Cantu M, Lindenfeld J, Hergott LJ, et al. Possible heart failure exacerbation associated with pregabalin: case discussion and literature review. *J Cardiovasc Med (Hagerstown).* 2008;9(9):922–925.
10. Macintyre PE. Safety and efficacy of patient-controlled analgesia. *Br J Anaesth.* 2001;87(1):36–46.
11. Bader P, Echtle D, Fonteyne V, et al. Guidelines to Pain Mangagement in Urology. http://www.uroweb.org/gls/pockets/english/Pain%20Management%20in%20Urology%202010.pdf
12. Little PJ, Sloper JS, de Wardener HE. A syndrome of loin pain and haematuria associated with disease of peripheral renal arteries. *Q J Med.* 1967;36:253.
13. Spetie DN, Nadasdy T, Nadasdy G, et al. Proposed pathogenesis of idiopathic loin pain-hematuria syndrome. *Am J Kidney Dis.* 2006;47:419.
14. Prager JP, DeSalles A, Wilkinson A, et al. Loin pain hematuria syndrome: pain relief with intrathecal morphine. *Am J Kidney Dis.* 1995;25:629.
15. Uzoh CC, Kumar V, Timoney AG. The use of capsaicin in loin pain-haematuria syndrome *BJU Int.* 2008;103:236.

16. Yatzidis H. Successful sodium thiosulphate treatment for recurrent calcium urolithiasis. *Clin Nephrol*. 1985;23:63.

17. Veith, FJ, Gupta, SK, Wengerter, KR, et al. Femoral-popliteal-tibial occlusive disease. In: Moore WS, ed., *Vascular Surgery: A Comprehensive Review*. Philadelphia: WB Saunders; 1991:364.

18. Walsh JA, Glynn CJ, Cousins MJ, Basedow RW. Blood flow, sympathetic activity and pain relief following lumbar sympathetic blockade or surgical sympathectomy. Anaesth Intensive Care 1985;13(1):18.

19. Horsch S, Claeys L. Epidural spinal cord stimulation in the treatment of severe peripheral arterial occlusive disease. *Ann Vasc Surg*. 1994;8:468.

20. Mingoli A, Sciacca V, Tamorri M, et al. Clinical results of epidural spinal cord electrical stimulation in patients affected with limb-threatening chronic arterial obstructive disease. *Angiology*. 1993;44:21.

21. Klomp HM, Spincemaille GH, Steyerberg EW, et al. Spinal-cord stimulation in critical limb ischemia. *Lancet*. 1999;353(9158):1040.

22. Docherty M, Jones R, et al. Managing pain in inflammatory bowel disease. *Gastroenterol Hepatol (NY)*. 2011;7(9):592–601.

23. Moulignier A, Authier FJ, Baudrimont M, et al. Peripheral neuropathy in human immunodeficiency virus–infected patients with the diffuse infiltrative lymphocytosis syndrome. *Ann Neurol*. 1997;41:438.

24. Ferrari A., Coccia CPR, Bertolini A, Sternieri E. Methadone—metabolism, pharmacokinetics and interactions. *Pharmacol Res*. 2004;50(6):551–559.

25. Wood MJ, Kay R, Dworkin RH, et al. Oral acyclovir therapy accelerates pain resolution in patients with herpes zoster: a meta-analysis of placebo-controlled trials. *Clin Infect Dis*. 1996;22:341.

26. Boulton AJ, Vinik AI, Arezzo JC, et al. Diabetic neuropathies: a statement by the American Diabetes Association. *Diabetes Care*. 2005;28:956.

27. Lawrence RC, Felson DT, Helmick CG, et al. Estimates of the prevalence of arthritis and other rheumatic conditions in the United States. Part II. *Arthritis Rheum*. 2008;58:26.

28. Goldenberg DL, Burckhardt C, Crofford L. Management of fibromyalgia syndrome. *JAMA*. 2004;292:2388.

Appendix 20.1 Pain Diary Form

Pain Diary for _____

Date & time	Pain score (0 to 10)	Where pain is and how it feels (ache, sharp, throbbing, shooting, tingling)	What I was doing when it began	Name and amount of medicine taken	Non-drug techniques I tried	How long the pain lasted	Other notes

Reprinted with permission from the American Cancer Society, 2012.

21

Management of Chronic Pain in Neurological Disorders

ALEXANDER FEOKTISTOV

KEY POINTS

- It is important to get familiar with diagnostic criteria of most common neurological conditions associated with chronic pain, such as multiple sclerosis, post-stroke pain, chronic migraine and medications overuse headaches, as well as complex regional pain syndrome.
- For inpatient treatment of these painful conditions it is important to use a multidisciplinary approach consisting of nonpharmacological treatment modalities (transcutaneous nerve stimulation, physical and occupational therapy, cognitive behavioral therapy), conservative medical management (use of antidepressants, anticonvulsants, various abortive medications), and interventional treatment. Therapy needs to be started conservatively using a multidisciplinary approach and treatment advanced on the basis of the patient's response.
- Acute on chronic pain may present as a leading symptom of exacerbation in these conditions or it may be found in the background of other neurological symptoms.
- Early recognition of acute pain in these chronic painful conditions can lead to their timely treatment, ultimately affecting patients' quality of life and overall treatment outcomes.

Introduction

Numerous neurological conditions present with chronic pain. In some of these conditions, pain may be the presenting or leading symptom while in others it may be found in the background. In either case, chronic pain that is frequently seen in neurological disorders represents a diagnostic and therapeutic challenge.

Multiple Sclerosis

Multiple sclerosis (MS) is the most common autoimmune inflammatory disorder of the central nervous system. It is one of the most significant neurological disorders, considering its high incidence and prevalence as well as its tendency to affect the most productive age group. Multiple sclerosis affects more females than males, with overall female incidence being 3.6 and male, 2.0 cases per 100,000 population per year.[1] Prevalence of multiple sclerosis varies from 30 to 300 per 100.000 population. In the United States the prevalence is 100 per 100,000, accounting for a total of 250,000 patients.[2]

Multiple sclerosis is a demyelinating disorder that affects primarily the central nervous system, with pathophysiological bases consisting of inflammation, demyelination, and axon degeneration. In MS it is very typical that the central nervous system lesions are disseminated in space and time, dictating characteristic clinical signs and flow. According to the McDonald criteria, these changes need to be verified by MRI findings revealing not only two to more lesions affecting periventricular, juxtacortical, infratentorial, or spinal cord areas but also presence of both gadolinium-enhancing and non-enhancing lesions.[3,4] Classic MS features include motor weakness, paresthesias, impaired vision, dysarthria, ataxia, and bladder dysfunction. It has been estimated that in addition to these neurological symptoms, 29% to 86% of patients may also suffer from acute and/or chronic pain.[5-7] About 80% of patients report having chronic pain.

The most common pain syndrome is dysesthesia; it is seen in more than 18% of patients. Dysesthesia is often described by patients as severe burning and tingling pain usually affecting the extremities (although it may affect any part of the body). It is typically worse at night. This type of pain responds to treatment with tricyclic antidepressants such as amitriptyline.[5,9] The treatment usually starts at 25 mg orally at night and is gradually increased to 150 mg at night as tolerated. Xerostomia, somnolence, and fatigue are the most common side effects. Other tricyclic antidepressants could also be used (nortriptyline, desipramine) and should be considered for patients not tolerating amitriptyline. Alternative treatment includes use of carbamazepine at dosages of 100–200 mg three times per day. Some patients may also respond to transcutaneous nerve stimulation methods.

Another common pain syndrome in MS is back pain. Its prevalence varies from 16%[8] to 40% of patients with MS.[7] The mechanism of this pain is likely related to spasticity, muscle weakness, and associated mechanical stress and eventually degenerative spine disease. In these cases generous use of muscle relaxants (which are also helpful in management of chronic spasticity, discussed later in the chapter), nonsteroidal anti-inflammatory drugs (NSAIDs), and physical therapy are indicated. For patients not responding to these modalities, opioid therapy should be considered. For chronic long-term management of chronic back pain tricyclic antidepressants (those just listed), duloxetine (30–60 mg per day)[14] and/or pregabalin (300–600 mg per day) could be used. In cases where there are signs of radiculopathy, spinal stenosis, or advanced facet arthropathy and these do not respond to medical management, interventional pain management treatment modalities (epidural steroids injections, facet medical branch nerve blocks, and radiofrequency ablations) are indicated.

Muscle spasticity is another major causative and contributing factor to chronic pain in MS. In most cases spasticity (and associated pain) is effectively treated with the muscle relaxants.[10] There are multiple muscle relaxant available that could be tried, but the most consistent results have been shown for baclofen and/or tizanidine. It is suggested that baclofen therapy be started at 5–10 mg orally every 8 hours. The dose should be gradually increased as tolerated, up to 120 mg per day. The most common side effects of baclofen are drowsiness, muscle weakness, ataxia, hypertension, and fatigue. In patients who do not respond to baclofen therapy a trial of tizanidine (instead or even in addition to baclofen) is recommended. Tizanidine should be started at a dose of 2–4 mg three to four times per day and the dose gradually increased to 36 mg per day total, as tolerated. The most common side effects are somnolence, xerostomia, muscle weakness, and hypotension. Occasionally, patients may also benefit from the addition of a small dose of benzodiazepines, such as diazepam 1–2 mg two to three times per day. In some cases, when oral forms of muscle relaxants are not sufficient (they are ineffective or use is limited by side effects), intrathecal baclofen administration can be considered. The doses used for spasticity treatment with intrathecal baclofen administration vary between 22 mcg and 1400 mcg per day, although most patients are adequately treated at doses between 90 and 703 mcg per day. Intrathecal baclofen should be titrated with great caution. It is very important to adjust doses (including discontinuation of the drug) gradually to avoid toxicity and potential withdrawal symptoms. Lhermitte's sign (painful electric shock–like sensations along the spine that occur with neck flexion), which affects 9% of patients with MS, and trigeminal neuralgia, which occurs in 2% of cases, usually respond to carbamazepine 100–200 mg two to three times per day[11] or phenytoin 100–200 mg two to three times per day. Another alternative is oxcarbazepine, which is similar in efficacy to carbamazepine but has a more favorable side-effect profile. The treatment is usually initiated with doses of 300 mg twice daily and increased weekly with 300 mg increments up to 1800 mg per day.[12] Muscle relaxants (such as baclofen) could also be used with benefit.[13] In patients with refractory trigeminal neuralgia pain trigeminal ganglion block and later radiofrequency ablation may also be considered.

Nonpharmacological methods of chronic pain management such as physical therapy, cognitive-behavioral therapy, massage, topical heat, and use of transcutaneous nerve stimulation (TENS units) should also be widely used for most of the chronic pain conditions described here.

Chronic Headache

Chronic daily headaches represent a large group of primary headache disorders, defined by headache frequency of at least 15 days per months for at least 3 months.[15] Chronic daily headache consists of the following: chronic migraine; chronic tension-type headache; medication overuse headache; hemicrania continua; new daily persistent headache; chronic cluster headaches (which must persist for at least a year without remission, or remission for less than 1 month); chronic paroxysmal hemicrania (which must persist for at least a year without remission, or remission for less than 1 month); hypnic headache; short-lasting, unilateral, neuralgiform headache attacks with conjunctival injection and tearing (SUNCT)/short-lasting unilateral neuralgiform headache attacks with cranial autonomic symptoms (SUNA); and primary stabbing headaches.

Of all of these chronic headaches forms chronic migraine and medication overuse headache are most commonly seen. We will focus here on management of these main headache types.

CHRONIC MIGRAINE

Chronic migraine is one of the most common and disabling medical conditions given its chronicity and severity. It has been estimated that chronic migraines affect 2% of the world's population.[16]

Diagnostic criteria for migraine and chronic migraines are presented in Box 21.1, Box 21.2, and Box 21.3.

Patients usually present with daily, constant, or nearly constant headache. If asked specifically to describe their headache they will usually talk about at least two different types of headaches—milder, constant background headache, and more severe exacerbations that may last for several days at a time. These patients frequently overuse pain medications (both over-the-counter and prescription drugs) and usually represent a therapeutic challenge. Two main therapeutic strategies are used: acute or abortive treatment, designed to help with current ongoing pain (immediate pain relief), and prophylactic or preventative treatment, geared toward preventing future headaches (long-term pain relief). It has been widely accepted that migraine is a chronic condition for which there is no cure. That said, frequency and severity of headache episodes and their impact on a patient's quality of life can be modified with treatment. Thus it is imperative to explain to a patient that the goal of treatment is not to cure or eliminate migraines but to reduce their frequency and severity, improve management, and, most importantly, to improve the patient's quality of life and functionality.

Acute migraine treatment consists of use of triptans (sumatriptan, almotriptan, zolmitriptan, rizatriptan, frovatriptan, eletriptan, and almotriptan). Although they all have a similar mechanism of action and have similar efficacy

Box 21.1 Diagnostic Criteria of Migraine without Aura

1.1 MIGRAINE WITHOUT AURA

A. At least five attacks fulfilling criteria B–D
B. Headache attacks lasting 4–72 hours (untreated or unsuccessfully treated)
C. Headache has at least two of the following four characteristics:
   1. Unilateral location
   2. Pulsating quality
   3. Moderate or severe pain intensity
   4. Aggravation by or causing avoidance of routine physical activity
D. During headache at least one of the following:
   1. Nausea and/or vomiting
   2. Photophobia and phonophobia
E. Not better accounted for by another ICHD-3 diagnosis

Box 21.2 Diagnostic Criteria of Migrate with Aura

1.2 MIGRAINE WITH AURA

A. At least two attacks fulfilling criteria B and C
B. One or more of the following fully reversible aura symptoms:
   1. Visual
   2. Sensory
   3. Speech and/or language
   4. Motor
   5. Brainstem
   6. Retinal
C. At least two of the following four characteristics:
   1. At least one aura symptom spreads gradually over >5 minutes, and/or two or more symptoms occur in succession.
   2. Each individual aura symptom lasts 5–60 minutes.
   3. At least one aura symptom is unilateral.
   4. The aura is accompanied, or followed within 60 minutes, by headache.
D. Not better accounted for by another ICHD-3 diagnosis, and transient ischemic attack has been excluded

---

Box 21.3 Diagnostic Criteria of Chronic Migraine

1.3 CHRONIC MIGRAINE

E. Headache (tension-type-like and/or migraine-like) on >15 days per month for >3 months and fulfilling criteria B and C

F. Occurring in a patient who has had at least five attacks fulfilling criteria B–D for 1.1 Migraine without Aura and/or criteria B and C for 1.2 Migraine with Aura

G. On >8 days per month for >3 months, fulfilling any of the following:
   5. Criteria C and D for 1.1 Migraine without Aura
   6. Criteria B and C for 1.2 Migraine with Aura
   7. Believed by the patient to be migraine at onset and relieved by a triptan or ergot derivative

H. Not better accounted for by another ICHD-3 diagnosis

---

and side-effect profile, there are differences regarding onset and duration of action that are worth noting (Table 21.1).

For migraines that tend to evolve over a short period of time and reach severe intensity in just 30–60 minutes, triptans with a rapid onset of action are preferred. For migraines that evolve over a period of 2–3 hours (slower evolving) and especially those that last for several days, longer-acting triptans are more beneficial. Another acute treatment alternative is ergotamine-containing medications, such as dihydroergotamine, which is most commonly used. It is available as a nasal spray and in oral and parenteral (IV and IM) forms. It is imperative that different forms of triptans, and triptans and ergotamine-containing medications not be used within 24 hours of each other, to prevent drug–drug interactions.

Table 21.1 **Triptans**

Name	Route	Half-life	Onset (50% Reduction)
Sumatriptan	sq, ns, po	2 hours	30 minutes, 30–60 minutes, 1–2 hours
Treximet	po	2 hours	1–2 hours
Zolmitriptan	ns, po, odt	3 hours	30–60 minutes, 1–2 hours
Rizatriptan	po, odt	1.5 hours	1–2 hours (highest %)
Naratriptan	po	5–6 hours	2–4 hours
Almotriptan	po	3 hours	2 hours
Eletriptan	po	3–6 hours	2 hours
Frovatriptan	po	26 hours	4 hours

Patients who do not respond to triptan and/or ergotamine treatment may benefit from a short course of corticosteroid therapy. We usually recommend using either dexamethasone or methylprednisolone, usually as a short 5–6 days' tapering course. If that treatment fails, hospital admission for parenteral medication administration is indicated. One of the most effective inpatient treatment regimens is DHE-45 protocol. This protocol consists of IV administration of 0.5–1.0 mg of dihydroergotamine every 8 hours for 9 doses total. One of the most common side effects is nausea, so all patients should be premedicated with an antiemetic (ondansetron, promethazine or metoclopromide). Other IV medications that may be beneficial are ketorolac (30 mg IV every 6 hours), orphenadrine (30–60 mg IV every 6 hours), diphenhydramine (50 mg IV every 6 hours), valproate sodium (500 mg every 8 hours), and magnesium sulfate (1000 mg every 12 hours). In those patients resistant to these therapies droperidol or chlorpromazine may be indicated. We recommend reserving opioid use only for patients who are not responding or have contraindications to or are unable to tolerate these therapies.

Prophylactic therapy consists of use of beta-blockers (metoprolol, propranolol). It is important to recognize that of beta-blockers need to be gradually increased on the basis of the patient's response. Discontinuation of beta-blockers also needs to be gradual.

Therapeutic effect of propranolol may occur at 160–240 mg per day dose range. Another effective treatment modality is topiramate. Treatment usually begins with 25–50 mg per day and is increased by 25–50 mg increments every week, up to a total daily dose of 100–200 mg.

Divalproex sodium may also be used in doses gradually titrated up to 1000 mg per day. Another alternative is a group of tricyclic antidepressants (amitriptyline, nortriptyline, protriptyline, desipramine). Treatment usually starts at doses of 10–25 mg per day that are gradually increased to 100–150 mg per day, if necessary. Finally, botulinum toxin type A has been shown to be effective in patients with chronic migraines. Recommended doses are 155–195 units per treatment and the treatment needs to be repeated every 3 months.

The choice of prophylactic therapy needs to be tailored for each patient, with consideration given to particular drug advantages and disadvantages. For example, for patients with chronic migraine and hypertension, the best starting prophylactic agent may be beta-blockers. Patients with coexisting depression may benefit from an antidepressant. Obese patients should be started on topiramate given its weight-lowering properties (and tricyclic antidepressant should be used with caution, given their weight-gaining potential). Patients should be educated that prophylactic therapy is supposed to be long term and that it usually takes 4–6 weeks before the desired outcome may be achieved.

Nonpharmacological treatment should include biofeedback, stress management, and physical therapy.

MEDICATION OVERUSE HEADACHE

Medication overuse headache is a primary chronic headache disorder that develops as a result of regular acute (abortive) medication overuse.[17,18] It affects about 1% of populations.[19] Most patients suffering from medication overuse headache have a history of another pre-existing primary headache disorder from which the medication overuse headache has evolved. The most common primary headache form that may evolve into medication overuse headache (in the presence of regular medication overuse) is migraine. Medication overuse headache is not drug-specific and may develop as a result of overuse of triptans, over-the-counter medications (acetaminophen, NSAIDs, etc.), opioids, ergotamine-containing medications, caffeine, and butalbital-containing medications. The diagnostic criteria for medication overuse headache are given in Box 21.4.

Patients should be considered overusing symptomatic or abortive medications if they take simples analgesics (for example, acetaminophen) or NSAIDs for at least 15 days per month for at least 3 months. With use of triptans, ergotamine-containing medications, opioids, and other prescription abortive medications, medication overuse should be suspected if the patient has been taking any of these medications for at least 10 days per month for at least 3 months. In cases of treatment with combinations of more than one rescue medication, medication overuse should be considered if the patient has been taking a combination of any of these abortive medications at least 15 days per month for at least 3 months. Usually a patient's history begins with a primary episodic headache form (most commonly migraine). Eventually (for various reasons), patients start overusing acute abortive medications and the pre-existing headache's frequency increases, gradually being "transformed" into a chronic medication overuse headache.[20] Along the way, some characteristic feature of that original pre-existing headache may be lost and the headache acquires more nonspecific symptoms and signs, making it present as a mixed headache syndrome.

When treating patients with medication overuse headache it is imperative to discontinue the medication(s) that the patient has been overusing. When discontinuing the drug it is important to avoid use of not only that particular drug but also the entire pharmacological family (NSAIDs, triptans, opioids, etc.).

Box 21.4 **Diagnostic Criteria of Medication Overuse Headache**

A. Headache occurring on >15 days per month in a patient with a pre-existing headache disorder
B. Regular overuse for >3 months of one or more drugs that can be taken for acute and or symptomatic treatment of headache
C. Not better accounted for by another ICHD-3 diagnosis

Discontinuation of the abortive medications the patient has been overusing not only reduces headache frequency but also positively affects prophylactic medication effectiveness. During the first few weeks the patient may notice worsening of his or her headaches. At the same time, while discontinuing the offending medicine new prophylactic therapy should be initiated.[21] Prophylactic and abortive therapy for medication overuse headache is similar to that used for chronic migraine treatment, with special attention paid to discontinuation of the abortive medications that led to development of the medication overuse headache.

Central Pain Syndrome

Central pain is a type of neuropathic pain resulted by central nervous system lesion. Most common causes of central pain are strokes (ischemic and hemorrhagic) especially in thalamic region, multiple sclerosis, cerebral and spinal cord injuries, tumors, Parkinson's disease.[22] The pain is usually described as severe, lacerating, burning, shooting, or freezing. In most cases central pain appears to be of moderate to severe intensity. It may occur immediately or several months after the inciting event (stroke, injury, etc.). The pain may be diffuse or localized and frequently associated with some type of loss of sensation in the affected area. The pain is aggravated by verity of non-noxious stimuli (hot or cold air, slight touch, etc.). It is frequently aggravated by emotions and emotional stress.[23,24]

Treatment of chronic central pain might be very challenging.[25] It recommended starting therapy with carbamazepine 100–200 mg three times daily and the dose may need to be increased up to 1200 mg per day. Rare but serious adverse events associated with carbamazepine use are agranulocytosis and aplastic anemia, thus complete blood count should be checked at baseline and closely monitored during therapy. Similarly to other types of chronic neuropathic pain treatment use of tricyclic antidepressant may of great value. Most commonly used antidepressant in that category is amitriptyline. Treatment usually starts at doses 10–25 mg at night and gradually increased to 100–150 mg at night. Most of tricyclic antidepressant are sedating (except protriptyline) and should be used at night. Other common side effects include xerostomia, constipation, tachycardia, orthostatic hypotension (especially in elderly) and weight gain.[26]

Antidepressants from the group of selective norepinephrine reuptake inhibitors such as duloxetine (30–60 mg per day) and venlafaxine (75–225 mg per day) could also be used.

Gabapentin has been shown to be beneficial in treatment of neuropathic pain and could be used in the management of central pain. Usual starting dose is 300 mg per day and it could be increased in 300 mg increments weekly up to a total daily dose of 3600 mg.[27] Lamotrigine has also been beneficial in treatment of central pain especially located in the face area.[22] Starting dose is 25 mg per day and it needs to be gradually increased over 5–6 weeks course up to 200 mg per day. Benzodiazepines (clonazepam 0.25 mg–6 mg per day) and topiramate (100–400 mg per day) have also been demonstrated beneficial.[26] Transcutaneous nerve stimulation may also be considered in most of the patients with central pain syndrome and used in combination with above mentioned medical treatment.[28] In patients not responding to conservative medical treatment modalities interventional/surgical approaches should be considered. Gasserian ganglion electrical stimulation was shown to be beneficial in patients with refractory central facial pain.[29] Finally spinal cord stimulation may be utilized in refractory cases especially for pain localized to a limited body area [30]. Deep brain stimulation and thalamotomy should only be considered as a last resort in most intractable cases.[22,30]

Complex Regional Pain Syndrome

Complex regional pain syndrome (CRPS) is a chronic, disabling pain disorder characterized by severe pain, localized edema, vasomotor and skin changes, decreased range of motion, and patchy bone mineralization.[31] There are two types of CRPS: CRPS type I (formerly known as reflex sympathetic dystrophy) and CRPS type II (formerly known as causalgia). The main differentiating factor in these two conditions is presence (in CRPS type II) or absence (in CRPS type I) of a definable nerve injury or trauma. CRPS is frequently preceded by an inciting event such soft tissues injury, fractures, medical interventions (such as arthroscopies), myocardial infarction, or stroke.[32] In some cases no particular inciting event can be identified.

CRPS usually affects the extremities (more commonly lower extremities), but ultimately it may affect any part of the body. The pain may migrate, occasionally involving an area that is distant from the inciting area. Patients usually present with localized, regional severe pain. They describe pain as burning, lancinating, throbbing, or shooting. Localized allodynia, edema, and usually purple skin discoloration are present. The affected area frequently feels cold to the touch, and atrophic skin changes and altered hair growth may be observed. A significant decrease in range of motion of the affected area is almost universally present. Over a period of time, muscle contractures may develop.

It has been suggested that CRPS prevention is the best management. It appears that early mobilization after stroke, trauma, and myocardial infarction may play an important role in preventing CRPS.[33]

CRPS management may be very frustrating and challenging. The most efficient therapeutic modality for patients with CRPS is a multidisciplinary approach consisting of rehabilitation, pain management, and psychological/behavioral therapy.[34] Cognitive behavioral therapy is found to be beneficial for most chronic pain conditions including CRPS. Patients may benefit from continuous physical and occupations therapy.[35] It appears that patients with CRPS benefit most from physical therapy when it has been initiated before significant limitations in range of motions have occurred.

Various conservative medical treatment modalities have described for CRPS, and the most successful approach included a combination of gabapentin with amitriptyline and an NSAID. In some instances an opioid could also be added for better pain control.[34] Sympathetically medicated pain seen in CRPS may also respond to the addition of alpha-1 adrenoceptor blocking agents, such as prazosin (1–6 mg per day). Patients who do not respond to these conservative treatment modalities may benefit from intravenous infusion of clonidine, lidocaine, or ketamine. In some studies use of calcitonin at doses of 300–400 international units per day administered via nasal spray was shown to be beneficial.[36] Sympathetic ganglion blocks (stellate ganglion block, lumbar sympathetic block) may provide short-term pain relief and provided help with mobilization during physical therapy. More refractory cases may benefit from epidural administration of clonidine.[37]

There is growing evidence supporting a beneficial role of spinal cord stimulation in treatment of refractory cases of CRPS.[38] Finally, sympathectomy could be used in patients for whom all of these treatment modalities are ineffective.[38]

Summary

Chronic pain conditions are very common in neurological practice. Early recognition and adequate therapy of these condition are very important in improving a patient's quality of life and overall treatment outcome. Considering that most neurological chronic pain conditions are very challenging to treat, it is important to use a multidisciplinary approach consisting of nonpharmacological treatment modalities (transcutaneous nerve stimulation, physical and occupational therapy, cognitive behavioral therapy), conservative medical management (use of antidepressants, anticonvulsants, various abortive medications), and interventional treatment.

References

1. Alonso A, Hernan MA. Temporal trends in the incidence of multiple sclerosis: a systematic review. *Neurology*. 2008;71(2):129–135.
2. Simpson S Jr, Blizzard L, Otahal P, Van der Mei I, Taylor B. Latitude is significantly associated with the prevalence of multiple sclerosis: a meta-analysis. *J Neurol Neurosurg Psychiatry*. 2011;82(10):1132–1141.

3. Swanton JK, Rovira A, Tintore M, et al. MRI criteria for multiple sclerosis in patients presenting with clinically isolated syndromes: a multicentre retrospective study. *Lancet Neurol.* 2007;6(8):677–686.

4. Montalban X, Tintoré M, Swanton J, et al. MRI criteria for MS in patients with clinically isolated syndromes. *Neurology.* 2010;74(5):427–434.

5. Clifford DB, Trotter JL. Pain in multiple sclerosis. *Arch Neurol.* 1984;41:1270–1272.

6. Archibald CJ, McGrath PJ, Ritvo PG, et al. Pain prevalence, severity and impact in a clinic sample of multiple sclerosis patients. *Pain.* 1994;58:89–93

7. Svendsen KB, Jensen SJ, Overvad K, Hansen HJ, Kock-Henriksen N, Back FW. Pain in patients with multiple sclerosis. *Arch Neurol.* 2003;60:1089–1094.

8. Solaro C, Brichetto G, Amato MP, et al. The prevalence of pain in multiple sclerosis: a multicenter cross-sectional study. *Neurology.* 2004;63(5):919–921.

9. Moulin DE, Foley KM, Evers GE. Pain syndromes in multiple sclerosis. *Neurology.* 1988;38:1830–1834.

10. Andersson PB, Goodkin DE. Current pharmacologic treatment of multiple sclerosis symptoms. *West J Med.* 1996;165(5):313–317.

11. Sweet WH. The treatment of trigeminal neuralgia (ticdouloureux). *N Engl J Med.* 1986;315:174–177.

12. Gronseth G, Cruccu G, Alksne J, et al. Practice parameter: the diagnostic evaluation and treatment of trigeminal neuralgia (an evidence-based review): report of the Quality Standards Subcommittee of the American Academy of Neurology and the European Federation of Neurological Societies. *Neurology.* 2008;71(15):1183–1190.

13. Fromm GH, Terrence CF, Chattha AS. Baclofen in the treatment of trigeminal neuralgia. Double-blind study and long-term follow-up. *Ann Neurol.* 1984;15:240–244.

14. Vollmer TL, Robinson MJ, Risser RC, Malcolm SK. A randomized, double-blind, placebo-controlled trial of duloxetine for the treatment of pain in patients with multiple sclerosis. *Pain Pract.* 2014;14(8):732–744.

15. Dodick DW. Clinical practice. Chronic daily headache. *N Engl J Med.* 2006;354(2):158–165.

16. Castillo J, Muñoz P, Guitera V, Pascual J. Kaplan Award 1998. Epidemiology of chronic daily headache in the general population. *Headache.* 1999;39(3):190–196.

17. Headache Classification Committee of the International Headache Society. The International Classification of Headache Disorders, 3rd edition (beta version). Cephalalgia. 2013;33(9):629–808.

18. Abrams BM. Medication overuse headaches. Med Clin North Am. 2013;97(2):337–352.

19. Pascual J, Colás R, Castillo J. Epidemiology of chronic daily headache. *Curr Pain Headache Rep.* 2001;5(6):529–536.

20. Diener HC, Limmroth V. Medication-overuse headache: a worldwide problem. *Lancet Neurol.* 2004;3(8):475–483.

21. Mathew NT, Kurman R, Perez F. Drug induced refractory headache—clinical features and management. *Headache.* 1990;30(10):634–638.

22. Boivie, J, Casey, KL. Central pain in the face and head. In: Olesen J, ed., *The Headaches.* Philadelphia: Lippincott Williams and Wilkins; 2006.

23. Tasker RR. Central pain states. In: Warfield CA, Bajwa ZH, eds., *Principles and Practice of Pain Medicine*, New York: McGraw-Hill; 2004.

24. Rowbotham MC. Mechanisms of neuropathic pain and their implications for the design of clinical trials. *Neurology.* 2005;65(12 Suppl 4):S66–73.

25. Tasker, RR, Watson, CPN. The treatment of central pain. In: Noseworthy JH, ed., *Neurological Therapeutics: Principles and Practice.* New York: Martin Dunitz; 2003.

26. Finnerup NB, Otto M, McQuay HJ, Jensen TS, Sindrup SH. Algorithm for neuropathic pain treatment: an evidence based proposal. *Pain.* 2005;118(3):289–305.

27. Backonja M, Glanzman RL. Gabapentin dosing for neuropathic pain: evidence from randomized, placebo-controlled clinical trials. *Clin Ther.* 2003;25(1):81.

28. Nnoaham KE, Kumbang J. Transcutaneous electrical nerve stimulation (TENS) for chronic pain. *Cochrane Database Syst Rev.* 2008;(3):CD003222.

29. Taub E, Munz M, Tasker RR. Chronic electrical stimulation of the gasserian ganglion for the relief of pain in a series of 34 patients. *J Neurosurg*. 1997;86(2):197–202.

30. Cruccu G, Aziz TZ, Garcia-Larrea L, Hansson P, et al. EFNS guidelines on neurostimulation therapy for neuropathic pain. *Eur J Neurol*. 2007;14(9):952–970.

31. Stanton-Hicks M, Jänig W, Hassenbusch S, Haddox JD, Boas R, Wilson P. Reflex sympathetic dystrophy: changing concepts and taxonomy. *Pain*. 1995;63(1):127–133.

32. Pak TJ, Martin GM, Magness JL, Kavanaugh GJ. Reflex sympathetic dystrophy. Review of 140 cases. *Minn Med*. 1970;53(5):507–512.

33. Petchkrua W, Weiss DJ, Patel RR. Reassessment of the incidence of complex regional pain syndrome type 1 following stroke. *Neurorehabil Neural Repair*. 2000;14(1):59–63.

34. Stanton-Hicks MD, Burton AW, Bruehl SP, et al. An updated interdisciplinary clinical pathway for CRPS: report of an expert panel. *Pain Pract*. 2002;2(1):1–16.

35. Oerlemans HM, Oostendorp RA, de Boo T, van der Laan L, Severens JL, Goris JA. Adjuvant physical therapy versus occupational therapy in patients with reflex sympathetic dystrophy/complex regional pain syndrome type I. *Arch Phys Med Rehabil*. 2000;81(1):49–56.

36. Gobelet C, Waldburger M, Meier JL. The effect of adding calcitonin to physical treatment on reflex sympathetic dystrophy. *Pain*. 1992;48(2):171–175.

37. Rauck RL, Eisenach JC, Jackson K, Young LD, Southern J. Epidural clonidine treatment for refractory reflex sympathetic dystrophy. *Anesthesiology*. 1993;79(6):1163–1169.

38. Kemler MA, De Vet HC, Barendse GA, Van Den Wildenberg FA, Van Kleef M. The effect of spinal cord stimulation in patients with chronic reflex sympathetic dystrophy: two years' follow-up of the randomized controlled trial. *Ann Neurol*. 2004;55(1):13–18.

22

Management of Chronic Pain in Hospitalized Patients with a History of Substance Abuse

EMAN NADA, NICOLE LABOR, AND DMITRI SOUZDALNITSKI

KEY POINTS

- Management of chronic pain in patients with a history of substance abuse who have been admitted to the hospital is a challenging task.
- Patient safety may be compromised by known interactions between substances abused and some of the pain medications. In addition, a number of medications used for pain control have potential for abuse. Patients may state that the substance they abuse can be helpful in self-medicating their pain.
- The strategies of helping these patients without compromising their safety while preserving their rights and autonomy depend on their stage of addiction (current addict, patient on replacement/maintenance medication, or remote drug abuse).
- Current drug abusers may be tolerant to opioid medications, which makes pain treatment difficult. Treating a patient with a drug of former abuse may result in relapse.
- It is extremely important to obtain a good history in which the patient is specifically asked about prior substance abuse and/or substance abuse treatment. If the patient has a history of substance abuse but is currently abstinent, it is incumbent upon the practitioner to obtain further information about the level of recovery.
- A patient abstaining from all substances may be at slightly lower risk of relapse than those patients abstaining from what they believe is their "drug of choice."
- Patients actively working a recovery program in conjunction with therapists, counselors, addiction specialists, and 12-step support groups are

---

294

less likely to relapse when prescribed addictive medications, especially when the support modalities are included in the treatment plan.
- It is very important to use multimodal analgesia with heavy use of regional analgesia, if applicable. Close communication with the patient's addictionologist or have one on board is necessary for successful treatment.

Introduction

Addiction affects people of all ages, all races, and all socioeconomic levels. Addictive disease is considered permanent, even after long periods of abstinence.[1] In 2011 in the United States, 20.7 million adults had a substance use disorder.[2] Taking care of these patients in the hospital setting is frequently a challenging task. Physicians and nurses should be cognizant of problems associated with substance abuse, including the epidemiology, pathology, and pharmacology of this common disorder. Pain medications are potentially addicting, and important drug interactions and a confounding clinical picture may affect care markedly. The pain practitioner should also be familiar with the terms used in pain and addiction medicine (Table 22.1).

Identification of the Patient with Substance Abuse: Privacy, Confidentiality, and Autonomy

Patients with substance abuse will not mention their problem easily and may even deny it. Notes in the medical records and abnormal laboratory drug screens in the chart are helpful ways to diagnose the problem.[8] For those with no history in medical records, a high index of suspicion is warranted. Clues to substance abuse problems include poor hygiene and numerous skin needle marks and scars.[9] In chronic pain patients abuse is suspected when a patient spontaneously increases the opioid dosage, reports increasing pain severity, seeks opioid prescriptions from multiple physicians, reports prescription or drug loss, and is unwillingness to switch to another drug.[10] It is extremely important to obtain a good history from patients that includes any past, even distant past, drug and alcohol treatment. Many times a patient with a history of past substance abuse will not be forthcoming in an initial history because the patient does not understand its relevance. It is paramount to ask specifically about any and all treatments received for substance abuse over a lifetime. To confirm suspicion of drug abuse a urine drug screen can be ordered, as it is the simplest and easiest way to test for abuse.[8]

Table 22.1 **Important Terminology Related to Substance Abuse**

Dependence	**Psychological dependence:** the need for a specific psychoactive substance either for its positive effects or to avoid negative psychological or physical effects associated with its withdrawal.[3] **Physical dependence:** a physiological state of adaptation to a specific psychoactive substance characterized by the emergence of a withdrawal syndrome during abstinence, which may be relieved in total or in part by readministration of the substance.[3]
Abstinence syndrome	Cessation of use of a psychoactive substance previously abused, or on which the user has developed drug dependence.[3]
Withdrawal syndrome	The onset of a predictable constellation of signs and symptoms involving altered activity of the central nervous system after the abrupt discontinuation of, or rapid decrease in, dosage of a drug.[3]
Drug-seeking behavior	Patient's requests for additional opioid. This term can be applied only when the patient's pain is adequately controlled, as this behavior may be an appropriate response to inadequately treated pain.[4]
Tolerance	Physiological adaptation to the effect of drugs, so as to diminish effects with constant dosages or to maintain the intensity and duration of effects through increased dosage.[3]
Opioid-induced hyperalgesia	A state of nociceptive sensitization caused by exposure to opioids which decreases the overall pain tolerance.[5]
Addiction	A chronic disorder characterized by the compulsive use of a substance, resulting in physical, psychological, or social harm to the user and continued use despite that harm.[3]
Pseudo-addiction	Pain relief–seeking behavior caused by inadequate pain control.[6]
Opioid rotation	A switch from one opioid to another in an effort to improve therapeutic response or reduce side effects.[7]

The label of being a drug user has huge implications for a patient's life. For this reason, drug addict medical records are protected by the Health Insurance Portability and Accountability Act (HIPAA). In addition, extra protection of medical records is provided in federally funded addiction specialty treatment programs. These programs cannot disclose any information about the patient without written consent, with only a few exceptions.[11]

Patients with a substance abuse problem have the same right as all other patients to receive non-punitive, respectful treatment. Addiction does not

Table 22.2 **Classes of Substances Abuse Medications**

Depressants	Alcohol, sedatives, hypnotics, opioids, and anxiolytics
Stimulants	Marijuana and nicotine
	Cocaine, amphetamines, and nicotine
Hallucinogens	**Psychedelic hallucinogens (psychotomimetics)** include lysergic acid diethylamide (LSD), psilocybin, mescaline, and 3,4-methylenedioxymethamphetamine (MDMA)
	Dissociative hallucinogens include dextromethorphan (DXM), phencyclidine (PCP), and ketamine.
	Deliriants: *Atropa belladonna, Datura stramonium*, and *Myristica fragran*; antihistamines such as diphenhydramine and dimenhydrinate
Inhalants	Anesthetics and solvents

preclude the patient from making autonomous decisions. Only when behavior is compromised is this ability limited.[12]

In general, three clinical scenarios relating to substance abuse are possible: patients with current drug abuse, patients on replacement/maintenance therapy, and patients in recovery. While all of these scenarios may require special management, the last two can be most challenging. Replacement/maintenance therapy can include buprenorphine, methadone, and naltrexone. Generally, these medications are stopped (if given in small doses) or converted to regular opioids (if given in high doses) prior to an elective surgical procedure (more details are given later in the chapter). Former drug addicts are at risk of relapse associated with hospital admission. The following suggestions may be helpful in management of this category of patients: initiate opioid therapy only if the potential benefits outweigh the risk, and use nonpharmacological pain control, non-opioid analgesics, and regional analgesia whenever possible.

Classes of substances commonly associated with abuse include depressants, stimulants, hallucinogens, and inhalants (Table 22.2). The management of pain in a patient with substance abuse depends on the class of the substance.

Management of Patients with Abuse of Depressants

ALCOHOL

Alcohol use disorder is a common disorder. In the United States, the 12-month prevalence of alcohol use disorder is estimated to be 8.5% among adults age 18 years and older.[13] It is important for the pain practitioner to be familiar with the clinical picture, treatments available, and drug interactions presented in Table 22.3.

Table 22.3 **Alcohol Abuse**

Clinical Picture and Intoxication	Withdrawal Syndrome	Treatment of Withdrawal and Alcohol Abuse	Drug Interactions in Pain Patient

• History of heavy drinking
• Smell of alcohol in breath
• Laboratory analysis of breath, blood, or urine
• Behavioral disinhibition: Initially euphoria or agitation and combativeness
• Flushed warm skin.
• Hypoglycemia may occur.
• Vasodilation, hypotension, and reflex tachycardia
• Severe intoxication results in central nervous system (CNS) depression and may cause respiratory depression and coma.[14]
	• **Early Manifestations:** Generalized tremors, nausea, vomiting, insomnia, and confusion with agitation
	• **Delirium tremens** (DT): hallucinations, disorientation, tachycardia, hypertension, fever, agitation[15]
		Treatment of Withdrawal
		• Substitute alcohol or use Benzodiazepines with slower onset as have less abuse potential[16]
		• Phenothiazines and haloperidol are used as adjuvants to benzodiazepines.
		• Beta-adrenergic blockers and clonidine reduce autonomic manifestations of withdrawal symptoms and convulsing activity[17]
		• Carbamazepine helps in reducing emotional distress[18]
		Treatment of Alcohol Abuse
		• **First-line treatment:** naltrexone, acamprosate
		• **Second-line treatments:** nalmefine disulfiram, chlordiazepoxide, topiramate, gabapentin, baclofen
			• Alcohol and sedatives: severe depression of the CNS[19]
			• Naltrexone and nalmefene: resistance to opioids
			• Disulfiram
			  • Induce sedation and hepatotoxicity
			  • Reduces the clearance of other drugs
			  • An altered response to sympathomimetic drugs[20]
			• Acetaminophen is safe in patients who chronically abuse, watch for abuse in a patient with active liver disease and chronic acetaminophen use[21]

Pain Patients with Active Alcohol Abuse Disorder

When treating these patients one must be aware of pain medications' interactions in an active alcohol abuser. It is also important to try to avoid withdrawal symptoms and to treat them if they do occur.[22] As already noted, pain practitioners need to be familiar with the patient's clinical picture, treatments, and potential drug interactions. Patients with a history of alcohol abuse who are currently not drinking may be triggered to start drinking again if prescribed addictive medication.

Chronic Pain Patients with Alcohol Abuse Disorder on Maintenance Therapy

Naltrexone is one of the first-line medications used to treat alcohol abuse. It is an opioid receptor antagonist usually taken orally, although intramuscular depot preparations are available to improve adherence to alcohol abstinence. Nalmefene is another opioid receptor antagonist used, but it is not available in some countries, including the United States.[23] In the setting of anticipated surgery, naltrexone should be discontinued 3 days and nalmefene 7 days before the surgical procedure.[24,25] If discontinuation is not possible, high doses of opioids are needed and close monitoring for side effects is mandatory. The mu receptors are upregulated and withdrawal of the opioid antagonists is associated with increased sensitivity to opioid agonists, resulting in a higher side-effect profile.[26]

Acamprosate is another first-line medication used for alcohol disorders. It decreases neuronal hyperexcitability by antagonizing the glutamate N-methyl-D-aspartate (NMDA) receptors.[27] Disulfiram, topiramate, gabapentin, and nalmefine are considered second-line treatments for alcohol abuse disorders.[23] Baclofen has been used with mixed results.[28]

Disulfiram inhibits aldehyde dehydrogenase and prevents the metabolism of alcohol's primary metabolite, acetaldehyde. Drinking alcohol while taking disulfiram results in the accumulation of acetaldehyde in the blood, which causes unpleasant effects.[29] Disulfiram should be stopped 10 days before any anticipated surgery.[30]

Regional Anesthesia

Patients should be carefully evaluated for disulfiram-induced polyneuropathy[31] and their coagulation profile should be assessed as well. Regional anesthesia may be accompanied by acute, unexplained hypotension that could reflect inadequate stores of norepinephrine due to disulfiram-induced inhibition of dopamine β-hydroxylase. This hypotension is better treated with direct-acting sympathomimetics such as phenylephrine.[32]

OPIOIDS

Over the past decade, rates of hospital admissions for treatment of prescription opioid misuse have steadily risen.[33] Heroin (diacetylmorphine) is another opioid that can be abused; it has a high street value.

Pain Patient with Current Opioid Abuse Disorder

A contract for addiction treatment must be established between the patient and healthcare staff. If the patient still does not consent to addiction treatment, he or she should not be prescribed opioids, except in an acute pain situation.[34] The key points in providing adequate pain management for these patients in the hospital are as follows:

- Multidisciplinary pain treatment including addiction specialists is especially important.
- Follow general guidelines for treatment of pain in an addict, and for an opioid-tolerant patient, tailor treatment according to this tolerance (see general guidelines for treatment of pain patients with a history of abuse).
- Avoid and treat withdrawal syndrome.

Pain Patient with Opioid Abuse Disorder on Replacement Therapy

Management of pain in patients on replacement therapy depends on the type of replacement/maintenance they are on. Replacement therapy can include buprenorphine (Subutex), buprenorphine with naloxone (Suboxone), methadone, or naltrexone.

BUPRENORPHINE

Also known as Subutex, buprenorphine is a partial mu-agonist that binds tightly to the receptor. Suboxone is a combination of buprenorphine and naloxone that is given orally. The naloxone has no effect orally and is intended to prevents misuse in case of injection.[35] The following treatment choices are suggested for management:

- For elective surgery the patient should be weaned off buprenorphine before the planned procedure. It is best if discontinued gradually over a 1- to 2-week period; if this is not possible or the dose of buprenorphine is low, discontinuation can take place over a period as short as 3–7 days.[36] If the dose of buprenorphine is high, a careful replacement with another opioid or methadone (the less preferable option) can be used in anticipation of hospitalization, for acute severe or postoperative pain.[37]
- With emergency surgery, buprenorphine can be continued if no severe acute pain is anticipated.[37] If there is severe pain, fentanyl is preferred because if its higher affinity to mu receptors. It can be titrated in a safe fashion, preferably in the intensive care setting, to overcome the buprenorphine blockade of the mu receptors.[38-40]

METHADONE

Methadone has a unique pharmacological profile (described in chapter 5). It is used in treatment of addiction because it blocks the euphoric effects and prevents withdrawal of opioids.[41] Patients maintained on methadone should be encouraged to continue their maintenance dose during the perioperative period, and additional opioids should be used during surgery and/or for breakthrough pain in the postoperative period. The dose of opioids needed to control the pain in an opioid-tolerant patient will be more than expected, thus postoperative monitoring for side effects, especially respiratory depression, is essential.[36]

NALTREXONE

Naltrexone is a pure opioid antagonist. It should be discontinued 3 days before surgery.[24] If this is not possible the amount of opioid analgesic required may be greater than usual because of opioid receptor upregulation.[37] To avoid respiratory depression following titration of opioids in a patient with naltrexone still in their system and suffering acute pain, a rapidly acting strong opioid analgesic like sufentanil, remifentanil, alfentanil, or fentanyl is preferred.[39]

Pain Patient with Former Opioid Abuse Problem

Former drug addicts are at risk of relapse,[1] thus the general principles of treating a patient with drug abuse apply here more than anywhere else. The general guideline is to maximize non-opioid treatment in general (pharmacological non-opioid, nonpharmacological, multimodal, and regional analgesia). Opioid therapy should be initiated only if the potential benefits outweigh the risk.[34,42]

BARBITURATES

Barbiturate abuse is a receding problem, as they were largely replaced by other medications with less abuse potential. They are abused for their euphoric effects, to treat insomnia, or to antagonize the stimulant effects of other drugs. They are also available in headache medications and easily available for purchase online.[43] Their abuse is especially high in individuals with ready access to drugs, such as healthcare providers. It is important for the pain practitioner to be familiar with the clinical picture, treatments available, and relevant drug interactions (Table 22.4).

BENZODIAZEPINES

Benzodiazepines are rarely preferred as the sole drug of abuse. Over 80% of benzodiazepine addicts have polysubstance abuse, most commonly with opioids. Benzodiazepine abuse is especially prevalent in patients who are taking methadone. Prescriptions constitute the primary source of supply for people who abuse benzodiazepines.[45] It is important for the pain practitioner to be familiar with the clinical picture, treatments, and relevant drug interactions (Table 22.5).

Table 22.4 **Barbiturate Abuse**

Clinical Picture and Intoxication	Withdrawal	Treatment of Withdrawal and Abuse	Important Drug Interactions in Pain Patient
• Euphoria, drowsiness. • Overdose results in CNS depression, including ventilatory depression	• Anxiety, skeletal muscle tremors, hyperreflexia • Tachycardia, and orthostatic hypotension, diaphoresis • Cardiovascular collapse, hyperthermia, and grand mal seizures	• Replace withdrawal with phenobarbital with a dose reduction of 10% per day • Benzodiazepines[44]	• Additive CNS depressant effects. Especially in alcoholics who use it to relieve their nervousness and tremors[19] • Chronic use results in cross-tolerance to other CNS depressants.[43]

Stimulants Abusers

TOBACCO

Smokers are known to have higher rates of other drug abuse.[46] They are more likely to experience pain, and they will also need more opioid analgesics.[47,48]

Table 22.5 **Benzodiazepines Abuse**

Clinical Picture and Intoxication	Withdrawal	Treatment of Withdrawal and Abuse	Drug Interactions
• Used to enhance the euphoria effects of opioids • To alleviate withdrawal syndromes • To temper cocaine highs, to augment alcohol **Intoxication:** • Depressant effect on the CNS, slow breathing to apnea[31]	• Anxiety, jitteriness, insomnia, seizures • These symptoms may not appear until the third day after cessation of the drug and may not reach their peak of severity until the fifth day.[31]	• Replace benzodiazepines and gradually taper them over a period of 1 to 2 weeks	• Interacts synergistically with other CNS depressants[31]

Although nicotine has analgesic properties in nonsmokers,[49,50] it increases pain perception in smokers. It is thought that the hypothalamic-pituitary-adrenal (HPA) axis is downregulated by smoking. The decreased sympathetic response increases pain perception. Smoking also accelerates degenerative changes and impairs bone healing.[51]

Nicotine patches should be applied in the postoperative period to prevent withdrawal and potentially to improve the patient's perception of recovery after surgery. Smokers deprived of nicotine in the postoperative period reported more pain and required a greater amount of opiates than did nonsmokers.[52,53] It is important for the pain practitioner to be familiar with the clinical picture, treatments, and relevant drug interactions when treating smokers with pain (Table 22.6).[54-57]

CANNABIS

Cannabis is the most common drug of abuse generally.[2] It is estimated that about 13% of pain patients take marijuana.[58] It inhibits glutamatergic transmission and antagonizes the NMDA glutamate receptor; both of these actions would be expected to inhibit pain. Cannabis may have an anti-inflammatory effect and may increase levels of endorphins.[59]

Table 22.6 **Tobacco Use Disorder**

Nicotine Clinical Picture and Intoxication	Withdrawal	Treatment of Withdrawal	Drug Interactions in Pain Patient
• History of smoking • Odor of tobacco smoke • Smoker's cough and voice • Face wrinkles • Yellow and brown teeth • Gingivitis and periodontitis • Complications like leukoplakia, certain cancers • Chronic obstructive pulmonary disease[65] • **Nicotine intoxication:** results in excessive CNS stimulation with tremor, insomnia, and nervousness; cardiac stimulation and arrhythmias; and respiratory paralysis[50]	• Irritability, frustration, or anger, anxiety, difficulty concentrating, increased appetite, restlessness, depressed mood, insomnia[66]	• Nicotine replacement products	Decreases the efficacy of hydorocodone and possibly other opioids[67]

Cannabinoids have a high fat solubility, which leads to rapid accumulation in adipose tissue. Marijuana users should be advised to avoid its use at least 7 days before surgery because of its long half-life.[60] As with pain treatment in the context of other substances, it is important for the pain practitioner to be familiar with the clinical picture, treatments available, and relevant drug interactions (Table 22.7).[61-65]

COCAINE AND AMPHETAMINES

Cocaine produces sympathetic nervous system stimulation by blocking the presynaptic uptake of norepinephrine and dopamine, thereby increasing the postsynaptic concentrations of these neurotransmitters and producing what is called a cocaine high.[66] Patients abusing cocaine will often state that cocaine can be helpful in self-medicating their pain. It is important for the pain practitioner to be familiar with the clinical picture, treatments and drug interactions (Table 22.8).[67-70]

Hallucinogens

Hallucinogen abusers get addicted to the "spiritual journeys" or the sense of detachment from the surrounding environment.[71] Hallucinogens are divided into three broad categories: psychedelics, dissociative, and deliriants.

PSYCHEDELICS

This group is also referred to as psychotomimetics or hallucinogens. They mainly stimulate 5-HT (2A) receptors, while some of them additionally

Table 22.7 **Marijuana Abuse**

Clinical Picture and Intoxication	Withdrawal	Treatment of Withdrawal	Drug Interactions in Pain Patient
• Abused because of the euphoriogenic effect • Signs of increased sympathetic nervous system activity • Drowsiness, red eyes, cannabis odor, yellowing of finger tips, chronic cough, loss of interest and motivation, and weight loss[49]	• Irritability, insomnia, diaphoresis • Nausea, vomiting, and diarrhea • Increased latency to fall asleep • Negative mood and behavioral symptoms[68]	• Tetrahydrocannabinol (THC) replacement[69] • Behavioral therapy • Treatment of concurrent nicotine addiction may help the individual stop marijuana. • Trazodone helps insomnia from Cannabis[68]	• Cross-tolerance with all CNS depressants • Cannabis is moderately efficacious for treatment of chronic pain, but beneficial effects may be offset by potentially serious harms.[70] • CNS depressants sedation • Disulfiram: hypomania • TCA: tachycardia: delirium • Anticholinergic agents: sedation[71]

Table 22.8 **Stimulant Abuse**

Clinical Picture and Intoxication	Withdrawal	Treatment of Withdrawal	Interactions Relevant to Pain Patient
Cocaine			

• Intense high followed by dysphoria sleeplessness, restlessness, anxiety, nasal damage, loss of appetite, chest pain, hypertension, myocardial infarction, life-threatening arrhythmia, seizures, sudden death from overdose[49]
 	
• **Treatment of overdose:** dexmeditomidine benzodiazepines[72]
	• Severe depression, fatigue for the drug	• Symptomatic treatment
		• Behavioral and social therapy[73]
			• Avoid using ketamine.
			• Persons with decreased plasma cholinesterase activity may be at risk of sudden death.
			• **Regional anesthesia**
			  • Patients may show combative behavior and altered pain perception.
			  • Cocaine-induced thrombocytopenia can occur.[74]
			• Refractory hypotension or bradycardia
			• Concurrent use of cocaine, Cannabis, amphetamines, MDMA, lidocaine, and carbamazepine may lead to large elevations in blood pressure and heart rate.[71,73,75]

Amphetamines			
• Increased cortical alertness, appetite suppression • With long-term amphetamine abuse: develop hypertension, arrhythmias, anxiety, violent behavior, psychosis, necrotizing arteritis, leading to cerebral hemorrhage and renal failure, death from overdose[49,50]	• Extreme lethargy, depression that may be suicidal, increased appetite, and weight gain	Symptomatic treatment	• Avoid using ketamine. • Reduce the morphine doses needed. • Refractory hypotension • Amitriptyline: hypertension, CNS stimulation[71]

stimulate dopamine D1 and D2 and adrenergic receptors. This group of drugs includes lysergic acid diethylamide (LSD), psilocybin, mescaline, and 3,4-methylenedioxymethamphetamine (MDMA).[72]

DISSOCIATIVE DRUGS

This group comprises NMDA receptor antagonists, including, dextromethorphan (DXM), phencyclidine (PCP), and ketamine.[73]

DELIRIANTS

The group includes tropanes and antihistamines. Tropanes are either naturally occurring, like Datura (jimson weed), or available as drugs—atropine, scopolamine, and hyoscyamine.

Antihistaminics include diphenhydramine (Benadryl), dimenhydrinate (Dramamine, Gravol), and cyclizine (Marezine or Marzine).[74,75] Chronic pain patients commonly get exposed to these medications for treating some of the side effect of opioids.

As always, it is important for the pain practitioner to be familiar with the clinical picture, treatments, and relevant drug interactions (Table 22.9).

Tricyclic Antidepressants

The tricyclic antidepressants (TCAs) are not uncommonly used to treat certain types of pain. It is important for the pain practitioner to be familiar with the clinical picture, treatments available and drug interactions (Table 22.10).

INHALANT ABUSE

This group includes anesthetics such as nitrous oxide, chloroform, diethyl ether, and industrial solvents.

Clinical Picture

Symptoms can include nausea, nose bleeds, headache, anemia, and drastic weight loss. There is a high risk of sudden death. Neurological symptoms include neuropathy; poor motor coordination; impaired vision, memory, and thought processes; and abusive, violent behavior. Many of these agents are toxic to the liver, kidneys, lungs, bone marrow, and peripheral nerves and cause brain damage in animals.[55,61]

Summary

Treating pain in a patient with a history of drug abuse can be challenging. Current drug abusers may be tolerant to opioid medication, while those in addiction treatment can be on multiple medications, such as agonists, partial agonists, or antagonists, which can make the treatment of pain difficult. Treating a patient with pain who previously abused substances may result in relapse. It is extremely important to obtain a good history in which the patient is specifically asked about prior substance abuse and/or substance abuse treatment. If the patient has a history of substance abuse but is currently abstinent, it is incumbent upon the practitioner to obtain further information about the level of recovery. A patient abstaining from all substances may be at slightly

Table 22.9 **Hallucinogen Abuse**

Clinical Picture and Intoxication	Withdrawal	Treatment of Withdrawal	Drug Interactions in Pain Patient
• Anticholinergic effect (tachycardia, hypertension, dilated pupils) • Hallucinogenic effect **Treatment:** • Benzodiazepines for control of agitation and anxiety reactions	• Psychological withdrawal • Physical symptoms are rare and occur after chronic abuse in the form of recurring experiences of flashbacks of going through a "trip." • Some chronic abusers develop diarrhea and chills.	• Hallucinogen rehabilitation program	• Exaggerated responses to sympathomimetic drugs are likely.
(LSD), Mescaline and Psilocybin • Hallucinations, illusions, mood swings, flashback, break from reality • Acute panic reaction, hyperactivity, in extreme cases, overt psychosis, seizures, coma and death			• Depressant effects of opioids are prolonged by LSD[32] • Seizures with TCA and serotonin reuptake inhibitors (SRRIs).

Table 22.9 **Continued**

Clinical Picture and Intoxication	Withdrawal	Treatment of Withdrawal	Drug Interactions in Pain Patient
Phencyclidine (PCP) • Slurred speech, blurred vision, nystagmus, marked hypertension, agitation, anxiety, depression, acute psychosis, convulsions		• Benzodiazepines for excitations and seizures	• PCP interacts with other central nervous system depressants and can lead to coma or accidental overdose. • Synergistic interaction with THC, may lead to production of strong hangover-like symptoms[75]
MDMA (ecstasy) • Used to enhance energy, endurance, sociability, and sexual arousal • **C/P:** Excessive thirst, hyponatremia and pulmonary or cerebral edema • Jaw clenching and tooth grinding[76] • Hyperthermia due to serotonin syndrome[61] • **Treatment** • Calm environment • Benzodiazepines for controlling agitation and anxiety reactions			• Hepatotoxic drugs. Serotonin syndrome with SSRI, tramadol, pethidine, or triptans[75]

Table 22.10 **Tricyclic Antidepressants Overdose**

Clinical Picture and Intoxication	Withdrawal	Treatment of Withdrawal	Drug Interactions
• Amitriptyline is misused for its euphoriogenic effect.[77] • **C/P:** Toxicity from its anticholinergic effect. Sinus tachycardia with prolongation of the PR interval, QRS and QTc, ventricular dysrhythmias, and myocardial depression • Seizures are not uncommon.	• Discontinuation of TCA results in cholinergic and adrenergic overdrive[78] • **C/P:** Nausea, vomiting. Anxiety, irritability, sleep disturbances, diaphoresis, headaches, dizziness, chills, gooseflesh, weakness, and delirium[79]	• In case of severe withdrawal reactions, reinstate the medication, and withdraw it more cautiously. • Symptoms can be treated symptomatically if they are of moderate severity. • Benzodiazepine for insomnia • Antimuscarinic agents for the gastrointestinal symptoms[80]	• Potentiates CNS depressant drugs

lower risk of relapse than patients abstaining from what they believe is their "drug of choice." Patients actively working a recovery program in conjunction with therapists, counselors, addiction specialists, and 12-step support groups are less likely to relapse when prescribed addictive medications, especially when the support modalities are included in the treatment plan. It is very important to use multimodal analgesia with heavy use of regional analgesia, if applicable. Additional tips for management of pain in patients with a history of substance abuse who are in the hospital setting is presented in Box 22.1.

Close communication with the patient's addictionologist or having one on board is of great importance for successful treatment.

Box 22.1 **Tips for Treatment of Pain in Patients with a History of Drug Abuse**

IDENTIFICATION OF A PATIENT WITH A HISTORY OF SUBSTANCE ABUSE

- Remember that substance abuse is common.
- Discuss privacy, confidentiality, and autonomy.
- Develop a good patient–physician relationship.
- Pay attention to the general appearance and manner of communication.
- Check for relevant notes in the medical records, including history of substance abuse, abnormal laboratory drug screen, repeated early refills, rapid escalation of opioid dose out of proportion with change in clinical picture, multiple telephone calls for requests to increase the dose of opioids, prescription problems (lost, stolen medications, or prescriptions), and multiple emergency rooms visits for pain-related issues.
- Check for state or federal,\ opioid prescription reports, if available, demonstrating multiple sourcing.
- Physical exam data (skin appearing to have numerous needle marks, skin abscesses, poor peripheral vein access, or disseminated superficial vein thrombosis)
- Repeat laboratory drug screen, pain medications panel
- Inform the patient that addiction history may complicate but not preclude adequate postoperative pain management.

DIFFERENTIATE VARIOUS TYPES OF CONDITIONS ASSOCIATED WITH SUBSTANCE USE DISORDER

- "Drug-seeking" patients should not be automatically assumed to be "drug abusers."
- Differentiate addiction and pseudo-addiction, opioid tolerance and pseudo opioid-tolerance, opioid-induced hyperalgesia, physical dependence, and

psychological dependence, and other conditions associated with substance use disorder.

- *Drug seeking* and other related terms can only be applied when the patient's pain is adequately controlled.
- Take universal precautions to reduce the risk of transmission of potentially life-threatening infectious diseases such as hepatitis B, hepatitis C, and human immunodeficiency virus (HIV) that accompany drug abuse.

MAINTAIN BASELINE OPIOID DOSE

- *Do not* attempt detoxification for *any* patient, whether they are abusing opioids or taking prescribed opioids.
- Make sure to uphold the baseline level of opioids.
- Keep in mind that patients may underreport or overreport opioid doses.
- Addicts' opioid requirements may be higher because of opioid receptor downregulation; side effects may be severe and prolonged.
- When opioids are to be administered, use scheduled rather than as-needed, long-acting medications, slow-onset medications. Try to avoid using intravenous boluses of undiluted opioids to prevent creating feelings of a sudden high.

MANAGEMENT OF PATIENTS PARTICIPATING IN SUBSTANCE ABUSE MAINTENANCE PROGRAMS

- Verify participation in these programs, as well as the methadone or buprenorphine doses, for patient safety.
- The intravenous baseline maintenance dose of methadone is typically half the oral methadone dose, which is taken by patients who are participating in these programs.
- Recovering opioid-abusers being maintained on buprenorphine may continue on this medication in the IV form for postoperative pain control (if the quality of analgesia provided by buprenorphine is inadequate, supplementation with methadone and morphine may be considered).

PREOPERATIVE MANAGEMENT OF PATIENTS TREATED WITH COMBINED AGONIST–ANTAGONIST AGENTS

- Combined formulations of opioids and opioid antagonists, and partial agonist-antagonists should be stopped before elective surgery because administration of opioids in the hospital setting may produce withdrawal symptoms.
- Naltrexone, a long-acting oral opioid antagonist sometimes used in recovering opioid-abusers, should also be discontinued at least 24 hours

prior to surgery. Buprenorphine should be discontinued or converted to other opioids 5–7 days before elective surgery.

- If buprenorphine was not discontinued before hospital admission, fentanyl can be effectively used for acute pain control; other opioids may produce a desirable clinical effect, but at significantly higher doses.

USE OF MIXED OPIOID AGONIST-ANTAGONIST DRUGS POSTOPERATIVELY

- Inform the surgical team that mixed agonists/antagonists opioids should not be used for substance abusers or opioid-dependent patients (agents such as nalbuphine, butorphanol, pentazocine, and tramadol)

CONSIDER MULTIMODAL REGIMENS BUT WATCH FOR COMORBIDITIES

- Some strategies may be useful to spare use of opioids: maximize use of multimodal, preemptive analgesia, local and regional anesthesia, and nonpharmacological methods whenever possible.
- Consider multiple comorbidities commonly accompanying substance abuse states, including viral or ETOH-related liver disease, HIV, lung disease (smoking is common in this patient population), encephalopathy, and psychiatric comorbidities.

ABUSE OF OTHER SUBSTANCES

- Substances other than opioids may complicate postoperative chronic pain management.
- Watch for ETOH abuse and withdrawal.
- Nicotine patches should be invariably applied to smokers to prevent withdrawal and to potentially improve their perception of recovery after surgery.

MANAGEMENT OF SUBSTANCE USE AT DISCHARGE

- Healthcare providers should address substance abuse issues in a conventional way, when the patient is stable and the pain tolerable.
- Standard pathways and recovery options should be offered to patients with a history of substance abuse, including abuse of ETOH and nicotine.
- Patients suffering from tobacco use disorder should be informed about the close association between chronic nicotine use and chronic back pain.
- The primary care provider, the addiction treatment maintenance program, and/or the prescribing physician of any opioids and benzodiazepines should be informed of medications given to the patient during

hospitalization because they may show up on routine urine drug screening. Clinicians should also be informed of the doses of these medications in order to provide effective continuous care.

Adapted from Souzdalnitski D, Walker J, Rosenquist RW. Chronic pain patient and other coexisting conditions (substance abuse, psychiatric). In: Urman R, Vadivelu N., eds., *Perioperative Pain Management*, 1st ed. New York: Oxford University Press; 2013:83–93.

References

1. Miller NS, Giannini AJ, Gold MS, Philomena JA. Drug testing: medical, legal, and ethical issues. *J Subst Abuse Treat*. 1990;7:239–244.
2. Substance Abuse and Mental Health Services Administration. Results from the 2012 National Survey on Drug Use and Health: Mental Health Findings, 2013 edition. Rockville, MD. http://archive.samhsa.gov/data/NSDUH/2k12MH_FindingsandDetTables/2K12MHF/NSDUHmhfr2012.htm.
3. Rinaldi RC, Steindler EM, Wilford BB, Goodwin D. Clarification and standardization of substance abuse terminology. *JAMA*. 1988;259:555–557.
4. Vukmir RB. Drug seeking behavior. *Am J Drug Alcohol Abuse*. 2004;30:551–575.
5. Angst MS, Clark JD. Opioid-induced hyperalgesia: a qualitative systematic review. *Anesthesiology*. 2006;104:570–587.
6. Weissman DE, Haddox JD. Opioid pseudoaddiction—an iatrogenic syndrome. *Pain*. 1989;36:363–366.
7. Knotkova H, Fine PG, Portenoy RK. Opioid rotation: the science and the limitations of the equianalgesic dose table. *J Pain Symptom Manage*. 2009;38:426–439.
8. Weaver MF, Jarvis ME. Substance use disorder: principles for recognition and assessment in general medical care. *UpToDate*. 2013. http://www.uptodate.com/contents/substance-use-disorder-principles-for-recognition-and-assessment-in-general-medical-care
9. Darke S, Ross J, Kaye S. Physical injecting sites among injecting drug users in Sydney, Australia. *Drug Alcohol Depend*. 2001;62:77–82.
10. Portenoy RK, Foley KM. Chronic use of opioid analgesics in non-malignant pain: report of 38 cases. *Pain*. 1986;25:171–186.
11. Hu LL, Sparenborg S, Tai B. Privacy protection for patients with substance use problems. *Subst Abuse Rehabil*. 2011;2:227–233.
12. Spriggs M. Can we help addicts become more autonomous? Inside the mind of an addict. *Bioethics*. 2003;17:542–554.
13. American Psychiatric Association. *Diagnostic and Statistical Manual of Mental Disorders*, 5th ed. (DSM-5). Arlington, VA: American Psychiatric Association; 2013.
14. Vonghia L, Leggio L, Ferrulli A, Bertini M, Gasbarrini G, Addolorato G. Acute alcohol intoxication. *Eur J Intern Med*. 2008;19:561–567.
15. Guthrie SK. The treatment of alcohol withdrawal. *Pharmacotherapy*. 1989;9:131–143.
16. Mayo-Smith MF. Pharmacological management of alcohol withdrawal. A meta-analysis and evidence-based practice guideline. American Society of Addiction Medicine Working Group on Pharmacological Management of Alcohol Withdrawal. *JAMA*. 1997;278:144–151.
17. Horwitz RI, Gottlieb LD, Kraus ML. The efficacy of atenolol in the outpatient management of the alcohol withdrawal syndrome. Results of a randomized clinical trial. *Arch Intern Med*. 1989;149:1089–1093.

18. Stuppaeck CH, Pycha R, Miller C, Whitworth AB, Oberbauer H, Fleischhacker WW. Carbamazepine versus oxazepam in the treatment of alcohol withdrawal: a double-blind study. *Alcohol Alcohol*. 1992;27:153–158.

19. Hall AJ, Logan JE, Toblin RL, Kaplan JA, Kraner JC, Bixler D, Crosby AE, Paulozzi LJ. Patterns of abuse among unintentional pharmaceutical overdose fatalities. *JAMA*. 2008;300:2613–2620.

20. Sellers EM, Holloway MR. Drug kinetics and alcohol ingestion. *Clin Pharmacokinet*. 1978;3:440–452.

21. Riordan SM, Williams R. Alcohol exposure and paracetamol-induced hepatotoxicity. *Addict Biol*. 2002;7:191–206.

22. Etherington JM. Emergency management of acute alcohol problems. Part 1: Uncomplicated withdrawal. *Can Fam Physician*. 1996;42:2186–2190.

23. Johnson BA. Pharmacotherapy of alcohol abuse disorder. *UpToDate*. 2014. http://www.uptodate.com/contents/pharmacotherapy-for-alcohol-use-disorder

24. Gonzalez JP, Brogden RN. Naltrexone. A review of its pharmacodynamic and pharmacokinetic properties and therapeutic efficacy in the management of opioid dependence. *Drugs*. 1988;35:192–213.

25. Selincro 18 mg film-coated tablet.The electronic Medicines Compendium (eMC) http://www.medicines.org.uk/emc/medicine/27609/SPC/Selincro+18mg+film-coated+tablets

26. Alford DP, Liebschutz J, Chen IA, Nicolaidis C, Panda M, Berg KM, Gibson J, Picchioni M, Bair MJ. Update in pain medicine. *J Gen Intern Med*. 2008;23:841–845.

27. Gass JT, Olive MF. Glutamatergic substrates of drug addiction and alcoholism. *Biochem Pharmacol*. 2008;75:218–265.

28. Addolorato G, Leggio L, Ferrulli A, Cardone S, Vonghia L, Mirijello A, Abenavoli L, D'Angelo C, Caputo F, Zambon A, Haber PS, Gasbarrini G. Effectiveness and safety of baclofen for maintenance of alcohol abstinence in alcohol-dependent patients with liver cirrhosis: randomised, double-blind controlled study. *Lancet*. 2007;370:1915–1922.

29. Fuller RK, Branchey L, Brightwell DR, et al. Disulfiram treatment of alcoholism. A Veterans Administration cooperative study. *JAMA*. 1986;256:1449–1455.

30. Fischer S, Bader A, Sweitzer B. Preoperative evaluation. In: Miller R, ed., *Miller's Anesthesia*, 7th ed. Philadelphia: Churchill Livingstone/Elsevier; 2010:1042.

31. Frisoni GB, Di Monda V. Disulfiram neuropathy: a review (1971-1988) and report of a case. *Alcohol Alcohol*. 1989;24:429–437.

32. Diaz JH, Hill GE. Hypotension with anesthesia in disulfiram-treated patients. *Anesthesiology*. 1979;51:366–368.

33. Manchikanti L, Helm S, 2nd, Fellows B, Janata JW, Pampati V, Grider JS, Boswell MV. Opioid epidemic in the United States. *Pain Physician*. 2012;15:ES9–E38.

34. Substance Abuse and Mental Health Services Administration, Center for Substance Abuse Treatment. Managing chronic pain in adults with or in recovery from substance use disorders. Revised 2013. http://store.samhsa.gov/shin/content//SMA12-4671/TIP54.pdf.

35. Orman JS, Keating GM. Buprenorphine/naloxone: a review of its use in the treatment of opioid dependence. *Drugs*. 2009;69:577–607.

36. Bryson EO. The perioperative management of patients maintained on medications used to manage opioid addiction. *Curr Opin Anaesthesiol*. 2014;27:359–364.

37. Alford DP, Compton P, Samet JH. Acute pain management for patients receiving maintenance methadone or buprenorphine therapy. *Ann Intern Med*. 2006;144:127–134.

38. Savage SR, Kirsh KL, Passik SD. Challenges in using opioids to treat pain in persons with substance use disorders. *Addict Sci Clin Pract*. 2008;4:4–25.

39. Mitra S, Sinatra RS. Perioperative management of acute pain in the opioid-dependent patient. *Anesthesiology*. 2004;101:212–227.

40. Laroche F, Rostaing S, Aubrun F, Perrot S. Pain management in heroin and cocaine users. Joint Bone Spine 2012; 79: 446–450.

41. Ling W, Charuvastra C, Kaim SC, Klett CJ. Methadyl acetate and methadone as maintenance treatments for heroin addicts. A Veterans Administration cooperative study. *Arch Gen Psychiatry*. 1976;33:709–720.

42. Souzdalnitski D, Halaszynski TM, Faclier G. Regional anesthesia and co-existing chronic pain. *Curr Opin Anaesthesiol*. 2010;23:662–670.

43. Morgan WW. Abuse liability of barbiturates and other sedative-hypnotics. *Adv Alcohol Subst Abuse*. 1990;9:67–82.

44. Olmedo R, Hoffman RS. Withdrawal syndromes. *Emerg Med Clin North Am*. 2000;18:273–288.

45. Longo LP, Johnson B. Addiction: Part I. Benzodiazepines—side effects, abuse risk and alternatives. *Am Fam Physician*. 2000;61:2121–2128.

46. Lai S, Lai H, Page JB, McCoy CB. The association between cigarette smoking and drug abuse in the United States. *J Addict Dis*. 2000;19:11–24.

47. Leboeuf-Yde C. Smoking and low back pain. A systematic literature review of 41 journal articles reporting 47 epidemiologic studies. *Spine (Phila Pa 1976)*. 1999;24:1463–1470.

48. Zvolensky MJ, McMillan K, Gonzalez A, Asmundson GJ. Chronic pain and cigarette smoking and nicotine dependence among a representative sample of adults. *Nicotine Tob Res*. 2009;11:1407–1414.

49. Souzdalnitski D, Lerman I, Chung K. Nicotine transdermal. In: Sinatra R, Jahr J, Watkins-Pitchford M, eds., *The Essence of Analgesia and Analgesics*, 1st ed. New York: Cambridge University Press; 2010:512–514.

50. Girdler SS, Maixner W, Naftel HA, Stewart PW, Moretz RL, Light KC. Cigarette smoking, stress-induced analgesia and pain perception in men and women. *Pain*. 2005;114:372–385.

51. Weingarten TN, Shi Y, Mantilla CB, Hooten WM, Warner DO. Smoking and chronic pain: a real-but-puzzling relationship. *Minn Med*. 2011;94:35–37.

52. Creekmore FM, Lugo RA, Weiland KJ. Postoperative opiate analgesia requirements of smokers and nonsmokers. *Ann Pharmacother*. 2004;38:949–953.

53. Biala G, Budzynska B, Kruk M. Naloxone precipitates nicotine abstinence syndrome and attenuates nicotine-induced antinociception in mice. *Pharmacol Rep*. 2005;57:755–760.

54. Usatine RP, Smith MA, Mayeaux EJ Jr, Chumley H, eds. Tobacco addiction. In: *The Color Atlas of Family Medicine*, 2nd ed. New York: McGraw-Hill; 2013.

55. Trevor AJ, Katzung BG, Kruidering-Hall MM, Masters SB, eds. Drugs of abuse. In: *Katzung and Trevor's Pharmacology: Examination & Board Review*, 10th ed. New York: McGraw- Hill; 2013:279–286.

56. American Psychiatric Association. Substance-related and addictive disorders. In: *Diagnostic and Statistical Manual of Mental Disorders*, 5th ed. Arlington, VA: American Psychiatric Association; 2013.

57. Ackerman WE 3rd, Ahmad M. Effect of cigarette smoking on serum hydrocodone levels in chronic pain patients. *J Ark Med Soc*. 2007;104:19–21.

58. Pesce A, West C, Rosenthal M, West R, Crews B, Mikel C, Almazan P, Latyshev S, Horn PS. Marijuana correlates with use of other illicit drugs in a pain patient population. *Pain Physician*. 2010;13:283–287.

59. Burns TL, Ineck JR. Cannabinoid analgesia as a potential new therapeutic option in the treatment of chronic pain. *Ann Pharmacother*. 2006;40:251–260.

60. May JA, White HC, Leonard-White A, Warltier DC, Pagel PS. The patient recovering from alcohol or drug addiction: special issues for the anesthesiologist. *Anesth Analg*. 2001;92:1601–1608.

61. Johnson MD, Heriza TJ, St Dennis C. How to spot illicit drug abuse in your patients. *Postgrad Med*. 1999;106:199–200, 203–206, 211–214 passim.

62. Greydanus DE, Hawver EK, Greydanus MM, Merrick J. Marijuana: current concepts. *Front Public Health*. 2013;1:42.

63. Levin FR, Mariani JJ, Brooks DJ, Pavlicova M, Cheng W, Nunes EV. Dronabinol for the treatment of cannabis dependence: a randomized, double-blind, placebo-controlled trial. *Drug Alcohol Depend*. 2011;116:142–150.

64. Martin-Sanchez E, Furukawa TA, Taylor J, Martin JL. Systematic review and meta-analysis of cannabis treatment for chronic pain. *Pain Med*. 2009;10:1353–1368.

65. Lindsey WT, Stewart D, Childress D. Drug interactions between common illicit drugs and prescription therapies. *Am J Drug Alcohol Abuse*. 2012;38:334–343.

66. Howell LL, Kimmel HL. Monoamine transporters and psychostimulant addiction. *Biochem Pharmacol*. 2008;75:196–217.

67. Menon DV, Wang Z, Fadel PJ, Arbique D, Leonard D, Li JL, Victor RG, Vongpatanasin W. Central sympatholysis as a novel countermeasure for cocaine-induced sympathetic activation and vasoconstriction in humans. *J Am Coll Cardiol*. 2007;50:626–633.

68. Vocci FJ, Montoya ID. Psychological treatments for stimulant misuse, comparing and contrasting those for amphetamine dependence and those for cocaine dependence. *Curr Opin Psychiatry*. 2009;22:263–268.

69. Kuczkowski KM. The cocaine abusing parturient: a review of anesthetic considerations. *Can J Anaesth*. 2004;51:145–154.

70. Dean A. Illicit drugs and drug interaction. *Pharmacist*. 2006;25(9):684–689. https://www.erowid.org/psychoactives/health/health_article1.pdf

71. Griffiths R, Richards W, Johnson M, McCann U, Jesse R. Mystical-type experiences occasioned by psilocybin mediate the attribution of personal meaning and spiritual significance 14 months later. *J Psychopharmacol*. 2008;22:621–632.

72. Nichols DE. Hallucinogens. *Pharmacol Ther*. 2004;101:131–181.

73. Nicholson KL, Hayes BA, Balster RL. Evaluation of the reinforcing properties and phencyclidine-like discriminative stimulus effects of dextromethorphan and dextrorphan in rats and rhesus monkeys. *Psychopharmacology (Berl)*. 1999;146:49–59.

74. Cox D, Ahmed Z, McBride AJ. Diphenhydramine dependence. *Addiction*. 2001;96:516–517.

75. de Nesnera AP. Diphenhydramine dependence: a need for awareness. *J Clin Psychiatry*. 1996;57:136–137.

76. Kalant H. The pharmacology and toxicology of "ecstasy" (MDMA) and related drugs. *CMAJ*. 2001;165:917–928.

77. Cohen MJ, Hanbury R, Stimmel B. Abuse of amitriptyline. *JAMA*. 1978;240:1372–1373.

78. Garner EM, Kelly MW, Thompson DF. Tricyclic antidepressant withdrawal syndrome. *Ann Pharmacother*. 1993;27:1068–1072.

79. Agbayewa MO. Symptoms of withdrawal from tricyclic antidepressants. *CMAJ*. 1981;125:420, 422.

80. Haddad PM, Anderson IM. Recognising and managing antidepressant discontinuation. *Adv Psychiatr Treat*. 2007;13:447–457.

23

Management of the Patients with Spinal Cord Stimulators and Intrathecal Pumps

SAMUEL W. SAMUEL AND KHODADAD NAMIRANIAN

KEY POINTS

- Spinal cord stimulation (SCS), dorsal root ganglion (DRG) stimulation, and peripheral nerve stimulation (PNS) are usually used for treating neuropathic pain, and intrathecal pumps (ITP) are used for nociceptive pain.
- The anesthesia management for these patients with already long-standing chronic pain relies on understanding the physiological and anatomical changes due to these implants.
- Except for the intrathecal baclofen pump, all other implantable devices are mainly for pain control and their cessation will not result in any life-threatening situation.
- The symptoms of baclofen overdose are dizziness, lightheadedness, and drowsiness progressing to somnolence, respiratory depression, hypothermia, seizures, hypotonia, and coma.
- Symptoms of baclofen withdrawal are seizures, high fever, exaggerated rebound spasticity and muscle rigidity that advances to rhabdomyolysis, multiple-organ failure, and death.
- SCS can be turned off before the procedure and turned on at the end of the procedure.
- Intrathecal pump infusion can be continued during the operation, and the postoperative pain regimen must be supplemented with other methods for analgesia.
- The implantable devices must be protected from electrocautery per the manufacturer's recommendation.
- The skin overlying the subcutaneous pocket of implantable pain management device must be well padded and protected during the perioperative period.
- Generally, MRI interferes with some SCS, but patients with ITP can be exposed to MRI with strength of magnetic field up to 1.5 Tesla.

Introduction

Spinal cord stimulation (SCS) and intrathecal pumps (ITP) have been used with increasing popularity for pain management given the current epidemic of chronic pain. The anesthesia management for these patients with already long-standing chronic pain is further complicated by the physiological and anatomical changes due to the implant. This chapter focuses on the perioperative management of patients with SCS and ITP. It discusses these devices and their indications as well as the resultant anatomical and physiological changes that need to be understood in order to provide safe and effective anesthesia care.

Implantable Devices for Pain Management

Neuropathic pain and nociceptive pain are the two main categories of pain. In *nociceptive pain*, the main injury occurs in the peripheral tissue from damage to the tissue. The nervous system is intact and transmits and perceives the pain. This type of pain is described mainly as sharp or achy. Acute postoperative pain is characteristic nociceptive pain. Opioids are indicated for the acute phase of nociceptive pain. *Neuropathic pain* occurs from damage to the structure in the nervous system and is described as burning or tingling pain. Postherpetic neuralgia and diabetic polyneuropathy are prototypes of neuropathic pain. This type of pain is managed mainly by antidepressant and anticonvulsants and is not satisfactorily responsive to opioids. Neurostimulation, including SCS as well as dorsal root ganglion (DRG) stimulation and peripheral nerve stimulation (PNS), is used to treat neuropathic pain. Intrathecal drug delivery, which uses an ITP, is used to treat nociceptive pain.

SPINAL CORD STIMULATION

Spinal cord stimulation (SCS), the prototype for neurostimulation, uses electrical stimulation for modulating the pain. SCS consists of an implantable pulse generator (IPG) and a single or several leads. The leads for SCS are placed in the epidural space either percutaneously or surgically for the paddle leads. The leads transmit the electrical pulses from the IPG to the epidural space and to the dorsal column of the spinal cord. IPG is implanted in a subcutaneous pocket in the gluteal area, in the lower back, or in the abdomen.

The exact mechanism of pain relief by SCS is not known, but it is believed that electrical stimulation of the descending inhibitory neurons in the posterior column modulates pain transduction in the spinal cord. The indications for SCS are failed back surgery syndrome, complex regional pain syndrome, phantom limb pain, and post-amputation stump pain.[1-3] SCS is also indicated for intractable angina pectoris and peripheral vascular disease with critical ischemia[4,5]; however, it is rarely implanted for these indications because of concurrent aggressive anticoagulation therapy.

DORSAL ROOT GANGLIA STIMULATION

Dorsal root ganglion, on the sensory dorsal root of the spinal nerves, is the home to sensory neuron cell bodies. DRG stimulator is a new mode of neurostimulation that delivers the electrical pulse to DRG. Its theoretical advantage is to cover the pain in locations that are difficult to manage with SCS, including groin and palm of foot [6]. DRG stimulator also consists of an IPG and leads. The leads are implanted in epidural space with the tip in close proximity to the DRG. DRG stimulator is widely used in Europe, and is awaiting FDA approval in USA. The anesthesia care for the patient with DRG stimulator is similar to that of SCS.

PERIPHERAL NERVE STIMULATION

Peripheral nerve stimulation (PNS) has been utilized for neuropathic pain related to cranial nerves or isolated nerves. The occipital nerve and cranial nerves are the main targets. Similar to the other modes of neurostimulation, an IPG and one to several leads are implanted. Since any nerve can be the target, there is significant variation in the location of the leads and IPG.[7] The anesthesia care for a patient with PNS is similar to that with SCS.

INTRATHECAL PUMPS

The intrathecal drug delivery system or intrathecal pump (ITP) delivers the medication directly to the cerebrospinal fluid (CSF). Via this method, the medication bypasses the blood-brain barrier and thus significantly less medication is needed, with fewer peripheral side effects. The ITP has two components, the catheter and the pump reservoir. The reservoir is filled with the solution containing the medications and the attached pump delivers a specific volume as a continuous flow. The catheter transports the medication to the CSF. Morphine, baclofen, and ziconotide are FDA approved for intrathecal use. Other medications commonly used intrathecally are hydromorphone, fentanyl, sufentanil, bupivacaine, and clonidine.[8]

The main indication for ITP is intrathecal (IT) baclofen pump for spasticity. Baclofen is a GABA-A agonist and is mainly used for treating spasticity. The continuous delivery of baclofen to the spinal CSF results in significantly improved symptom relief with fewer side effects and reduced medication dose. The symptoms of baclofen overdose are dizziness, lightheadedness, and drowsiness progressing to somnolence, respiratory depression, hypothermia, seizures, hypotonia, and coma. Symptoms of baclofen withdrawal are pruritus, seizures, high fever, exaggerated rebound spasticity and muscle rigidity that may advance to rhabdomyolysis, multiple-organ failure, and death. Differential diagnoses for baclofen withdrawal are malignant hyperthermia, neuroleptic malignant syndrome, autonomic dysreflexia, sepsis, meningitis, and seizures. Baclofen withdrawal is life-threatening and must be treated with aggressive supportive therapy, reinstitution of intrathecal baclofen, and control of seizure with benzo-diazepines. The conversion rate of IT to oral baclofen is estimated at about 1:300; however, baclofen withdrawal due to IT baclofen cessation may not be respon-sive to even very high doses of oral baclofen (>120 mg/day in divided doses).[9]

The other main indication for ITP is severe chronic pain, mainly nocicep-tive pain. Patients with advanced cancer pain (with life expectancy of more than 3 months) and those with long-standing chronic pain who cannot tolerate the peripheral side effects of oral medication may benefit from ITP. The more hydrophilic opioids, like morphine and hydromorphone (medium hydrophilic), have longer half-lives in the CSF compared to more hydrophobic opioids, such as fentanyl and sufentanil, and thus will provide longer pain relief along with the increased risk of delayed respiratory depression.

Ziconotide (Prialt®) is noncompetitive blocker of N-type voltage-sensitive calcium channels. There is no reported dependency or tolerance induced by this medication, and no life-threatening emergency due to abrupt discontinuation has been reported. The main side effect of ziconotide is neurological and psy-chological disturbances. Other medications, such as local anesthetics (bupiva-caine) and α2-adrenergic agonists (clonidine), are also used in combination with opioids.[8]

Pain Control in Inpatients with Implanted Devices

Patients with implantable devices for pain (SCS, DRG stimulator, PNS, or ITP) are essentially patients with chronic pain who have an implanted device. Basic oper-ative management of the patients with chronic pain applies to these patients. These patients usually need anesthesia care for operations that are unrelated to their chronic pain symptoms. They became candidates for implantable devices when all conservative approaches, interventions, injections, and surgery failed and usually are not candidates for any further surgery related to their original chronic pain.

The anesthesia management must also accommodate these implants. For these implants, these patients have endured prolonged therapy, numerous trials, and significant cost so in order to receive pain relief. Therefore, extreme caution must be used to keep these implants safe, especially from infection and electro-magnetic interference. With the exception of the baclofen pump, these implants can be turned off during surgery, as they are mainly for pain control and their off-state will not result in any life-threatening situations.

The anatomical location of the leads or catheter may interfere with the axial (epidural or spinal) anesthesia plan, since the leads or catheters are implanted in close proximity to the spinal cord. Patients with chronic pain are more likely to have poor postoperative pain control,[10] and the postoperative pain is aggravated by succinylcholine-induced myalgia, deconditioning due to loss of muscle tone during anesthesia, and immediate postoperative immobilization. Therefore, postoperative pain is likely to be undertreated in these patients and any option, including epidural or regional anesthesia, for pain control is encouraged. If an axial technique is to be used, strict aseptic technique must be used. The IT catheter is in direct communication with the intrathecal space and any contamination is carried directly to the intrathecal space and CNS. Fluoroscopy must be used for identifying the SCS leads or ITP catheter and blind techniques must be avoided. If the IPG or pump reservoir interferes with the surgical approach, they may need to be transferred to another subcutaneous pocket. For this reason, coordination and consultation with an interventional pain specialist, a neurosurgeon, or an experienced general surgeon is required.

The magnetic field used in MRI and many other surgical operations can interfere with the implants. Thermal energy is induced in the SCS leads by the magnetic fields and can be transferred to the spinal cord, causing permanent neurological damage. Therefore, many patients with SCS should avoid exposure to strong magnetic fields. Some of the newer leads can be conditionally used in MRI, such as an MRI-compatible lead for MRI with less than 1.5 Tesla or brain MRI in patients with lumbar SCS. The details must be verified with the manufacturer and discussed with the radiologist. The intrathecal catheter is made of silicone and does not interact with the magnetic fields. Therefore a, patients with ITP can be exposed to magnetic fields. However, the currently available pumps stall temporarily in strong magnetic fields and restart within 24 hours. Patients with an ITP pump can receive MRI; however, the manufacturer recommends investigating the pump after MRI to ensure that the pump has resumed function.

PREOPERATIVE PERIOD

Perioperative management starts with a detailed evaluation and consultation, including history of medications, surgeries, prior procedures, prior anesthesia, psychiatric issues, and substance abuse. A significant number of these patients may still take oral opioids chronically or as needed, in addition to having ITP or SCS. The details of the chronic pain symptoms must be obtained from the patient. Consultation with a chronic pain team may be needed at hospital admission or in the preoperative period.

The evaluation must also focus on the implanted device, including the indication for placement, location of the IPG and leads, the model, manufacturer, and program. Any recommendations must be obtained from the practitioner who implanted the device and from the device's manufacturing company. The detailed procedure notes, relevant imaging, and the history of the device must be reviewed. The medication and dosage used in ITP are of extreme importance. Any interruption in the baclofen pump is dangerous and must be avoided. If opioids are part of treatment, the dosage must be known since opioid underdosing induces withdrawal symptoms, and overdosing carries the risk of respiratory depression and death.

These patients usually have neuropathy due to extensive spine surgeries, other comorbidities (cancer, obesity, diabetes), or medications. Detailed neurological symptoms as well as motor, sensory, and reflexes must be documented. The SCS leads may migrate, and the anesthesia team must document the coverage provided by SCS before and after the surgical procedure. Patients tend to describe the SCS coverage area as having a pleasant tingling sensation.

The implants must be assessed by the manufacturer representative or by a healthcare provider with relevant experience. Three companies, Boston Scientific (previously Advanced Bionics, Inc., Natick, MA), Medtronic, Inc. (Minneapolis, MN), and St. Jude's Medical (previously Advanced Neuromodulation Systems, St. Paul, MN) are the major manufacturers of SCS in the United States. Most of the available intrathecal pumps are manufactured by Medtronic, Inc. (Minneapolis, MN).

A multimodality approach to acute pain is encouraged, using a regimen of drugs targeting other pathways, such as acetaminophen, NSAIDs, NMDA antagonist (ketamine, magnesium, methadone), α2-adrenergic agonists (clonidine and dexmedetomidine), or calcium channel blockers (gabapentin and pregabalin). Regional anesthesia is strongly encouraged. The anesthesia plan must be discussed preoperatively with the patient to decrease his or her anxiety and develop realistic expectations.

INTRAOPERATIVE CONSIDERATIONS

We recommend that SCS be turned off before the procedure and turned on at the conclusion of anesthesia. The patient or the healthcare provider can turn SCS on and off. SCS is mainly implanted for neuropathic pain that is usually of much less intensity than the surgical pain. Also, the electrical stimulation of SCS may intensify when patients are lying flat.

We strongly recommend that ITP infusion be continued during the operation. The postoperative pain regimen must be supplemented with other methods for analgesia, including oral and intravenous opioids. Abrupt cessation of the baclofen pump is life-threatening. If intrathecal opioids are discontinued, the pain, usually extremely severe, returns and opioid withdrawal syndrome occurs.

Table 23.1 **Table for Converting Opioid from Intrathecal to Oral Form**

Opioid	Oral	Parenteral	Epidural	Intrathecal
Morphine (mg)	300	100	10	1
Hydromorphone (mg)	60	20	2	0.2
Meperidine (mg)	3000	1000	100	10
Fentanyl (mg)	—	1	0.1	0.01
Sufentanil (mg)	—	0.1	0.01	0.001

Sufficient intravenous or oral opioids must be provided to cover the surgical and original pain. The conversion rate of intrathecal morphine to oral morphine is 1:300 (Table 23.1).

The available ITPs cannot be stopped and can only be programmed to run at the lowest possible rate. Increasing the rate of an ITP is not advised due to the increased risk of respiratory depression.

The delicate electronic structures of the IPG or pump reservoir make them prone to interference and possible damage from electrocautery. It is recommended that bipolar electrocautery be used; if unipolar electrocautery is needed, the returning pad must be applied so that the current will be as far from the SCS components as possible. The energy must be set to the lowest setting clinically indicated. The presence of a subcutaneous IPG or pump reservoir must be taken into account at the time of positioning and the site must be well padded to prevent any skin breakdown.

POSTOPERATIVE CONSIDERATIONS

If an epidural catheter is used for postoperative anesthesia, frequent neurological examination (not less than every 2 hours) is needed to detect early signs of space-occupying epidural lesions. This is important since the epidural leads and subarachnoid catheters make patients more susceptible to the deleterious effects of a space-occupying lesion. At the conclusion of anesthesia, the device must be assessed and reprogrammed to the original setting.

Summary

Patients with implantable devices for pain (SCS, DRG stimulator, PNS, or ITP) are essentially patients with chronic pain who have an implanted device. The basic operative management of patients with chronic pain applies to these patients. Multimodal analgesia as well as regional anesthesia is strongly recommended. Preoperatively, details of the device as well as the chronic pain symptoms must be investigated. Intraoperatively, these devices must be protected from the electrocautery and magnetic fields per manufacturer's recommendation. Fluoroscopy must be used for axial techniques and blind techniques must be avoided. Cessation of baclofen pump may result in seizures, high fever, exaggerated rebound spasticity, and muscle rigidity that advances to rhabdomyolysis, multiple-organ failure, and death. Intrathecal opioid infusion is better continued during surgery, and the postoperative pain regimen must be supplemented with other methods for analgesia, including oral and intravenous opioids. SCS may be turned off before the procedure and turned on at the conclusion of anesthesia.

References

1. Kemler MA, Barendse GA, van Kleef M, et al. Spinal cord stimulation in patients with chronic reflex sympathetic dystrophy. *N Engl J Med*. 2000;343(9):618–624.
2. North RB, Kumar K, Wallace MS, et al. Spinal cord stimulation versus re-operation in patients with failed back surgery syndrome: an international multicenter randomized controlled trial (EVIDENCE study). *Neuromodulation*. 2011;14(4):330–335; discussion 335–336.
3. Kumar K, Taylor RS, Jacques L, et al. Spinal cord stimulation versus conventional medical management for neuropathic pain: a multicentre randomised controlled trial in patients with failed back surgery syndrome. *Pain*. 2007;132(1-2):179–188.
4. Klomp HM, Spincemaille GH, Steyerberg EW, Habbema JD, van Urk H. Spinal-cord stimulation in critical limb ischaemia: a randomised trial. ESES Study Group. *Lancet*. 1999;353(9158):1040–1044.
5. Ubbink DT, Spincemaille GH, Prins MH, Reneman RS, Jacobs MJ. Microcirculatory investigations to determine the effect of spinal cord stimulation for critical leg ischemia: the Dutch multicenter randomized controlled trial. *J Vasc Surg*. 1999;30(2):236–244.
6. Deer TR, et al. A prospective study of dorsal root ganglion stimulation for the relief of chronic pain. *Neuromodulation*. 2013;16(1):67–71; discussion 71–72.
7. Hong J, Ball PA, Fanciullo GJ. Neurostimulation for neck pain and headache. *Headache*. 2014;54(3):430–444.
8. Deer TR, Prager J, Levy R, et al. Polyanalgesic Consensus Conference 2012: recommendations for the management of pain by intrathecal (intraspinal) drug delivery: report of an interdisciplinary expert panel. *Neuromodulation*. 2012;15(5):436–464; discussion 464–466.
9. Coffey RJ, Edgar TS, Francisco GE, et al. Abrupt withdrawal from intrathecal baclofen: recognition and management of a potentially life-threatening syndrome. *Arch Phys Med Rehabil*. 2002;83(6):735–741.
10. Pizzi LT, Toner R, Foley K, et al. Relationship between potential opioid-related adverse effects and hospital length of stay in patients receiving opioids after orthopedic surgery. *Pharmacotherapy*. 2012;32(6):502–514.

Part V

PERIOPERATIVE CHRONIC
PAIN MANAGEMENT

24

Preoperative Chronic Pain Management: Coordination of Surgical and Anesthesiology Services in Preparation for Surgery

SHERIF ZAKY, STEVEN ROSENBLATT, AND SALIM HAYEK

KEY POINTS

- Chronic pain patients presenting for surgical procedures represent a genuine challenge to healthcare providers.
- Despite the long-standing recognition of the prevalence of postoperative pain, 20% to 30% of patients continue to experience moderate to severe pain after surgery.
- Three steps are important for an efficient pain management plan regarding the chronic pain patient: system preparation, patient evaluation, and preoperative optimization.
- Education and training of healthcare providers, building an acute pain management service, and establishing metrics for outcomes are important components of system preparation.
- Patient evaluation includes a thorough history and physical examination, a psychological evaluation, a review of previous images, and discussion of previous and existing medications and treatment interventions.
- Preoperative optimization entails education, preoperative adjustment of medication, and treatment of pre-existing pain conditions.
- As part of a multimodal perioperative analgesia plan, premedication and the use of regional anesthesia, preferably with perineural catheters when possible, will optimize postoperative analgesia in this difficult patient population. Additional tips for preoperative preparation of chronic pain patients are presented in Box 24.1.

Introduction

Chronic pain patients represent a unique population as they share a complex biological, psychological, and social state. They pose a real challenge to healthcare providers when they present for surgery.[1] Chronic pain patients are frequently treated with opioids, non-steroidal anti-inflammatory drugs (NSAIDs), antidepressants, and anticonvulsants. Such patients suffer from prolonged inactivity or from neurological deficits, which may be associated with complications and adverse effects resulting from perioperative treatment. Inappropriate or excessive medication is a commonly observed problem among patients with chronic pain.[2]

System Preparation, Patient Evaluation, and Preoperative Optimization

Despite the long-standing recognition of postoperative pain as both prevalent and undertreated, 20% to 30% of patients continue to experience moderate to severe pain after surgery.[3,4] High levels of postoperative pain are associated with an increased risk of pulmonary and cardiovascular complications and are the most common reason for delayed discharge or for unexpected hospital admission after ambulatory surgery. Inadequate pain control is responsible for prolonged convalescence after inpatient surgery and for increased healthcare costs.[5-11]

The association between preoperative opioid use and ineffective postoperative pain control has been demonstrated in the literature. De Leon-Casasola et al.[12] studied 116 patients with cancer and reported that subjects who chronically consumed opioids (daily oral morphine dose 90–360 mg) required more than three times as much morphine given via a continuous epidural infusion and more than four times as much morphine as an intermittent intravenous bolus for breakthrough pain after surgery compared with opioid-naive patients. The severity of postoperative pain in chronically opioid-consuming patients prolonged the need for epidural analgesia by a factor of 3 (9 days versus 3 days). A case-controlled retrospective analysis done by Rapp et al. on 360 patients who experienced malignant or nonmalignant pain reported a threefold greater postoperative opioid requirement in chronically opioid-consuming patients.[13]

The need for increasing doses of opioid medication is often attributed to the development of tolerance. However, dose escalation can be the result of other factors, such as the progression of the underlying disease that causes the chronic pain. This development is particularly true in patients with cancer pain and less likely in those with chronic non-cancer pain.

The American Society of Anesthesiologists (ASA) has published practice guidelines for acute pain management in the perioperative setting[14] and for chronic pain management.[15] These recommendations have recently been updated[16,17] to reflect the most recent relevant data. However, these protocols do not cover patients with chronic pain presenting for surgery. In this chapter we will examine this specific situation, which is seen by healthcare providers with increasing frequency.

Three steps are important for an efficient pain management plan for the chronic pain patient: system preparation, patient evaluation, and preoperative optimization.

SYSTEM PREPARATION

System preparation includes the following:

• Education and training of healthcare providers
• Acute pain management team
• Establishing metrics to evaluate patient outcomes

With the increasing awareness of pain control as an essential part of hospital HCAHPS scores, which reflect in many ways on the hospital performance and reimbursement, it has become crucial for each hospital to develop protocols and strategies to improve each patient's pain experience. The most challenging population involves patients with pre-existing pain conditions. Hospital performance depends on collaboration between the different members of the perioperative surgical team to improve the patient pain outcome. This team includes the surgery, anesthesiology, nursing, and acute and chronic pain management services. The relationship between these providers should be set up within hospital policy through protocols that focus on the patient. The first link in the chain should concentrate on education and training of healthcare providers in pain management concepts, safety, and evaluation techniques.

Anesthesiologists offering perioperative analgesia services should provide ongoing education and training to ensure that hospital personnel are knowledgeable and skilled with regard to the effective and safe use of the available treatment options within the institution. Education can be provided through different materials, including lectures, online videos, and mandatory courses. A pain pioneer or champion from the nursing team can function as a crucial member of the team to make sure that pain is adequately evaluated and managed on his or her own floor. These floor advocates can be a reference for other nursing or midlevel providers for immediate help with acute pain issues. This system improves patient satisfaction, as the ongoing presence of such proponents on the floor provides assurance to patients—even while the pain-managing physician is busy with a large pool of patients. Observational studies suggest that education and training of healthcare providers are associated with decreased pain levels,[18-21] and improved patient satisfaction.[21]

Establishing a dedicated acute pain management service capable of providing both interventional and non-interventional pain techniques is very important to optimize the patient perioperative pain experience. A plan should be formulated between the patient and the acute pain management, chronic pain management, and surgical teams. As there is no accurate predictor of postoperative pain experience, regular follow-up with the inpatient pain management service can ensure that the plan is effectively executed, and any changes can be made as needed. Studies have clearly demonstrated that acute pain services are associated with a reduction in perioperative pain.[22-30]

Outcome metrics should be established and collected routinely by the hospital and utilized by healthcare providers to review their performance and help improve areas of deficiency in pain control. Comparing hospital length of stay for different pain approaches (e.g., epidural versus intravenous patient-controlled analgesia, or transversus plane block versus subcutaneous catheters) can help tailor and ultimately optimize patients' experience. Studies assessing postoperative care indicate that pain outcomes are not fully documented in patient records.[31-37] The conversion to electronic medical records will hopefully improve immediate as well as historical documentation.

PREOPERATIVE EVALUATION

Preoperative Evaluation by the Surgical Team

Patients with a history of chronic pain should first be identified during their preoperative visit with their surgeon. Each institution should have its own criteria to identify these patients based on preselected criteria, which include the chronic use of opioids, a history of difficulty with pain control during previous operations, multiple allergies or reactions to most of the common pain medications, and existing implantable pain devices such as an intrathecal pump or spinal cord stimulator. Once such patients are identified, the surgical team should discuss with them in detail the risks and benefits of the upcoming surgery, including the increased potential of prolonged postoperative pain and anticipated difficulty with pain control using conventional treatment.

If regional anesthesia and analgesia can be employed on the basis of type of surgery, these options should be suggested as the preferred perioperative plan. A discussion regarding the feasibility of regional anesthesia should be initiated at the surgeon's office and clearly documented in the medical record. A clear communication about anesthesia and postoperative preferences or limitations should be clearly noted. The final decision regarding the modality of pain control should be that of the anesthesia/acute pain management team on the day of the procedure, in consultation with the surgical team. Communication is of great importance since in certain situations, the surgical team might prefer to avoid regional anesthesia due to the need to monitor nerve function periopera- tively when there is risk of potential nerve injury or a pre-existing one. Similarly, the need for early anticoagulation after the surgical procedure and its impact on the ability to manipulate or remove neuroaxial or peripheral nerve catheters is another important consideration.

Consultation with the pain management service for evaluation and optimiza- tion is absolutely crucial preoperatively. Patients with chronic pain conditions typically have complex physical, psychological, and social factors affecting their pain state. A preoperative assessment by a pain specialist should examine these different dimensions of preexisting pain, which are often beyond the recogni- tion of the surgical services.

Preoperative Evaluation by Pain Management Service

The goal of the preoperative visit to the pain management service is to:

1. Evaluate the type and extent of the preexisting pain condition.
2. Treat or optimize the chronic pain condition.
3. Formulate a perioperative pain control plan with the patient and the family.
4. Discuss a follow-up schedule to help assist the patient's return back to preop- erative baseline.

This consultation should take into consideration the type of surgery, the expected severity of postoperative pain, pre-existing chronic pain conditions, and previous experiences with pain control after prior surgeries.

HISTORY

A comprehensive medical history with emphasis on conditions that can cause or affect pain condition is crucial. Other elements to be included in the patient's history are as follows:

- A complete pain history that contains information about the onset, quality, intensity, distribution, duration, course, and sensory and affective compo- nents of the pain as well as details about exacerbating and relieving factors
- Additional information on new sensory, motor, or autonomic changes
- Constitutional symptoms such as bowel or bladder incontinence
- Previous diagnostic studies, such as imaging, lab work, and drug screen tests
- Previous as well as current therapies that focus on opioid usage and its dos- age. A review of prescription monitoring program data is helpful to assess accuracy of opioid consumption and potential preoperative opioid acquisition from multiple prescribers. Review of previous urine drug screen results, if available, helps in identifying patients with a history of substance abuse.

- Review of previous medical records with focus on historical substance use or misuse, current or previous litigations related to work injury or compensation
- Review of medical, surgical, social, and family history
- Review of systems

PHYSICAL EXAMINATION

The physical examination should include a general physical review as well as a thorough neurological and musculoskeletal evaluation. The focused exam should include sensory and motor examination, evaluation of reflexes and gait, as well as provocative tests specific to the pain condition tested.

The goal of the sensory examination is to determine which fibers or neuronal tracts are involved in the transmission of the patient's pain. A-δ fibers are responsible for transmission of fast pain signals and are tested with pinprick and cold. C-fibers are responsible for slow pain signal transmission and are evaluated by using both pinprick and warm temperature. Isolated decreased sense to warm and cold temperature is an early finding in small fiber neuropathy. A-β fibers are examined through light touch, vibration, and joint position. Isolated decreased vibratory sense is an early finding of large fiber neuropathy. Sensory dissociation in which patients report sharp sensation to pinprick in an area without fine touch or proprioception can occur with lesions that interrupt fibers at the spinal cord level (e.g., syrinx).

Anatomically, lesions can be divided into central (brain and spinal cord), spinal nerve root (dermatomal), and peripheral nerve lesions.

The motor examination begins with careful assessment. Inspection can reveal hypertrophy, atrophy, and fasciculations. Hypertrophy is a sign of overuse, while atrophy and fasciculations are manifestations of lower motor neuron disorders. Palpation is valuable in identifying pain generators such as trigger points. Muscle tone examined through resistance to manipulation of the range of motion can be described as hypotonic (decreased) or hypertonic (increased). Hypertonia is further divided into spasticity (velocity-dependent increase in tone) and rigidity (generalized increase). Spasticity is commonly seen after brain or spinal cord injury because of loss of the descending inhibitory control, while rigidity is seen with extrapyramidal diseases due to lesions in the nigrostrial system.

Deep tendon reflexes serve as a guide to the anatomical location of any lesions. Nerve root levels for commonly tested reflexes are biceps reflex C5-C6, triceps reflex C7-C8, patellar reflex L3-L4, and Achilles reflex S1-S2. Clonus might be indicative of upper motor neuron lesion. Babinski's sign usually indicates upper motor neuron disease but can be normal in infants up until the age of 18 months. In the upper extremity, Hoffman's sign is indicative of upper motor neuron disease or myelopathy. Coordination and equilibrium are functions of the cerebellum. Coordination can be tested by finger-nose-finger, and heel-knee-shin tests. Gait, heel, and toe walking and tandem gait testing can be used to assess equilibrium.

Gait can be divided into two phases, swing and stance. From a pain perspective gait can be described as normal, antalgic, or abnormal. An antalgic gait is characterized by avoidance of weight bearing on the affected limb secondary to pain. An abnormal gait is a broad category that includes balance, musculoskeletal, and neurological disorders.

A brief mental examination can be assessed while obtaining the history. This evaluation includes (1) orientation to time, place, and person; (2) ability to name objects, (3) memory at 1 and 5 minutes; (4) ability to calculate serial 7s; and (5) signs of cognitive deficit or aphasia.[38]

Multiple provocative tests have been described to confirm or point to a specific diagnosis—for example, a positive Faber test with sacroiliac joint dysfunction, or a positive straight leg raise test in the case of spinal stenosis. The validity of these tests is questionable, but they serve as an additional tool during physical examination to evaluate the source of pain.

PSYCHOSOCIAL EVALUATION

A comprehensive, multidisciplinary assessment may be necessary in order to develop a treatment plan for patients with chronic pain who are about to undergo a surgical procedure. Psychological evaluation is necessary to evaluate the emotional, behavioral, and social factors that must be considered in the treatment plan. The psychosocial evaluation should include information about the presence of psychological symptoms (e.g., anxiety, depression, or anger), psychiatric disorders, personality traits, and coping mechanisms. The assessment should determine the impact of chronic pain on a patient's ability to perform daily activities as well as the influence of pain on mood, sleep, and appetite. Focus should concentrate on legal, vocational, or substance issues that can influence the patient's desire or motivation to improve.

Conclusions from the patient history, physical examination, and psychological and diagnostic evaluation should be used as the basis for an individualized treatment plan focused on optimization of the risk–benefit ratio, with an appropriate progression of treatment from a lesser to greater degree of invasiveness.

PREOPERATIVE OPTIMIZATION

Preoperative optimization includes following:

- Preoperative adjustment of medication
- Preoperative treatment to treat pre-existing pain conditions
- Premedication before surgery as a part of a multimodal analgesia
- Preoperative evaluation of patients with implantable pain devices
- Patient and family education

Chronic pain patients are typically treated with medications that belong to one or more categories: (1) anticonvulsants, (2) antidepressants, (3) benzodiazepines, (4) N methyl-D-aspartate (NMDA) receptor antagonists, (5) non steroidal anti inflammatory drugs (NSAIDs), (6) opioids, (7) skeletal muscle relaxants, and (8) topical agents. Techniques to optimize the preoperative pain medication regimen include review of current and previous pain medications, review of the patient's previous history of pain control after prior surgeries, and knowledge of the efficacy of different medications used previously in terms of pain control.

Adjustment of pain medications should ensure continuation of medications whose sudden cessation can precipitate a withdrawal syndrome. Most pain adjuvants can be safely continued in the perioperative period. However, physicians must be very cognizant that some drugs may cause serious interactions with other medications provided in the perioperative period. Tramadol added for postoperative pain in a patient taking selective serotonin reuptake inhibitors (SSRIs), for example, can precipitate serotonergic syndrome. Similarly, patients on monoamine oxidase (MAO) inhibitors can develop serious cardiovascular reactions when these are combined with sympathomimetic agents. Antidepressants in general should not be stopped preoperatively even if the patient is NPO. These medications can usually be administered orally or enterally via a feeding tube.

Nonpharmacological treatment for patients with chronic pain includes interventional treatment, psychotherapy, and behavioral therapy. Further modalities, such as joint injections, epidural steroid injection, and tunneled epidural, intrathecal or peripheral nerve catheters, can be employed by the pain physician as needed before surgery to optimize relief in chronic pain conditions.

Summary

Perioperative management of chronic pain patients is challenging. System preparation, patient evaluation by both surgical and pain management teams, and preoperative optimization are paramount. Education and training of healthcare providers, building an acute pain management service, and establishing metrics for outcomes are important components of system preparation. Patient evaluation includes a thorough history and physical examination, a psychological evaluation, a review of previous images, and discussion of previous and existing medications and treatment interventions. Preoperative optimization entails education, preoperative adjustment of medication, and treatment of preexisting pain conditions. As part of a multimodal perioperative analgesia plan, premedication and the use of regional anesthesia, preferably with perineural catheters when possible, will optimize postoperative analgesia in this difficult patient population. Additional tips for preoperative preparation of chronic pain patients are presented in Box 24.1.

Box 24.1 **Practice Tips for Preoperative Preparation of Chronic Pain Patients**

FOR HEALTH SYSTEM/HEALTHCARE PROVIDERS

- Provide adequate education and training on pain management concepts, safety, and evaluation techniques.
- Establish an inpatient pain management service capable of using interventional and noninterventional pain management techniques.
- Establish outcomes metrics collected routinely for each floor, service, and providers.

FOR THE SURGICAL TEAM

- Identify the high-risk patient during the preoperative visit.
- Discuss with the patient the higher risk of prolonged pain after surgery and difficulty with pain control.
- Discuss with the patient regional anesthesia options, if applicable, and document that in the patient's chart.

FOR PAIN MANAGEMENT SERVICE

- Review previous medical records with a focus on pain history.
- Consider preoperative pain interventions, as needed.
- If regional techniques are considered, avoid stopping preoperative long-acting opioids.
- Expect chronic pain patients to have opioid demand two to four times that of an opioid-naïve patient.
- Convert long-acting oral opioids to intravenous route for medium and major surgeries.
- Consider opioid rotation in case of continuous opioid escalation.
- Consider intra- or postoperative ketamine infusion for patients with significant tolerance to opioids.
- Consider switching route for opioid administration to intrathecal or epidural if systemic opioids fail to provide adequate analgesia.

References

1. Kopf A, Banzhaf A, et al. Perioperative management of the chronic pain patient. *Best Pract Res Clin Anaesthesiol.* 2005;19(1):59–76.
2. Bigal ME, Rapoport AM, et al. Transformed migraine and medication overuse in a tertiary headache centre—clinical characteristics and treatment outcomes. *Cephalalgia.* 2004;24(6):483–490.
3. Michel MZ, Sanders MK. Effectiveness of acute postoperative pain management. *Br J Anaesth.* 2003;91:448–449.

4. Dolin SJ, Cashman JN, Bland JM. Effectiveness of acute postoperative pain management: I. Evidence from published data. *Br J Anaesth*. 2002;89:409–423.

5. Shea RA, Brooks JA, Dayhoff NE, Keck J. Pain intensity and postoperative pulmonary complications among the elderly after abdominal surgery. *Heart Lung*. 2002;31:440–449.

6. Gust R, Pecher S, Gust A, Hoffmann V, Bohrer H, Martin E. Effect of patient-controlled analgesia on pulmonary complications after coronary artery bypass grafting. *Crit Care Med*. 1999;27:2218–2223.

7. Puntillo K, Weiss SJ. Pain: its mediators and associ- ated morbidity in critically ill cardiovascular surgical patients. *Nurs Res*. 1994;43:31–36.

8. Pavlin DJ, Horvath KD, Pavlin EG, Sima K. Preincisional treatment to prevent pain after ambulatory hernia surgery. *Anesth Analg*. 2003;97:1627–1632.

9. Capdevila X, Barthelet Y, Biboulet P, Ryckwaert Y, Rubenovitch J, d'Athis F. Effects of perioperative analgesic technique on the surgical outcome and duration of rehabilitation after major knee surgery. *Anesthesiology*. 1999;91:8–15.

10. Poobalan AS, Bruce J, Smith WC, King PM, Krukowski ZH, Chambers WA. A review of chronic pain after inguinal herniorrhaphy. *Clin J Pain*. 2003;19:48–54.

11. Tsui SL, Law S, Fok M, Lo JR, Ho E, Yang J, Wong J. Postoperative analgesia reduces mortality and morbidity after esophagectomy. *Am J Surg*. 1997;173:472–478.

12. de Leon-Casasola OA, Myers DP, Donaparthi S, Bacon DR, Peppriell J, Rempel J, Lema MJ. A comparison of postoperative epidural analgesia between patients with chronic cancer taking high doses of oral opioids versus opioid-naive patients. *Anesth Analg*. 1993;76:302–307.

13. Rapp SE, Ready LB, Nessly ML. Acute pain management in patients with prior opioid consumption: a case-controlled retrospective review. *Pain*. 1995;61:195–201.

14. Practice guidelines for acute pain management in the perioperative setting. A report by the American Society of Anesthesiologists Task Force on Pain Management, Acute Pain Section. *Anesthesiology*. 1995;82(4):1071–1081.

15. Practice guidelines for chronic pain management. A report by the American Society of Anesthesiologists Task Force on Pain Management, Chronic Pain Section. *Anesthesiology*. 1997;86(4):995–1004.

16. Practice guidelines for acute pain management in the perioperative setting. An updated report by the American Society of Anesthesiologists Task Force on Acute Pain Management. *Anesthesiology*. 2012;116:248–273.

17. Practice guidelines for chronic pain nanagement. An updated report by the American Society of Anesthesiologists Task Force on Chronic Pain Management and the American Society of Regional Anesthesia and Pain Medicine. *Anesthesiology*. 2010;112:810–833.

18. Coleman SA, Booker-Milburn J. Audit of postoperative pain control: influence of a dedicated acute pain nurse. *Anaesthesia*. 1996;51:1093–1096.

19. Harmer M, Davies KA. The effect of education, assessment and a standardised prescription on postoperative pain management. The value of clinical audit in the establishment of acute pain services. *Anaesthesia*. 1998;53:424–430.

20. Rose DK, Cohen MM, Yee DA. Changing the practice of pain management. *Anesth Analg*. 1997;84:764–772.

21. White CL. Changing pain management practice and impacting on patient outcomes. *Clin Nurse Spec*. 1999;13:166–172.

22. Bardiau FM, Taviaux NF, Albert A, Boogaerts JG, Stadler M. An intervention study to enhance postoperative pain management. *Anesth Analg*. 2003;96:179–185.

23. Gould TH, Crosby DL, Harmer M, Lloyd SM, Lunn JN, Rees GA, Roberts DE, Webster JA. Policy for controlling pain after surgery: effect of sequential changes in management. *BMJ*. 1992;305:1187–1193.

24. Mackintosh C, Bowles S. Evaluation of a nurse-led acute pain service. Can clinical nurse specialists make a difference? *J Adv Nurs*. 1997;25:30–37.

25. Miaskowski C, Crews J, Ready LB, Paul SM, Ginsberg B. Anesthesia-based pain services improve the quality of postoperative pain management. *Pain*. 1999;80:23–29.

26. Pesut B, Johnson J. Evaluation of an acute pain service. *Can J Nurs Admin*. 1997;10:86–107.
27. Sartain JB, Barry JJ. The impact of an acute pain service on postoperative pain management. *Anaesth Intensive Care*. 1999;27:375–380.
28. Stacey BR, Rudy TE, Nelhaus D. Management of patient-controlled analgesia: a comparison of primary surgeons and a dedicated pain service. *Anesth Analg*. 1997;85:130–134.
29. Stadler M, Schlander M, Braeckman M, Nguyen T, Boogaerts JG. A cost-utility and cost-effectiveness analysis of an acute pain service. *J Clin Anesth*. 2004;16:159–167.
30. Tighe SQ, Bie JA, Nelson RA, Skues MA. The acute pain service: effective or expensive care? *Anaesthesia*. 1998;53:397–403.
31. Briggs M, Dean KL. A qualitative analysis of the nursing documentation of post-operative pain management. *J Clin Nurs*. 1998;7:155–163.
32. Camp LD, O'Sullivan PS. Comparison of medical, surgical and oncology patients' descriptions of pain and nurses' documentation of pain assessments. *J Adv Nurs*. 1987;12:593–598.
33. Clarke EB, French B, Bilodeau ML, Capasso VC, Edwards A, Empoliti J. Pain management knowledge, attitudes and clinical practice: the impact of nurses' characteristics and education. *J Pain Symptom Manage*. 1996;11:18–31.
34. Davis BD, Billings JR, Ryland RK. Evaluation of nursing process documentation. *J Adv Nurs*. 1994;19:960–968.
35. Ehnfors M, Smedby B. Nursing care as documented in patient records. *Scand J Caring Sci*. 1993;7:209–220.
36. Idvall E, Ehrenberg A. Nursing documentation of postoperative pain management. *J Clin Nurs*. 2002;11:734–742.
37. Salanteïa S, Lauri S, Salmi TT, Aantaa R. Nursing activities and outcomes of care in the assessment, management, and documentation of children's pain. *J Pediatr Nurs*. 1999;14:408–415.
38. Fuller G. Mental state and higher function. In: Fuller G, ed., *Neurological Examination Made Easy*, 2nd ed. London: Churchill Livingston; 1999:19–34.

25

General and Regional Anesthesia for Patients with Pre-existing Chronic Pain

DMITRI SOUZDALNITSKI, MICHAEL P. SMITH,

YILI HUANG, AND MAGED GUIRGUIS

KEY POINTS

- A significant number of patients with chronic pain present to the hospital for surgical treatment. A large percentage of these patients are on long-term opioid therapy for non-cancer or cancer-associated pain.
- Tolerance to opioids represents a major challenge in perioperative pain control. Therefore, special attention to the perioperative care of patients with chronic pain is imperative.
- This chapter provides an overview of considerations regarding patients with chronic pain undergoing general anesthesia or regional anesthesia.

Introduction

General anesthesia (GA) is defined as a drug-induced central nervous system depression that renders the subject unconscious and unresponsive to all external stimuli. It is important to understand that this is a broad definition and does not necessarily include all of the aspects of the anesthetic state, which consists of unconsciousness, amnesia, immobility, attenuation of autonomic response to noxious stimuli, and, of course, analgesia. For example, barbiturates can provide GA without providing analgesia.[1] This is a very important distinction for chronic pain patients because it is well established that the presence of chronic pain increases perioperative analgesic requirements.[2] Patients with chronic pain frequently have coexisting depression or take antidepressant medications, which may increase their anesthetic requirements.

Regional anesthesia (RA) techniques have been available for patients with chronic pain since the last century. The number of surgeries in which RA is applicable is continuing to grow, as is the role of RA in perioperative pain control, because of the advantages of targeted pain interventions over systemic pharmacological therapy. The role of RA in pediatric and geriatric patient population will also increase with growing debates over the consequences of GA in these age groups. RA has been shown to provide improved outcomes of thoracic, gynecological, orthopedic, and certain general surgery procedures, as well as to reduce morbidity and mortality following a major surgery in high-risk patients.[3]

General Anesthesia in Patients with Chronic Pain

Intraoperative anesthetic management is affected by the presence of chronic pain and relevant chronic pain medications. The spectrum of medications affected range from opioids to calcium channel blockers to antidepressants. Administration of these medications is associated with alterations in minimum alveolar concentration (MAC) requirement during general anesthesia. Therefore, it is important to identify these patients before surgery and to exercise special precautions during their anesthetic care.

Preoperative considerations, including evaluation, education, and treatment, are very important[4] and are discussed elsewhere in this book (see Chapter 24).

MONITORING CONSIDERATIONS

Standard American Society of Anesthesiologist (ASA) monitors should be used at a minimum for all GA techniques, and an anesthesia provider must be present for the duration of the anesthetic. Monitors should measure oxygenation, ventilation, circulation, and temperature. Additional monitors should be considered for chronic pain patients undergoing a variety of surgical procedures common in the patient population. A variety of techniques, for example, bispectral index (BIS), may be considered to monitor level of consciousness in chronic pain patients, as they may be more tolerant to analgesics because of chronic exposure to opioid, antidepressant, and anti-anxiety drugs. But even use of a BIS may not eliminate the risk of awareness under anesthesia for patients on chronic opioid medications.[5,6] In addition to routine monitoring, continuous arterial pressure monitoring can be useful in procedures during which perfusion maintenance is important, such as in spine surgery. Further, these arterial lines may provide beat-to-beat blood pressure monitoring and thus facilitate management of the intraoperative stress response. While intraoperative neurophysiological monitoring can be useful in spine surgery to help avoid potentially devastating postoperative neurological deficits,[7] it is important to keep in mind that monitoring of somatosensory evoked potential (SSEP) and motor-evoked potential (MEP)

Table 25.1 **Effects of Anesthetics on Somatosensory- and Motor-Evoked Potentials**

	SSEP	MEP
Inhaled anesthetics	Decrease in amplitude and increase in latency	Decrease in amplitude and increased latency
IV anesthetics	Propofol/thiopental—decrease in amplitude, increase in latency Ketamine/etomidate—increase in amplitude	None
Muscle relaxants	None	Suppresses

MEP, motor evoked potential; SSEP, somatosensory evoked potential.

may be altered by general anesthetics and adjunct medications, such as ketamine, that may be used to complement GA for chronic pain patients.[8] (Table 25.1).

INTRAOPERATIVE CONSIDERATIONS

MAC is defined as the concentration of inhaled anesthetics in the lungs that will prevent movement in 50% of subjects in response to surgical stimulus. Decreased MAC means that a subject will require less inhaled anesthetics for surgery, while increased MAC means the subject will require more. Acute administration of sedating drugs such as opioids, gabanoids, calcium channel blockers, and α_2-agonists decreases MAC; chronic administration of these medications increases MAC. Conversely, administration of drugs that increase synaptic catecholamine availability, such as serotonin reuptake inhibitors (SSRIs), serotonin norepinephrine reuptake inhibitors (SNRIs), and tricyclic antidepressants (TCAs), can increase MAC (Table 25.2).

INTRAOPERATIVE DRUG CHOICE AND POSTOPERATIVE PAIN CONTROL

General anesthesia choices may also influence postoperative pain management. Some anesthetic agents and analgesics produce improved conditions for perioperative pain management more than others. Intraoperative administration of

Table 25.2 **Effect of Selected Drugs on MAC Level**

Decrease MAC	Increase MAC
Acute opioid use	Chronic opioid use
Calcium channel blockers (ziconotide)	SSRIs
α-agonists (clonidine, tizanidine)	SNRIs
Gabapentin/pregabalin	Tricyclic antidepressants

medications with NMDA receptor antagonist properties has been shown to produce postoperative opioid-sparing effect. These include ketamine,[9] magnesium salts,[10] and methadone.[11] Nitrous oxide, an inhalation anesthetic, may have similar effects. Nitrous oxide was found to be an effective inhibitor of the NMDA receptors, even in subanesthetic concentrations. Intraoperative nitrous oxide has been shown to reduce the risk of chronic postsurgical pain.[12] Propofol-based general anesthesia tends to be associated with decreased acute and chronic postoperative pain.[13] In one study patients anesthetized with propofol appeared to experience less pain compared with patients anesthetized with sevoflurane.[14] One meta-analysis demonstrated that total intravenous anesthesia appeared to produce better patient satisfaction among those in ambulatory settings than did inhalational general anesthesia.[15] Another drug, a short-acting beta-blocker, esmolol, has been shown to have not only antinociceptive properties but also intraoperative anesthetic-sparing effects and perioperative opioid-sparing effects.[16] In addition to peripheral analgesic effects, realized through the sympathetic nervous system, it is potentially involved in pain modulation, hypnosis, and memory function. Along with intravenous infusion of esmolol, a neuraxial route of administration has been discussed as a potentially novel treatment strategy for perioperative pain.[17]

Some agents produce less ideal conditions for postoperative pain control than others. For example, the effects of the ultra-short-acting opioid remifentanil, which is frequently used in spine surgery, wear off very quickly, exposing patients with chronic pain to a sudden drop in opioid concentration and the likelihood of severe pain during emergence from surgery. It has been shown that opioid-dependent patients require much higher doses of remifentanil—up to 30 times that of opioid-naive patients—to control their pain in outpatient settings.[18] While remifentanil is not associated with development of opioid-induced hyperalgesia (OIH) and acute opioid tolerance in opioid-naive patients, [19] it is unclear if remifentanil increases tolerance and/or OIH in opioid-dependent patients. Clinical observations suggest that remifentanil may cause acute opioid tolerance in opioid-dependent patients after surgery, rendering them with reduced responsiveness to longer-acting opioids.

There are many aspects to consider when providing GA for chronic pain patients. When approached with caution and with careful perioperative planning for medication, education, monitoring, and maintenance, the anesthesiologist can provide each chronic pain patient with a safe, individualized, and complete general GA experience.

Regional Anesthesia in Patients with Chronic Pain

BENEFITS OF REGIONAL ANESTHESIA IN PATIENTS WITH CHRONIC PAIN

Hospitalized chronic pain patients with multiple comorbidities also benefit greatly with RA. When anesthetic concerns such as morbid obesity, obstructive sleep apnea, and a potentially difficult airway are present in a patient with chronic opioid consumption, RA often provides an advantage over GA. Additional benefits of RA may be seen in the setting of OIH. While the risk of OIH remains controversial in opioid-naive patients, the risk of OIH is better described in association with chronic pain. Therefore, the OIH risk may be reduced with the application of non-opioid alternative techniques such as RA, to control severe acute on chronic pain. Following are advantages of RA in hospitalized chronic pain patients:

1. RA may be opioid sparing. There is normally a two to four times increase in opioid requirements in chronic pain patients perioperatively. By decreasing opioid use, RA may lead to improved patient safety.
2. RA may provide improved pain relief and management.
3. Patient satisfaction is increased. Because of the increased demand for analgesia in patients with chronic pain, the patient care team may be better able to reach pain control targets with RA.
4. RA may prevent the development of chronic postoperative pain. Persistent pain requiring heightened analgesic amounts are among the factors leading to development of chronic postsurgical pain.
5. RA may help promote improved mobilization and active engagement in physical rehabilitation therapy and may thus improve surgical outcome. Restriction in patient mobility is a known factor leading to disability.
6. RA is associated with a reduced need for sedatives/hypnotics, less anesthetic consumption during GA, and reduced opioid requirements. Effective RA, together with multimodal analgesia, may help reduce the MAC requirement during GA and, therefore, its associated side effects. RA may also be associated with less cognitive dysfunction compared to that with GA. This is an important consideration for children and older adults with chronic pain, as these patients are more likely to have surgery than those in these age groups who have no chronic pain.
7. RA may be associated with decreased surgical stress in patients with significant comorbidities (cardiovascular disease, respiratory disease, etc.).
8. RA allows for improved control of acute on chronic pain and thus may decrease the risk of catastrophic cardiovascular events and iatrogenic respiratory depression.
9. RA is shown to reduce the stress response in cancer patients. More than half of all cancer patients struggle with chronic pain. A decreased surgical stress response is currently being explored as a factor that may prevent further dissemination of the cancer.
10. There are economic benefits of RA associated with ambulatory surgery: shorter recovery time, improved pain control, and less opioid use. These are important factors for patients with chronic pain, as uncontrolled acute pain leads to prolonged recovery and overall hospital stay. Further,

avoiding a two to four times increase in opioid dose (typically required otherwise) may prevent the need for monitored unit admission such as telemetry/step-down or ICU admission. Lastly, RA may lead to a reduced need for hospital admission or readmission of patients with poorly controlled pain.

11. RA techniques can be flexible: peripheral nerve or nerve plexus can be blocked at various locations. If implanted pain management devices are present in the chronic pain patient (opioids, baclofen pump, spinal cord stimulator, etc.), alternative RA techniques may be employed (paravertebral blocks for thoracic surgery, peripheral nerve blocks, or supplemental local infiltrate for other surgeries).

12. Prevention of OIH: OIH is a significant clinical problem in patients with coexisting chronic pain and is associated with opioid dose escalation (this may not be relevant for opioid-naïve patients).

13. RA is a useful option in the elderly because of improved pain control without opioid-related side effects, and use of RA hastens the rehabilitation process, leading to decreased muscle mass loss, venous thromboembolism, and cutaneous pressure ulcers.

14. The positive impact of RA on morbidity and mortality after hip surgery has been demonstrated. Uncontrolled pain may prove detrimental to these patients, who often also present with coronary artery disease, diabetes mellitus, and other comorbidities prevalent in the elderly (67% prevalence of coexisting pain in the elderly).

15. RA and labor pain: data have indicated a 17 times higher mortality rate in parturients with GA versus RA administration. Application of supplemental to neuraxial RA techniques (i.e., transverses abdominis plane [TAP] block) is possible if needed. Management of chronic pain patients on the labor and delivery unit is discussed in detail elsewhere in this book (see Chapter 10).

16. Potential benefits of use of RA in children with acute on chronic pain are probably the similar to those for adults; however; they are not well described.

With the growth in RA popularity and knowledge, requests for this service will likely increase.

REGIONAL ANESTHESIA RISKS IN PATIENTS WITH CHRONIC PAIN

While case reports on RA complications are reported in the literature, the actual incidence of RA complications can only be calculated from large samples or over a long period of time because they are quite rare. In addition, application of neurostimulation, ultrasound, echogenic and stimulating needles and catheters, and newer local anesthetics in the last two decades has significantly improved RA safety, although the exact figures and data have not been documented in the literature yet to a full extent.[20] The rates for complications of neuraxial anesthesia, peripheral nerve blocks, local anesthetic toxicity, and malpractice/litigation issues are similar for both the general surgical population and chronic pain patients. The incidence of infection associated with neuraxial RA has been quoted as 1.1 in 100,000 spinal applications, and in 1 in 1930 epidurals. Patients with coexisting chronic pain are noted to have an impaired immune system. However, the rate of infectious complications from interventional pain management in this category of patients is similarly low.[19]

Some reports suggest that neuraxial blocks should be contraindicated in certain categories of patients with chronic pain (for example, intravenous drug users) because of the high risk of infectious complications. The infections associated with neuraxial interventions are usually related to skin and nasal microbial flora, most commonly *Staphylococcus aureus* and *Staphylococcus epidermidis*.[19]

Based on the data provided, prophylactic use of antibiotics (if not administered for the surgery) in immunocompromised patients with coexisting chronic pain may be applied so that these patients are not deprived of the benefits of RA. Observation of strict aseptic precautions by RA providers is mandatory.

Peripheral nerve or spinal cord injuries are a rare consequence of RA. The most common peripheral nerve block adverse event described in the literature is paresthesias. This complication was noted in 10% to 15% of patients and it resolved completely in 99% of patients within 1 year. The more recent data demonstrated a significantly lower risk of nerve injury with contemporary RA techniques less than 0.5%.[19]

There are reasons to believe that transient neurological symptoms, observed in about 3% of patients, are one of the more common complications of RA. They are strongly associated with the use of lidocaine, independent of its concentration. While most peripheral nerve block malpractice claims involving this technique are associated with temporary injuries, the major cause of death or brain damage in these claims is associated with local anesthetic toxicity. While common precautions in the use of local anesthetic apply to patients with chronic pain, additional caution may be required.[19]

One of the downsides of RA is that sometimes it may not work. Absence of or decreased sensitivity to certain local anesthetics is known to exist in patients with chronic pain. It is also important to differentiate true technical failures from those that are perceived by the chronic pain patient, who may continue to be uncomfortable after successful RA. These patients frequently have to undergo GA or require deep sedation, even after a successful nerve blockade. This is probably secondary to a higher level of anxiety, which creates suboptimal operative conditions for the surgical team. The high level of anxiety in this category of patients is likely in part associated with fear of worsening of their pain. There may also be a pathophysiological basis for their response, stemming from the fact that chronic pain produces structural and functional changes not only at the level of impairment but also at multiple levels in the central nervous system.

Many anesthesiologists would take the additional risks of GA to supplement RA in order to decrease the excessive opioid associated with life-threatening adverse events.

Summary

Tolerance to opioids and decreased pain threshold are notable challenges in intra-operative and perioperative management of patients with chronic pain pathology. Therefore, special attention to the perioperative care of these patients and utilization of applicable techniques and technologies of GA and RA are of great importance.

References

1. Jewett BA, Gibbs LM, Tarasiuk A, Kendig JJ. Propofol and barbiturate depression of spinal nociceptive neurotransmission. *Anesthesiology*. 1992;77(6):1148–1154.
2. Althaus A, Hinrichs-Rocker A, Chapman R, et al. Development of a risk index for the prediction of chronic post-surgical pain. *Eur J Pain*. 2012;16(6):901–910.
3. Kooij FO, Schlack WS, Preckel B, Hollmann MW. Does regional analgesia for major surgery improve outcome? Focus on epidural analgesia. *Anesth Analg*. 2014;119(3):740–744.
4. Livbjerg AE, Froekjaer S, Simonsen O, Rathleff MS. Pre-operative patient education is associated with decreased rate of arthrofibrosis after total knee arthroplasty: a case control study. *J Arthroplasty*. 2013;28(8):1282–1285.
5. Sandhu K, Dash H. Awareness during anaesthesia. *Indian J Anaesth*. 2009;53(2):148–157.
6. Rampersad SE, Mulroy MF. A case of awareness despite an "adequate depth of anesthesia" as indicated by a Bispectral Index monitor. *Anesth Analg*. 2005;100(5):1363–1364.
7. Glover CD, Carling NP. Neuromonitoring for scoliosis surgery. *Anesthesiol Clin*. 2014;32(1):101–114.
8. Loftus RW, Yeager MP, Clark JA, et al. Intraoperative ketamine reduces perioperative opiate consumption in opiate-dependent patients with chronic back pain undergoing back surgery. *Anesthesiology*. 2010;113(3):639–646.
9. Yamauchi M, Asano M, Watanabe M, Iwasaki S, Furuse S, Namiki A. Continuous low-dose ketamine improves the analgesic effects of fentanyl patient-controlled analgesia after cervical spine surgery. *Anesth Analg*. 2008;107(3):1041–1044.
10. Oguzhan N, Gunday I, Turan A. Effect of magnesium sulfate infusion on sevoflurane consumption, hemodynamics, and perioperative opioid consumption in lumbar disc surgery. *J Opioid Manag*. 2008;4(2):105–110.
11. Gottschalk A, Durieux ME, Nemergut EC. Intraoperative methadone improves postoperative pain control in patients undergoing complex spine surgery. *Anesth Analg*. 2011;112(1):218–223.
12. Chan MT, Wan AC, Gin T, Leslie K, Myles PS. Chronic postsurgical pain after nitrous oxide anaesthesia. *Pain*. 2011;152(11):2514–2520.
13. Ogurlu M, Sari S, Küçük M, Bakis M, et al. Comparison of the effect of propofol and sevoflurane anaesthesia on acute and chronic postoperative pain after hysterectomy. *Anaesth Intensive Care*. 2014;42(3):365–370.
14. Tan T, Bhinder R, Carey M, Briggs L. Day-surgery patients anesthetized with propofol have less postoperative pain than those anesthetized with sevoflurane. *Anesth Analg*. 2010;111(1):83–85.

15. Leonova M. Souzdalnitski D. Patient satisfaction is higher with TIVA than with inhalational anesthesia for ambulatory surgery. http://www.asaabstracts.com/strands/asaabstracts/abstractList.htm;jsessionid=8A584C6412A12B1CCAFCD29295CB52ED?year=2010&index=1

16. Celebi N, Cizmeci EA, Canbay O. Intraoperative esmolol infusion reduces postoperative analgesic consumption and anaesthetic use during septorhinoplasty: a randomized trial. *Braz J Anesthesiol*. 2014;64(5):343–349.

17. Kim YH. The antinociceptive effect of esmolol. *Korean J Anesthesiol*. 2010;59(3):141–143.

18. Hay JL, White JM, Bochner F, Somogyi AA. Antinociceptive effects of high-dose remifentanil in male methadone-maintained patients. *Eur J Pain*. 2008;12(7):926–933.

19. Angst MS, Chu LF, Tingle MS, Shafer SL, Clark JD, Drover DR. No evidence for the development of acute tolerance to analgesic, respiratory depressant and sedative opioid effects in humans. *Pain*. 2009;142(1-2):17–26.

20. Souzdalnitski D, Halaszynski TM, Faclier G. Regional anesthesia and co-existing chronic pain. *Curr Opin Anaesthesiol*. 2010;23(5):662–670.

26

Postoperative Pain Management

DMITRI SOUZDALNITSKI, IMANUEL R. LERMAN,

AND SAMER NAROUZE

KEY POINTS

- Postoperative pain control is a common concern of patients with chronic pain and may be associated with substantial adverse outcomes.
- Escalation of the opioid dose by as much as a factor of 2–4 from baseline is frequently required to control acute postoperative pain superimposed on chronic pain in opioid-dependent patients because of opioid tolerance.
- Improved postoperative experience of patients with chronic pain can be achieved using regional anesthesia and analgesia, non-opioid analgesics, adjunct medications, and peripherally acting opioid receptor antagonists.

Introduction

It is estimated that 234.2 million major surgical procedures are carried out worldwide every year.[1] More than 51 million inpatient surgical procedures are performed in the United States on an annual basis.[2] The prevalence of chronic pain is 34.3% in women and 26.7% in men.[3] A key fear for patients undergoing surgery is poor pain control after the operation. Their apprehension is reasonable because these patients are more likely to have inadequate pain control and may experience an exacerbation of their pre-existing chronic pain condition in the postoperative period.[4]

This chapter will focus on postoperative pain management. It is important to note, however, that satisfactory postoperative pain control is highly dependent on comprehensive preoperative preparation and on intraoperative management. In addition to obtaining a detailed history of medication use, past surgeries, prior anesthetics, prior procedures, psychiatric history, and any history of substance abuse, a physical examination should be conducted, available data reviewed, and use of implanted pain management devices verified. The plan of postoperative pain control should be discussed with the patient. This may help to decrease any preconceived fear and to form realistic expectations about what to expect after the surgery. On the morning of surgery, the patient should take his or her usual morning dose of opioids. Buprenorphine should be weaned off of or replaced by other opioids 5–7 days before the surgery. If a fentanyl transdermal opioid delivery system is in use, it should be maintained. If the patient fails to take the usually scheduled morning opioid dose, it should be replaced with an equivalent dose of opioids before the surgery with either an oral medication (with a sip of water up to 2 hours prior to the surgery) or intravenous opioids during induction of anesthesia.[5] In addition, intraoperative management should be discussed with the patient because chronic administration of certain medications used to treat chronic pain may influence intraoperative management.

The objective of this chapter is to provide readers with an overview of tools used to optimize postoperative pain management in patients with pre-existing chronic pain. The main issue in postoperative pain control in opioid-dependent patients remains accurate and adequate opioid management.

Postoperative Opioid Dosing and Patient Monitoring

Despite a lack of evidence for the benefit of long-term opioid use, the routine use of opioids for non-cancer pain remains quite common.[6] Large doses of opioids are usually required to achieve satisfactory postoperative pain control.[7] Independent from the pre-admission dose, these patients frequently require an increase in opioid dose by 200% to 400%, likely due to downregulation of opioid receptors.[8] Opioid dose escalation may result in untoward side effects. Specifically, these patients may experience severe postoperative pain but also be at risk of opioid overdose due to high opioid requirements. Therefore, judicious use of high-dose opioid therapy in the postoperative period remains challenging. Predicting the intensity of postoperative pain in opioid-dependent patients may be accomplished using a variety of nociceptive stimulation methods, including heat injury, pressure algometry, and electrical stimulation. [9]

It is recommended that the same type of opioid be continued, including the morning of the surgical procedure, as the need for conversion and rotation of opioids during the postoperative period is very likely. Widely available conversion tables can be used to estimate the perioperative opioid dose. One of these tables is presented in the Appendix A. There are differing opinions, however, about the conversion of oral to intravenous opioids and vice versa and about opioid rotation.[10] Most of the time intravenous or intramuscular doses of opioids are lower than oral doses because parenteral administration bypasses gastrointestinal absorption, first-pass hepatic clearance, and metabolism. For example, oral morphine has a bioavailability and systemic potency that is three times less than equipotent intravenous doses. An exception is oxycodone, which has an intravenous bioavailability less than that of an equivalent oral dose; therefore, it is not routinely used intravenously. Most importantly, individual patient characteristics need to be accounted for when converting between routes and dosages of opioid medications using conversion tables. These variables, including concomitant use of other medications, especially sedatives; patient comorbidities; age; and sex, may change the pharmacokinetics and pharmacodynamics of opioids and may result in an inappropriate dose estimate.

An early initiation of intravenous patient-controlled analgesia (PCA) decreases the likelihood of inadequate postoperative pain control. Basal intravenous PCA infusions can also be helpful in achieving successful postoperative analgesia. Some sources, however, recommend avoiding basal infusions via PCA because of safety concerns. This strategy may cause severe postoperative pain when intraoperative anesthesia and analgesia start to wear off. Therefore, we recommend use of basal infusions in opioid-tolerant patients, especially with newer PCA devices, which allow exhaled CO_2 monitoring. A continuous intravenous PCA opioid infusion rate established on the basis of the patient's preoperative opioid dose requirement is advisable in most cases. This basal rate should be supplemented with on-demand PCA boluses. A higher than normal on-demand bolus dose is typically required to compensate for the patient's opioid tolerance. It is common that the the intravenous PCA opioid dose is 200% to 400% higher than the baseline dose. However, it is possible to gain an equivalent therapeutic effect at much lower doses when opioid-sparing strategies are implemented, as discussed in the next section.

Intravenous (IV) PCA settings should be reassessed frequently during the first 24 hours after surgery according to the type of opioid used and effectiveness of pain control. The reassessment should allow for adjustment of the opioid regimen until an adequate opioid dose for pain relief is established. The ratio of patient demand to frequency of delivery of opioids should not exceed 2 to 1, to avoid undertreatment of postoperative pain. For example, undertreatment is likely if the PCA log demonstrates that the patient pressed the PCA button 80 times during the selected time interval, but the actual delivery of medicine happened only 20 times. Preferably, the ratio of these two has to match at 1–2:1.

How long should PCA be used? Ideally, IV PCA should be continued until a satisfactory level of postoperative pain control has been reached. Then the PCA dose should be converted to oral opioids if the patient can tolerate PO medications.

Despite tolerance to analgesic effects of opioids, excessive sedation and respiratory depression are common in opioid-dependent patients. Close monitoring of these patients should be implemented during the postoperative period, when high doses of opioids are used for analgesia. The risk of respiratory depression significantly increases with concomitant administration of even small doses of anxiolytics or sedatives. The respiratory rate and level of sedation should be monitored routinely. Capnography may be quite helpful if significant sedation is expected.

Opioid-Sparing Strategies in the Postoperative Period

USE OF NONSTEROIDAL ANTI-INFLAMMATORY DRUGS

Patients should remain on their non-steroidal anti-inflammatory drugs (NSAIDs) until the surgery (including the morning dose) unless contraindicated (certain cardiovascular and kidney diseases) or advised otherwise by the surgical team. This strategy may help to reduce inflammatory reactions to surgical injury and to spare use of opioids. Patients are commonly advised to stop NSAIDs prior to surgery because of concerns of blood loss related to antiplatelet effects of NSAIDs. This concern, however, is not uniformly supported by the literature. A systematic review and meta-analysis of randomized controlled trials showed that there is no increase in perioperative bleeding with use of ketorolac.[11] At the same time, patients can expect meaningfully lower opioid needs and better pain scores throughout the postoperative course.[12] One study showed that NSAIDs can reduce pain by 30% and the total amount of morphine required over 48 hours postoperatively by 40% compared to placebo with the number needed to treat of 3 for at least 50% pain relief.[13] Current guidelines on the application of regional anesthesia techniques suggested that NSAIDs could be used along with regional anesthesia, including neuraxial anesthesia.[14] Further studies, however, are needed to confirm safe use of NSAIDs in the setting of neuraxial analgesia, especially when catheter techniques are utilized (Box 26.1).

MEMBRANE STABILIZERS

Membrane stabilizers, or anticonvulsants, are commonly used to treat chronic myofascial or neuropathic pain. These medications should be continued postoperatively if there are no contraindications, because rapid withdrawal from these drugs may prompt seizures, anxiety, and worsening of pain. Gabapentin and pregabalin have been successfully used as adjuncts for postoperative pain control. Patients who start these medications in the acute perioperative period should be counseled about their possible side effects, including increased suicidal risks in younger and older patients, patients with mood disorders, and patients with epilepsy or seizures.[15]

NONSTEROIDAL ANTI-INFLAMMATORY DRUGS AND ACETAMINOPHEN

- Continue oral or intravenous NSAIDs or acetaminophen after the surgery unless contraindicated or opposed by the surgeon.

MEMBRANE STABILIZERS

- Continue antiepileptics if the patient takes these medications for chronic pain, neuropathy, or seizure disorder and if there are no contraindications.
- Consider use of pregabalin or gabapentin for preemptive analgesia.
- Rapid withdrawal from antiepileptics may trigger seizures, anxiety, and depression.

ANTIDEPRESSANTS AND ANTIPSYCHOTICS

- Continue TCAs, SSRIs, and SNRIs in the perioperative period unless contraindicated.
- Watch for adverse effects of TCAs (sedation, delirium, or other anticholinergic effects, particularly in elderly patients).
- Continue antipsychotics and monitor for signs of neuroleptic malignant syndrome in the acute postoperative setting (hyperthermia, hypertonicity of skeletal muscles, fluctuating levels of consciousness, and autonomic nervous system instability).
- Avoid meperidine in combination with SSRIs (paroxetine, fluoxetine, sertraline, citalopram, and others) and MAOI antidepressants (phenelzine, selegiline, tranylcypromine and others), as these combinations may produce "serotonin syndrome."

ANXIOLYTICS

- Anti-anxiety medications should be continued before and after surgery.
- When considering clonidine or dexmedetomidine, continue the preadmission dose of benzodiazepines in the postoperative period to avoid withdrawal symptoms.
- Watch for excessive sedation, potentiated by an escalation in the opioid dose.

OTHER ADJUNCTIVE MEDICATIONS

- Alpha-2-receptor agonists (dexmedetomidine, clonidine)

- NMDA receptor antagonists (ketamine, methadone, potentially nitrous oxide and magnesium)
- Cholinergic receptor agonists (nicotine, neostigmine)
- Corticosteroids

OTHER ADJUNCTIVE STRATEGIES

- Identification of dose, type of opioid (and other pain management medications), history of substance abuse, quality of previous anesthesia
- Education of patient and surgical team on postoperative chronic pain management and preemptive analgesia (premedication, preemptive local anesthetic infiltration, preemptive epidural), multimodal postoperative chronic pain management
- Complement the preoperative discussion with multimedia information
- Pre-rehabilitation: the augmenting of functional capacity before the surgery
- Early rehabilitation
- Effective use of regional anesthesia and analgesia

MAOIs, monoamine oxidase inhibitors; NMDA, N-methyl-D-aspartate; NSAIDs, nonsteroidal anti-inflammatory drugs; SNRIs, serotonin/norepinephrine reuptake inhibitors; SSRIs, selective serotonin reuptake inhibitors; TCAs, tricyclic antidepressants.

Adapted from Souzdalnitski D, Walker J, Rosenquist RW. Chronic pain patient and other coexisting conditions (substance abuse, psychiatric). In: Urman R, Vadivelu N, eds. *Perioperative Pain Management*. New York: Oxford University Press; 2013:83–93.

ACETAMINOPHEN

Acetaminophen is the active metabolite of phenacetin. Despite the fact that this medicine has been used since 1893, its mechanism of action remains unclear. It appears to serve as a reversible inhibitor of cyclooxygenase in the central nervous system, interfering with prostaglandin synthesis and, therefore, inhibiting synthesis of various pain mediators. Oral and intravenous acetaminophens are commonly used as adjuncts to opioids for postoperative pain control. In two studies patients who received a perioperative multimodal regimen including acetaminophen had a significant reduction in opioid consumption, pain scores, nausea, and drowsiness and had less pain interference with walking, coughing, and deep breathing.[16,17] This medicine should be carefully used in patients with a history of alcohol abuse because these patients have a higher chance of hepatotoxicity or nephrotoxicity. These untoward effects are due to depletion of glutathione accompanying the accumulation of metabolites of acetaminophen.

ANXIOLYTICS

About 10% of surgical patients take anxiolytic mediations for their chronic pain, even though these medications are not indicated.[18] Yet, these medications should not be withdrawn in patients with pre-existing chronic pain, to avoid worsening of their anxiety in the postoperative period. In addition, it is advisable to continue the pre-admission dose of benzodiazepines in the postoperative period so that withdrawal symptoms are avoided. Patients should be monitored for oversedation, which may be worsened with escalation of the opioid dose postoperatively.

ANTIDEPRESSANTS AND ANTIPSYCHOTICS

Many antidepressant medications have analgesic effects and are thus used for chronic pain management. Not surprisingly, up to 25% of surgical patients take antidepressants.

Selective serotonin reuptake inhibitors (SSRIs), tricyclic antidepressants (TCAs), and serotonin/norepinephrine reuptake inhibitors (SNRIs) should be continued, if there are no contraindications, in the postoperative period to avoid worsening of pain or depression. Patients taking TCAs should be monitored for sedation and delirium or other anticholinergic effects and should be used with caution, if used at all, in elderly patients. Meperidine should not be used in combination with SSRIs (citalopram, paroxetine, fluoxetine, and others) or monoamine oxidase inhibitors (MAOIs), including phenelzine, selegiline, tranylcypromine, and others MAOI antidepressants. These combinations may cause hyperreflexia, myoclonus, ataxia, fever, shivering, diaphoresis, diarrhea, anxiety, salivation, and/or confusion, often described as "serotonin syndrome."

It is also advisable that pre-admission antipsychotics be continued postoperatively.[19] In addition, antipsychotics are sometimes used to prevent postoperative nausea and vomiting, or even postoperative delirium in certain patient populations.[20] It is not advisable, however, to use these medications as adjuncts for postoperative pain control or anxiety because they lack analgesic properties. Patients taking antipsychotics in the perioperative period should be closely monitored because of the possibility (less than 1%) of neuroleptic malignant syndrome. This syndrome may present as hyperthermia, hypertonicity of muscles, and evidence of central and autonomic nervous system instability.

α2 AGONISTS

Postoperative α2 agonists demonstrate analgesic, opioid-sparing effect, and decreased nausea.[21] One example is clonidine, which can be administered orally, intravenously, or as a transdermal patch (0.1–0.3 mg/day). In addition, it has been used epidurally with doses of 1.5 mcg/kg for opioid-sparing effects. Another α2 agonist, dexmedetomidine, was found to be an effective adjunct to morphine-based intravenous PCA at doses of 0.4 mcg/kg/hour for 24 hours. Its use reduced about one-third of the total morphine PCA dose.[22] In addition, dexmedetomidine was found to be an effective adjunct to peripheral nerve and neuraxial blockade.[23,24] Patients receiving α2 agonists must be monitored for hypotension, bradycardia, and excessive sedation.

NMDA RECEPTOR ANTAGONISTS

NMDA receptors have been implicated in the mechanisms of opioid-induced hyperalgesia, which appears to be a significant barrier to satisfactory postoperative pain control. Ketamine, an NMDA receptor antagonist, has been shown to produce opioid analgesic and opioid-sparing effect for up to 6 weeks postoperatively. Subanesthetic doses of ketamine—for example, a 50–100 mcg/kg/hour ketamine infusion preceded by a loading dose of 1 mg/kg—showed opioid-sparing effect when used in conjunction with opioid-based intravenous PCA.[25] Use of ketamine as an adjunct to postoperative opioid-based analgesia was favorably evaluated by nursing staff because it made it easier to care for opioid-dependent patients with chronic pain.[26] It is advisable to have a dedicated intravenous line for postoperative ketamine infusion in order to avoid boluses, which may be associated with mental status change and sympathetic stimulation. Ketamine infusion should be carefully used in patients with advanced cardiovascular disease.[27] Other NMDA receptor antagonists, including magnesium and methadone, have been associated with better perioperative pain control.[28]

CHOLINERGIC RECEPTOR AGONISTS

Cholinergic receptors may potentially be involved in the central regulation of pain.[29] Chronic use of a well-known cholinergic agonist, nicotine, is linked to chronic lower back pain.[30] Nicotine has been found to serve as an adjunct to opioids in nonsmokers in postoperative pain management. Nicotine withdrawal may worsen perioperative pain. Therefore, a nicotine patch should be used if not contraindicated for postoperative management. The analgesic effects of nicotine have been elucidated by a variety of pathophysiological mechanisms, including stimulation of the central nervous system and increase of dopamine in the mesolimbic system, as well as α2 adrenergic receptor stimulation (similar to clonidine) and induction of production of endogenous analgesics, β-endorphin and enkephalins. Morphine and other opioids produce analgesia, in part, by releasing acetylcholine and stimulating acetylcholine receptors. Nicotine stimulates the same acetylcholine receptors as well.

CORTICOSTEROIDS

While there are theoretical concerns over the increased risks of infections associated with postoperative corticosteroid use, they can potentially be used in postoperative acute on chronic pain management because of their anti-inflammatory effects and, according to some studies, opioid-sparing effects.[31]

Postoperative Regional Anesthesia and Analgesia

The benefits of intraoperative regional anesthesia for chronic pain patients admitted to the hospital were discussed in detail in previous chapter of this book (see Chapter 25). Postoperative regional anesthesia and analgesia have been associated with better pain control, opioid-sparing effects, reduced costs, improved patient satisfaction, improved surgical outcomes, and reduced morbidity and mortality, especially for major surgeries in high-risk patients.

NEURAXIAL BLOCKADE

Postoperative spinal or epidural analgesia has been found to be suitable for patients undergoing a variety of surgeries. The benefits of neuraxial anesthesia are related to the fact that intrathecal and epidural doses of opioids are approximately 100 and 10 times more effective, respectively, than the same opioid doses injected intravenously. The doses of local anesthetics, administered via intrathecal or epidural route, are similar in both opioid-dependent and opioid-naïve patients.[32] However, as with oral and intravenous administration, because of downregulation of opiate receptors, doses of neuraxial opioids, used for postoperative pain control in patients with chronic pain, are two to three times higher than in patients naïve to opioids. However, neuraxial opiate administration may not be safe when long-acting formulations are used.[33] In one study, the shorter-acting opioid fentanyl, administered intrathecally (15 mcg), produced a significant decrease in postoperative pain scores, delay of the first on-demand intravenous PCA bolus, and an almost 50% reduction of the total PCA morphine dose compared to placebo, without respiratory compromise.[34] More research is needed to determine a safety margin of neuraxial opioid dose escalation. The combination of neuraxial and supplemental oral or parenteral opioid administration is commonly required for postoperative management of opioid-dependent patients because even with an effective opioid-based neuraxial anesthesia, the centrally administered opioid dose may not prevent acute withdrawal triggered by deprivation of peripheral opioid receptors.

Epidural Anesthesia and Analgesia
Epidural analgesia has been shown to improve postoperative pain control, reduce opioid consumption compared to patient-controlled intravenous analgesia, and

decrease intravenous opioid administration as rescue analgesia. It is also associated with a quicker return to consumption of solid foods and less nausea and, in many studies, it did not cause any complications.[35-37] If continuous epidural infusion is not feasible, a single-dose epidural administration of local anesthetics and opioids can be employed.

WOUND INFILTRATION AND PERINEURAL CATHETERS

Wound infiltration as well as perineural and subcutaneous catheters are used for postoperative pain control in patients with pre-existing chronic pain.[38] These techniques appear to provide adequate pain control in the general patient population. For example, compared to intravenous PCA, continuous infusion of 0.5% bupivacaine via an elastomeric pump into the wound resulted in 35% lower pain scores and reduced opioid demand by about half within the first few days after surgery.[39] In addition, there was a lower incidence of nausea, early ambulation and first bowel movement, and, overall, accelerated functional recovery. Additional benefits included reduced total opioid requirement and shortened hospital stay by 2 days. No complications were associated with this technique.[40] The use of continuous local anesthetic infusion may help in alleviating postoperative pain, even beyond the acute postoperative phase. [41]

Early Rehabilitation

The early postoperative period has been suggested to be a very important time of postoperative intervention.[42] While having a positive impact on outcomes, early postoperative rehabilitation may worsen chronic pain and thus reduce patient satisfaction with postoperative pain control. It is advisable, therefore, to use early rehabilitation as part of a comprehensive postoperative pain management. Compared to conventional treatment, a comprehensive postoperative rehabilitation and pain approach has been shown to significantly expedite recovery.[43] Such a program includes prehabilitation (physical reconditioning *before* the surgery), patient-controlled epidural analgesia, early mobilization, and dietary supplements. This program was shown to decrease postoperative hospital length of stay and improve patient satisfaction. In addition, postoperative TENS therapy may reduce postoperative demand for analgesics during the postoperative period and has no systemic side effects.[44] Psychological interventions have also been found to be beneficial in some studies.[45] Even with successful application of multimodal postoperative analgesia, including neuraxial administration of opioids and continuing opioid analgesia at doses at least half the pre-admission maintenance dose, it is advisable that withdrawal from opioids be prevented in opioid-dependent patients.

Summary

Postoperative pain control in patients with pre-existing chronic pain is exceedingly challenging, mainly because of the opioid dose escalation often required due to tolerance in opioid-dependent patients, which may be associated with excessive sedation and respiratory depression. The opioid dose may have to be increased by as much as a factor of 2–4 in order to control acute postoperative pain superimposed on chronic pain. The use of non-opioid analgesics, adjuncts, peripherally acting opioid receptor antagonists, and regional anesthesia and analgesia creates an opportunity for improving postoperative pain control in patients with chronic pain.

References

1. Weiser TG, Regenbogen SE, Thompson KD, Haynes AB, Lipsitz SR, Berry WR, Gawande AA An estimation of the global volume of surgery: a modelling strategy based on available data. *Lancet*. 2008;372(9633):139–144.
2. FactStats: Inpatient Surgery. http://www.cdc.gov/nchs/fastats/inpatient-surgery.htm
3. Johannes CB, Le TK, Zhou X, Johnston JA, Dworkin RH. The prevalence of chronic pain in United States adults: results of an Internet-based survey. *J Pain*. 2010;11(11):1230–1239.
4. Erlenwein J, Schlink J, Pfingsten M, et al. Pre-existing pain as comorbidity in postoperative acute pain service. *Anaesthesist*. 2013;62(10):808–816.
5. Kopf A, Banzhaf A, Stein C. Perioperative management of the chronic pain patient. *Best Pract Res Clin Anaesthesiol*. 2005;19(1):59–76.
6. Kissin I. Long-term opioid treatment of chronic nonmalignant pain: unproven efficacy and neglected safety? *J Pain Res*. 2013;6:513–529.
7. Souzdalnitski D, Halaszynski TM, Faclier G. Regional anesthesia and co-existing chronic pain. *Curr Opin Anaesthesiol*. 2010;23(5):662–670.
8. Mitra S, Sinatra RS. Perioperative management of acute pain in the opioid-dependent patient. *Anesthesiology*. 2004;101(1):212–227.
9. Werner MU, Mjobo HN, Nielsen PR, Rudin A. Prediction of postoperative pain: a systematic review of predictive experimental pain studies. *Anesthesiology*. 2010;112(6):1494–1502.
10. Knotkova H, Fine PG, Portenoy RK. Opioid rotation: the science and the limitations of the equianalgesic dose table. *J Pain Symptom Manage*. 2009;38(3):426–439.
11. Gobble RM, Hoang HL, Kachniarz B, Orgill DP. Ketorolac does not increase perioperative bleeding: a meta-analysis of randomized controlled trials. *Plast Reconstr Surg*. 2014;133(3):741–755.
12. Cassinelli EH, Dean CL, Garcia RM, Furey CG, Bohlman HH. Ketorolac use for postoperative pain management following lumbar decompression surgery: a prospective, randomized, double-blinded, placebo-controlled trial. *Spine (Phila Pa 1976)*. 2008;33(12):1313–1317.
13. Jirarattanaphochai K, Thienthong S, Sriraj W, et al. Effect of parecoxib on postoperative pain after lumbar spine surgery: a bicenter, randomized, double-blinded, placebo-controlled trial. *Spine (Phila Pa 1976)*. 2008;33(2):132–139.
14. Horlocker TT, Wedel DJ, Rowlingson JC, et al. Regional anesthesia in the patient receiving antithrombotic or thrombolytic therapy: American Society of Regional Anesthesia and Pain Medicine evidence-based guidelines (third edition). *Reg Anesth Pain Med*. 2010;35(1):64–101.
15. Patorno E, Bohn RL, Wahl PM, et al. Anticonvulsant medications and the risk of suicide, attempted suicide, or violent death. *JAMA*. 2010;303(14):1401–1409.

16. Tzortzopoulou A, McNicol ED, Cepeda MS, Francia MB, Farhat T, Schumann R. Single dose intravenous propacetamol or intravenous paracetamol for postoperative pain. *Cochrane Database Syst Rev*. 2011;(10):CD007126.

17. Rajpal S, Gordon DB, Pellino TA, et al. Comparison of perioperative oral multimodal analgesia versus IV PCA for spine surgery. *J Spinal Disord Tech*. 2010;23(2):139–145.

18. Walid MS, Robinson JS 3rd, Robinson ER, Brannick BB, Ajjan M, Robinson JS Jr. Comparison of outpatient and inpatient spine surgery patients with regards to obesity, comorbidities and readmission for infection. *J Clin Neurosci*. 2010;17(12):1497–1498.

19. Seidel S, Aigner M, Ossege M, Pernicka E, Wildner B, Sycha T. Antipsychotics for acute and chronic pain in adults. *J Pain Symptom Manage*. 2010;39(4):768–778.

20. Hirota T, Kishi T. Prophylactic antipsychotic use for postoperative delirium: a systematic review and meta-analysis. *J Clin Psychiatry*. 2013;74(12):e1136–1144.

21. Blaudszun G, Lysakowski C, Elia N, Tramèr MR. Effect of perioperative systemic α2 agonists on postoperative morphine consumption and pain intensity: systematic review and meta-analysis of randomized controlled trials. *Anesthesiology*. 2012;116(6):1312–1322.

22. Sadhasivam S, Boat A, Mahmoud M. Comparison of patient-controlled analgesia with and without dexmedetomidine following spine surgery in children. *J Clin Anesth*. 2009;21(7):493–501.

23. Wiesmann T, Steinfeldt T, Wagner G, Wulf H, Schmitt J, Zoremba M. Supplemental single shot femoral nerve block for total hip arthroplasty: impact on early postoperative care, pain management and lung function. *Minerva Anestesiol*. 2014;80(1):48–57.

24. Mohamed AA, Fares KM, Mohamed SA. Efficacy of intrathecally administered dexmedetomidine versus dexmedetomidine with fentanyl in patients undergoing major abdominal cancer surgery. *Pain Physician*. 2012;15(4):339–348.

25. Yamauchi M, Asano M, Watanabe M, Iwasaki S, Furuse S, Namiki A. Continuous low-dose ketamine improves the analgesic effects of fentanyl patient-controlled analgesia after cervical spine surgery. *Anesth Analg*. 2008;107(3):1041–1044.

26. Souzdalnitski D, Vadivelu N, Chung KS. Low-dose ketamine as an adjunct to routine pain practice: are we ready yet? *Pain Pract*. 2009;9(5):405–406.

27. Timm C, Linstedt U, Weiss T, Zenz M, Maier C. Sympathomimetic effects of low-dose S(+)-ketamine. Effect of propofol dosage. *Anaesthesist*. 2008;57(4):338–346.

28. Oguzhan N, Gunday I, Turan A. Effect of magnesium sulfate infusion on sevoflurane consumption, hemodynamics, and perioperative opioid consumption in lumbar disc surgery. *J Opioid Manag*. 2008;4(2):105–110.

29. Souzdalnitski D, Lerman I, Chung KS. Nicotine transdermal. In Sinatra R, Jahr J, Watkins-Pitchford, eds., *The Essence of Analgesia and Analgesics*, 1st ed. New York: Cambridge University Press; 2010:512–514.

30. Shiri R, Karppinen J, Leino-Arjas P, Solovieva S, Viikari-Juntura E. The association between smoking and low back pain: a meta-analysis. *Am J Med*. 2010;123(1):87.e7–87.35.

31. Jirarattanaphochai K, Jung S, Thienthong S, Krisanaprakornkit W, Sumananont C. Peridural methylprednisolone and wound infiltration with bupivacaine for postoperative pain control after posterior lumbar spine surgery: a randomized double-blinded placebo-controlled trial. *Spine (Phila Pa 1976)*. 2007;32(6):609–616.

32. Ziegeler S, Fritsch E, Bauer C, et al. Therapeutic effect of intrathecal morphine after posterior lumbar interbody fusion surgery: a prospective, double-blind, randomized study. *Spine (Phila Pa 1976)*. 2008;33(22):2379–2386.

33. Gehling M, Tryba M. Risks and side-effects of intrathecal morphine combined with spinal anaesthesia: a meta-analysis. *Anaesthesia*. 2009;64(6):643–651.

34. Chan JH, Heilpern GN, Packham I, Trehan RK, Marsh GD, Knibb AA. A prospective randomized double-blind trial of the use of intrathecal fentanyl in patients undergoing lumbar spinal surgery. *Spine (Phila Pa 1976)*. 2006;31(22):2529–2533.

35. Milbrandt TA, Singhal M, Minter C, et al. A comparison of three methods of pain control for posterior spinal fusions in adolescent idiopathic scoliosis. *Spine (Phila Pa 1976)*. 2009;34(14):1499–1503.

36. Cata JP, Noguera EM, Parke E, et al. Patient-controlled epidural analgesia (PCEA) for postoperative pain control after lumbar spine surgery. *J Neurosurg Anesthesiol.* 2008;20(4):256–260.

37. Ukita M, Sato M, Sato K, et al. Clinical utility of epidural anesthesia during and after major spine surgery. *Masui.* 2009;58(2):170–173.

38. Ganapathy S, Brookes J, Bourne R. Local infiltration analgesia. *Anesthesiol Clin.* 2011;29(2):329–342.

39. Elder JB, Hoh DJ, Wang MY. Postoperative continuous paravertebral anesthetic infusion for pain control in lumbar spinal fusion surgery. *Spine (Phila Pa 1976).* 2008;33(2):210–218.

40. Elder JB, Hoh DJ, Liu CY, Wang MY. Postoperative continuous paravertebral anesthetic infusion for pain control in posterior cervical spine surgery: a case-control study. *Neurosurgery.* 2010;66(3 Suppl Operative):99–106; discussion 106–107.

41. Singh K, Phillips FM, Kuo E, Campbell M. A prospective, randomized, double-blind study of the efficacy of postoperative continuous local anesthetic infusion at the iliac crest bone graft site after posterior spinal arthrodesis: a minimum of 4-year follow-up. *Spine (Phila Pa 1976).* 2007;32(25):2790–2796.

42. Sipko T, Chantsoulis M, Kuczynski M. Postural control in patients with lumbar disc herniation in the early postoperative period. *Eur Spine J.* 2010;19(3):409–414.

43. Nielsen PR, Jorgensen LD, Dahl B, Pedersen T, Tonnesen H. Prehabilitation and early rehabilitation after spinal surgery: randomized clinical trial. *Clin Rehabil.* 2010;24(2):137–148.

44. Unterrainer AF, Friedrich C, Krenn MH, Piotrowski WP, Golaszewski SM, Hitzl W. Postoperative and preincisional electrical nerve stimulation TENS reduce postoperative opioid requirement after major spinal surgery. *J Neurosurg Anesthesiol.* 2010;22(1):1–5.

45. Tefikow S1, Rosendahl J, Strauß B. Psychological interventions in surgical care: a narrative review of current meta-analytic evidence. *Psychother Psychosom Med Psychol.* 2013;63(6):208–216.

Part VI

PATIENT SATISFACTION AND QUALITY MANAGEMENT OF HOSPITALIZED CHRONIC PAIN PATIENTS

27

Prevention of Chronic Postoperative Pain after Hospitalization: Myth or Reality?

HARSHA SHANTHANNA, HARI KALAGARA,

AND LORAN MOUNIR SOLIMAN

KEY POINTS

- Between 10% and 50% of patients suffer from chronic postsurgical pain (CPSP) due to various surgeries.
- Pre-existing chronic pain near the surgical site and pain elsewhere in the body are recognized as key predictors for CPSP.
- Current knowledge of the nature and cause of CPSP is not adequate for effective prediction and hence prevention.
- Current knowledge of CPSP supports a multifaceted but individually tailored approach.
- It is important to identify risk factors and use multiple strategies.
- It is crucial to effectively treat acute postsurgical pain, along with continuing treatment for pre-existing pain.
- Supportive evidence exists for use of thoracic epidural for thoracotomies, paravertebral block for breast cancer surgeries, and ketamine to alleviate pain.
- Use of pregabalin and gabapentin has a good rationale but mixed evidence for their use in reducing CPSP.

Introduction

Chronic postsurgical pain (CPSP) is a well-recognized entity. The term refers to the presence of persistent pain at or near the surgical area for a period of 4–6 months or more.[1] Recent epidemiological studies have highlighted the prevalence and significance of this condition: the incidence of CPSP is in the range of 10%–50%, the wide range accounting for differences in measurement of pain

and the applied criteria for diagnosis. CPSP has been observed in patients undergoing a wide variety of surgeries. It impairs quality of life, prolongs hospitalization and recovery, and involves increased resource utilization and costs. To be diagnosed with CPSP there should be a definite temporal association with a perioperative event, along with site-specific pain, distinguishing this from any pre-existing chronic pain (PCP) that a patient might have had. Considering the increasing prevalence of patients with chronic pain, estimated to be around 19%[2] to 50%,[3] the chances of a patient with pre-existing pain presenting for surgery have increased significantly. PCP around the surgical site or elsewhere in the body has been considered a predisposing factor for CPPP.[4,5]

This chapter explores the available preventive strategies one can use to minimize development of CPSP, more specifically as it applies to patients with PCP.

Pre-existing Chronic Pain as a Contributing Factor in Chronic Postsurgical Pain

The etiopathogenesis of CPSP includes several interacting factors which could be categorized as patient factors (presurgical)—genetic susceptibility, age and sex, psychological factors, social factors, preceding pain in the surgical site, presence of chronic pain; and surgical factors—type of surgery, tissue injury and dissection,[6] severity and duration of acute postsurgical pain, choice of anesthesia, type of postoperative analgesia, and others.

PCP as an important factor in the development of CPSP has been highlighted across various surgeries such as hernia repair,[4] breast surgeries,[7] and others.[8] For post-thoracotomy pain syndrome (PTPS), overall there is less information on the role of pre-existing pain because most studies have excluded such patients.[9]

In the risk assessment score for CPSP, developed by Althaus et al.,[10] preoperative pain in the operating field and other chronic preoperative pain were identified as separate predictive factors among the five identified by multivariate logistic regression analysis. Chronic pain alters several components involved in the processing and modulation of pain. Most of these changes are maladaptive and further increase the chances of developing CPSP. Figure 27.1 illustrates the various aspects which independently, or as coexisting factors predispose a patient with PCP to developing CPSP.

In general, the severity of pain could be greater after a second insult, possibly reflecting a role of central sensitization.[11]

A study by Chapman and colleagues showed that postoperative pain in patients with PCP resolved at a slower rate; beyond that, patients on chronic opioids had higher pain scores during the entire period of pain resolution, even though the rate of resolution was similar to that for patients not on opioids.[8] This probably reflects opioid-induced hyperalgesia. A similar finding was observed by Keller et al. for PTPS.[12]

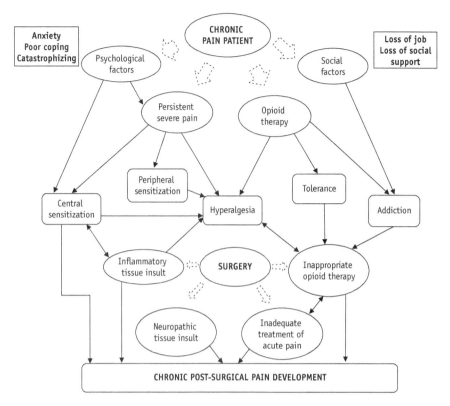

Figure 27.1 Possible factors playing a role in the development of CPSP in a chronic pain patient.

Considerations for Prevention of Chronic Postsurgical Pain in Chronic Pain Patients

Given the presently available evidence, it is uncertain whether we can predictably prevent the development of CPSP. This is even more the case for PCP patients. The most important barrier to preventing CPSP is that we still do not fully understand the nature and definitive pathogenesis of CPSP. As highlighted, multiple factors are involved. Given their independent and interdependent effects, which are complex and individually variable, it is challenging to establish which aspects play a prominent role in a particular patient. Keeping this in mind, strategies aimed at prevention of CPSP must be multifaceted and individually tailored (Figure 27.2). In order to establish a practical strategy, these preventive strategies could be conceived of as various categories that need to be focused on. All of these factors may or may not be applicable to all patients. Individual considerations merit a clear, specific strategy. For example, a patient with predominantly psychological factors may need formal psychiatric input, whereas a patient on high doses of opioids might need opioid titration and adjustments. Prevention begins from the time of first contact when one establishes a PCP patient as being

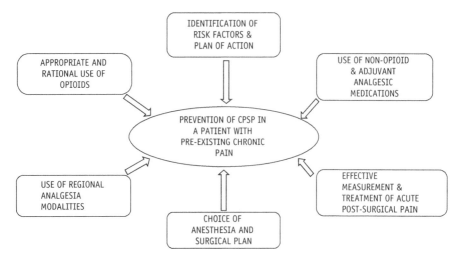

Figure 27.2 Strategies aimed at prevention of CPSP in a patient with pre-existing chronic pain.

predisposed to CPSP. Aspects of prevention and therapy go together. Some of these considerations may also apply to any significant hospitalization (without a surgical procedure) in a patient with PCP.

Identification of Risk Factors and Plan of Action

The development of CPSP cannot be easily predicted. However, there are several patient-specific factors which are correlated with the development of CPSP. Although they may not have a casual relationship, they have to be identified and considered for modification.

One patient-specific factor is psychosocial predisposition. Anxiety and fear of surgery have been found to correlate with severity of acute surgical pain but not directly with CPSP. According to a recent review, depression, psychological vulnerability, stress, and late return to work were found to correlate positively with CPSP.[13] Depending on the necessity, a formal psychological evaluation and involvement may need to be planned.

Another aspect is quantitative sensory functioning, which tests for abnormalities in the processing of afferent signals within the nervous system. The value of identifying the presence of neuropathic pain and opioid-induced hyperalgesia is to predict the development of CPSP, help with stratification, and guide treatment choices.[14] The cold pressor test is claimed to better identify the hyperalgesic component.[15] Others feel that DNIC (diffuse noxious inhibitory control) testing might enable stratification of at-risk individuals for effective prevention.[16] Although future studies may identify specific components of quantitative sensory testing associated with CPSP,[17] there are no present guidelines for such formal testing.

Formulating a plan of action involves suitable anesthetic and surgical care pathways, including the special needs for postoperative analgesia.

Effective Measurement and Treatment of Acute Postsurgical Pain

The intensity and impact of postsurgical pain is recognized as the most important factor in the development of CPSP.[1,14] Studies have found a consistent and strong correlation between severity of postoperative pain and the development of CPSP, although not all patients with inadequately treated pain develop CPSP. In particular, overall severity over the first 7 days was a better predictor than the maximum pain score. Inadequate treatment of postoperative pain also results from inappropriate measurements for pain severity. A single-dimension pain intensity score, such as a visual analogue or numerical scale, has been criticized as oversimplistic. Less than 50% of studies on analgesia measure postoperative pain with mobilization, even though it has been shown that evoked pain possibly correlates more with functional recovery and individual satisfaction. For prevention of CPSP, acute postsurgical pain must be effectively treated using a multimodal approach, with more appropriate and multidimensional measurements of pain.

APPROPRIATE AND RATIONAL USE OF OPIOIDS

Patients on chronic opioid treatment pose many problems for addressing their pain control. Important considerations to bear in mind are physical dependence leading to possible withdrawal symptoms; psychological dependence, with or without a diagnosed addiction; and opioid-induced tolerance (OIT) and opioid-induced hyperalgesia (OIH). These patients will need adjustment of ongoing opioid dosing and higher than usual perioperative opioid treatment, due to tolerance.[15,18] Tolerance can be illustrated by a right-shifting dose–response curve; there is decreased drug effect after prolonged intake that is overcome by increasing the drug dose. Hyperalgesia is an enhanced response to a stimulus that is not usually painful. Tolerance and hyperalgesia are distinct but possibly overlapping phenomena that have to be factored into the overall equation of pain control. In opioid rotation, an opioid is replaced by another from the same group (e.g., morphine to hydromorphone) or from a different group (e.g., morphine to buprenorphine), with the rationale of minimizing the effects of tolerance.[19] Establishing the right dose, means of drug administration, and other specific considerations are important in carrying out opioid rotation.[19-21]

Beyond this, an opioid-dependent patient may also have addiction issues.[20] The patient may be on a methadone maintenance program or could require initiation of methadone to help with pain and OIH. Considerations regarding perioperative opioid treatment, including methadone and buprenorphine, are discussed in detail elsewhere in this book (see Chapters 24–26).

USE OF NON-OPIOID AND ADJUVANT ANALGESIC MEDICATIONS

There are several groups of non-opioid analgesics. Some of them are commonly used for acute postsurgical pain, and others are typically used in chronic pain settings. Incorporating the use of these medications within a multimodality approach has several advantages due to their independent actions: they are opioid sparing, provide anti-inflammatory effects, treat neuropathic pain and hyperalgesia, inhibit sensitization, improve sleep, reduce depression, and are effective for OIH (Table 27.1).

Ketamine

Ketamine has been shown to decrease the use of opioids perioperatively. A small dose of ketamine is safe and is a useful adjunct, as shown in a systematic review.[22] Suggested ketamine dosing is bolus 0.5–1 mg/kg, followed by infusion 10–20 mcg/kg/minute (0.6–1.2 mg/kg/hour).[23] Ketamine has been observed to be effective using different routes, including continuous infusion, bolus IV doses, epidural, and as PCA. A recent Cochrane review also found some evidence for its benefit in preventing CPSP.[25]

Anticonvulsants

Anticonvulsants have been widely used for treating neuropathic pain. Although we still do not know the nature of CPSP, it demonstrates features of nervous system plasticity leading to sensitization. With this rationale, both gabapentin and pregabalin have been used and studied for the prevention of CPSP. Systematic reviews are still unclear regarding their efficacy in the prevention of CPSP. Clarke et al. showed that both were effective in preventing CPSP,[24] but a recent Cochrane review did not find enough convincing evidence to support this claim.[25]

Lidocaine

Lidocaine is known to have analgesic, anti-hyperalgesic, and anti-inflammatory actions apart from their well-known local anesthetic properties. Its perioperative intravenous use has been the subject of many randomized control trials (RCT).[26] In most studies, lidocaine has been shown to provide analgesia and decrease opioid need for 24–72 hours. However, only a single small RCT studied its effect on CPSP, with positive results.[27]

USE OF REGIONAL ANALGESIC MODALITIES

Regional anesthesia/analgesia (RA) can involve neuraxial blockade (spinal or epidural), major nerve or plexus blockade, or local infiltration or intra-articular injections. Apart from effective pain relief, the advantages of RA also include significant opioid sparing and better functional recovery with fewer side effects.

Table 27.1 **Non-Opioid and Adjuvant Analgesics**

Class	Mechanisms	Clinical Effects	Commonly Used Drugs and Doses	Remarks
Paracetamol	Analgesic mechanism not known	Mild analgesia; opioid sparing	Paracetamol: 350–950 mg	Potential for hepatotoxicity
Nonsteroidal anti-inflammatory drugs (NSAIDs)	Anti-inflammatory	Opioid sparing; anti-hyperalgesia	Naproxen: 250–500mg/day Naproxen: 375–500 mg (max: 1000 mg/day); Ketorolac: 15–30 mg/day (max: 120 mg/day) Celecoxib: 100–400 mg (max: 400mg/day for 7 days)	Consider relative contraindications and procedure-specific considerations
Tricyclic antidepressants	Stabilization of nerve membrane; Inhibition of reuptake of serotonin and norepinephrine	Anti-neuropathic pain; decreases signs of sensitization; normalizes sleep patterns	Amitryptline and nortryptline: 50–75mg/day; maintenance doses are less for chronic pain then for depression	Continue as normal; discontinuation could be associated with delirium, confusion, and depression
Serotonin nor-epinephrine reuptake inhibitors (SNRIs)	Inhibition of reuptake of serotonin and norepinephrine	Anti-neuropathic pain; decreases signs of sensitization; antidepressant	Duloxetine: 30–60 mg/day; Venlafaxine: 25–75 mg/day	Continue as normal; potential for serotonin syndrome and drug interactions
Anticonvulsants	Blockage of voltage-gated calcium channels; sodium channel blockade; GABA potentiation; decreased glutamate transmission	Anti-neuropathic pain; decreases signs of sensitization; opioid sparing; prevents CPSP? (there is some direct but limited evidence)	Gabapentin: 600–1200 mg/day Pregabalin: 150–300 mg/day Doses in single or divided doses; initiated in preoperative period and continued postoperatively	Must continue as withdrawal symptoms are reported; perioperatively initiated therapy also has benefits with minor side effects
Local anesthetics (as infusions)	Membrane stabilization; sodium channel blockade	Anti-neuropathic pain; anti-hyperalgesia; anti-inflammatory; local anesthetic	Lidocaine: 1.5 mg/kg and infusion as 1–2 mg/kg/hour	Could be used both intra- and postoperatively
NMDA antagonists	NMDA antagonism	Anti-neuropathic pain; decreases sensitization of pain; decreases OIH; opioid sparing	Ketamine: 0.5 mg/kg as bolus and 2 mcg/kg/minute as infusion	Can be used intra- and postoperatively; may require additional monitoring

It has been widely appreciated that RA is very effective at preventive analgesia, a concept of attenuating the peripheral noxious input, irrespective of its perioperative timing.[28] Secondary sensitization of nociceptive surgical inputs is recognized as an important link in the development of CPSP. Although provision of regional analgesia can conceptually decrease the incidence of CPSP, there is no convincing evidence for this from the literature. The depth of afferent blockade, achieved even with neuraxial techniques, is not complete, and most studies do not measure this.[1] Surgical insult and inflammation also produce humoral signals that may not be amenable to blockade by RA.[29] However, there is supporting evidence (in RCTs) for epidural analgesia for thoracotomies (three studies) and paravertebral block for breast cancer surgery (two studies).[30] Despite the current lack of evidence for their use in addressing CPSP, there are relatively more gains with RA procedures, and these should be used whenever appropriate.

CHOICE OF ANESTHESIA AND SURGICAL TECHNIQUE

Although still inconclusive, some surgical techniques may be associated with a greater possibility of CPSP developing. Longer-duration surgeries (>3 hours), open surgeries, repeat hernia surgeries, nerve-cutting surgeries, and axillary node dissection[6] have more chances of surgical insult, nerve injury, and possible sensitization to and development of neuropathic pain. Although the choice of anesthetic drugs has not been thought to make a difference in this regard, there are limited studies addressing this issue. Nitrous oxide is an analgesic and also has NMDA antagonistic action. Its use may be associated with a reduced occurrence of CPSP.[32] Anesthesia with propofol has been shown to improve pain scores over those with sevoflurane anesthesia.[33]

Summary

Chronic postsurgical pain has been observed to develop in up to half of patients after various surgeries. Recent evidence supports the belief that preexisting chronic pain (PCP) near the surgical site or elsewhere in the body is an important determining factor. There are several maladaptive changes in a patient with PCP that contribute to the development of CPSP. Lack of understanding of the etiology and pathogenesis of CPSP has been a major obstacle in finding preventive strategies. Given the variable, individual, and interdependent factors that play a role in CPSP, preventive strategies to minimize the chances of CPSP developing must be multifaceted. A patient-centered, and the use of non-opioid analgesics individually tailored pathway should include preoperative identification and stratification, appropriate titration of opioid analgesics, and use of non-opioid adjuvant analgesics and regional analgesic modalities. All of these factors must be directed toward effective treatment of acute postsurgical pain with minimal compromise. Presently, only epidural analgesia for thoracic surgeries and paravertebral block for breast surgeries are supported with clear but limited evidence. Among pharmacological modalities, use of ketamine has been shown to prevent CPSP. Despite the lack of a good rationale, the use of gabapentin or pregabalin to prevent CPSP is supported by mixed evidence.

References

1. Kehlet H, Jensen TS, Woolf CJ. Persistent postsurgical pain: risk factors and prevention. *Lancet*. 2006;367(9522):1618–1625.
2. Reid KJ, Harker J, Bala MM, Truyers C, Kellen E, Bekkering GE, Kleijnen J. Epidemiology of chronic non-cancer pain in Europe: narrative review of prevalence, pain treatments and pain impact. *Curr Med Res Opin*. 2011;27(2):449–462.
3. Clark JD. Chronic pain prevalence and analgesic prescribing in a generalmedical population. *J Pain Symptom Manage*. 2002;23(2):131–137.
4. Aasvang EK, Gmaehle E, Hansen JB, Gmaehle B, Forman JL, Schwarz J, Bittner R, Kehlet H. Predictive risk factors for persistent postherniotomy pain. *Anesthesiology*. 2010;112(4):957–969.
5. Johansen A, Schirmer H, Stubhaug A, Nielsen CS. Persistent post-surgical pain and experimental pain sensitivity in the Tromsø study: comorbid pain matters. *Pain*. 2014;155(2):341–348.
6. De Oliveira GS Jr, Chang R, Khan SA, Hansen NM, Khan JH, McCarthy RJ, Apkarian AV. Factors associated with the development of chronic pain after surgery for breast cancer: a prospective cohort from a tertiary center in the United States. *Breast J*. 2014;20(1):9–14.
7. Gärtner R, Jensen MB, Nielsen J, Ewertz M, Kroman N, Kehlet H. Prevalence of and factors associated with persistent pain following breast cancer surgery. *JAMA*. 2009;302(18):1985–1992.
8. Chapman CR, Davis J, Donaldson GW, Naylor J, Winchester D. Postoperative pain trajectories in chronic pain patients undergoing surgery: the effects of chronic opioid pharmacotherapy on acute pain. *J Pain*. 2011;12(12):1240–1246.
9. Wildgaard K, Ravn J, Kehlet H. Chronic post-thoracotomy pain: a critical review of pathogenic mechanisms and strategies for prevention. *Eur J Cardiothorac Surg*. 2009;36(1):170–180.
10. Althaus A, Hinrichs-Rocker A, Chapman R, Arránz Becker O, Lefering R, Simanski C, Weber F, Moser KH, Joppich R, Trojan S, Gutzeit N, Neugebauer E. Development of a risk index for the prediction of chronic post-surgical pain. *Eur J Pain*. 2012;16(6):901–910.
11. Brennan TJ, Kang S. Is second pain worse than the first? *Pain*. 2014;155(1):2–3.
12. Keller SM, Carp NZ, Levy MN, Rosen SM. Chronic post thoracotomy pain. *J Cardiovasc Surg (Torino)*. 1994;35(6 Suppl 1):161–164.
13. Hinrichs-Rocker A, Schulz K, Järvinen I, Lefering R, Simanski C, Neugebauer EA. Psychosocial predictors and correlates for chronic post-surgical pain (CPSP)—a systematic review. *Eur J Pain*. 2009;13(7):719–730.
14. Lavand'homme P. The progression from acute to chronic pain. *Curr Opin Anaesthesiol*. 2011;24(5):545–550.
15. Huxtable CA, Roberts LJ, Somogyi AA, MacIntyre PE. Acute pain management in opioid-tolerant patients: a growing challenge. *Anaesth Intensive Care*. 2011;39(5):804–823.
16. Yarnitsky D, Crispel Y, Eisenberg E, Granovsky Y, Ben-Nun A, Sprecher E, Best LA, Granot M. Prediction of chronic post-operative pain: pre-operative DNIC testing identifies patients at risk. *Pain*. 2008;138(1):22–28.

17. Granot M. Can we predict persistent postoperative pain by testing preoperative experimental pain? *Curr Opin Anaesthesiol.* 2009;22(3):425–430.
18. Hadi I, Morley-Forster PK, Dain S, Horrill K, Moulin DE. Brief review: perioperative management of the patient with chronic non-cancer pain. *Can J Anaesth.* 2006;53(12):1190–1199.
19. Eipe N, Penning J. Opioid conversions and patient-controlled analgesia parameters in opioid-dependent patients. *Can J Anaesth.* 2010;57(12):1129–1130.
20. Richebé P, Beaulieu P. Perioperative pain management in the patient treated with opioids: continuing professional development. *Can J Anaesth.* 2009;56(12):969–981.
21. Ripamonti C, Groff L, Brunelli C, Polastri D, Stavrakis A, De Conno F. Switching from morphine to oral methadone in treating cancer pain: what is the equianalgesic dose ratio? *J Clin Oncol.* 1998;16(10):3216–3221.
22. Subramaniam K, Subramaniam B, Steinbrook RA. Ketamine as adjuvant analgesic to opioids: a quantitative and qualitative systematic review. *Anesth Analg.* 2004;99(2):482–495.
23. Koppert W, Schmelz M. The impact of opioid-induced hyperalgesia for postoperative pain. *Best Pract Res Clin Anaesthesiol.* 2007;21(1):65–83.
24. Clarke H, Bonin RP, Orser BA, Englesakis M, Wijeysundera DN, Katz J. The prevention of chronic postsurgical pain using gabapentin and pregabalin: a combined systematic review and meta-analysis. *Anesth Analg.* 2012;115(2):428–442.
25. Chaparro LE, Smith SA, Moore RA, Wiffen PJ, Gilron I. Pharmacotherapy for the prevention of chronic pain after surgery in adults. *Cochrane Database Syst Rev.* 2013;7:CD008307.
26. McCarthy GC, Megalla SA, Habib AS. Impact of intravenous lidocaine infusion on postoperative analgesia and recovery from surgery: a systematic review of randomized controlled trials. *Drugs.* 2010;70(9):1149–1163.
27. Grigoras A, Lee P, Sattar F, Shorten G. Perioperative intravenous lidocaine decreases the incidence of persistent pain after breast surgery. *Clin J Pain.* 2012;28(7):567–572.
28. Barreveld A, Witte J, Chahal H, Durieux ME, Strichartz G. Preventive analgesia by local anesthetics: the reduction of postoperative pain by peripheral nerve blocks and intravenous drugs. *Anesth Analg.* 2013;116(5):1141–1161.
29. Samad TA, Moore KA, Sapirstein A, Billet S, Allchorne A, Poole S, Bonventre JV, Woolf CJ. Interleukin-1 beta-mediated induction of Cox-2 in the CNS contributes to inflammatory pain hypersensitivity. *Nature.* 2001;410(6827):471–475.
30. Andreae MH, Andreae DA. Regional anaesthesia to prevent chronic pain after surgery: a Cochrane systematic review and meta-analysis. *Br J Anaesth.* 2013;111(5):711–720.
31. Kehlet H, Dahl JB. Assessment of postoperative pain—need for action! *Pain.* 2011;152(8):1699–1700.
32. Chan MT, Wan AC, Gin T, Leslie K, Myles PS. Chronic postsurgical pain after nitrous oxide anesthesia. *Pain.* 2011;152(11):2514–2520.
33. Tan T, Bhinder R, Carey M, Briggs L. Day-surgery patients anesthetized with propofol have less postoperative pain than those anesthetized with sevoflurane. *Anesth Analg.* 2010;111(1):83–85.

28

Patient Satisfaction

DMITRI SOUZDALNITSKI, RICHARD W. HOHAN,

CARMEN V. NATALE, AND BETH MINZTER

KEY POINTS

- Acceptable pain control remains challenging when treating hospitalized patients with chronic pain. These patients have more hospital admissions, longer hospital stays, and avoidable trips to the emergency department.
- Higher doses of analgesics were associated with lower patient satisfaction scores.
- Pain scores themselves were not predictive of higher patient satisfaction scores.
- Increased patient satisfaction, however, is associated with higher mortality, along with other negative outcomes.
- Exploring the mechanisms of anger and dissatisfaction in pain sufferers might improve patient experience and provide evidence for more effective pain management.
- Suggested approaches to balancing adequate pain control with patient satisfaction include expectation management, use of clear algorithms of care, active patient involvement in decisions regarding their pain control, attention to nurses' job satisfaction, and the early involvement of comprehensive inpatient pain management and expert resources, such as pain services.

Introduction

Results of the Hospital Consumer Assessment of Healthcare Providers and Systems Survey (HCAHPS) show that only 7 out of 10 hospitalized patients reported that their pain was well controlled[1] (Figure 28.1). Acceptable pain control remains even more challenging in hospitalized patients with pre-existing chronic pain, despite extensive research aimed toward better understanding

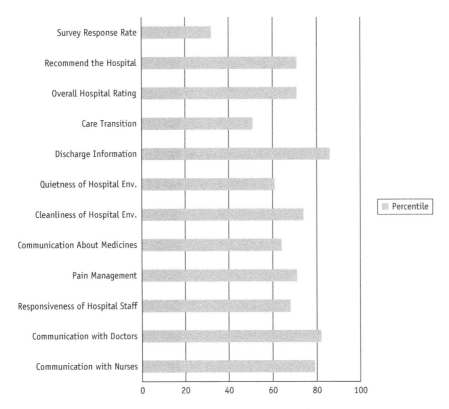

Figure 28.1 A Sample of Summary of HCAHPS Survey results. Adapted from Summary of HCAHPS Survey Results. HCAHPS Percentiles. Centers for Medicare Medicaid Services, Baltimore, MD. Originally posted December, 2014. Available at: www.hcahpsonline.org.

the needs of these patients and the development of new treatments modalities. Chronic pain patients have more hospital admissions, longer hospital stays, and multiple trips to the emergency department (ED), most or all of which can be avoided.[2]

While the satisfaction with pain control during hospital admission is measurable and the results are publically available, the intrinsic subjectivity of pain makes the problem of its assessment and treatment quite complex. As a result, despite significant efforts over the last few years to improve patient satisfaction, one study reported only a 3% increase in the number of patients who rated their pain as always well controlled.[3] The use of increased doses of analgesics to improve patient satisfaction has been associated with routine as well as with life-threatening side effects. Contrary to expected outcomes, higher doses of analgesics were associated with worse patient satisfaction.[4–6] Moreover, the pain scores themselves were not predictive of increased patient satisfaction.[7] There was a lack of association between Press Ganey patient satisfaction scores and administration of analgesic medications in the ED.[8]

This chapter examines available literature on inpatient satisfaction regarding pain control with the goal of elucidating the factors that may have an impact on inpatient pain control in patients with pre-existing chronic pain and the relationship of these factors to patient satisfaction. In addition, we will discuss management of complaints, grievances, and risks related to inpatient pain control.

Hospital Consumer Assessment of Healthcare Providers and Systems (HCAHPS) Survey and Pain Management

Traditionally, individual healthcare providers, as well as hospitals, have looked for the most effective and safe techniques to help their patients and to assess the practical outcomes of their treatments. The need to manage and compare healthcare quality, as well as The Patient Protection and Affordable Care Act (PPACA) of 2010, led to the implementation of the Centers for Medicare and Medicaid Services (CMS) Hospital Inpatient Value-Based Purchasing program (HIVBP).[9] Patient satisfaction became a major component of this program because results from previous research had identified a strong association between patient outcomes and patient satisfaction scores. Therefore, the CMS positioned patient satisfaction as one of the important determinants of the quality of care and designated satisfaction an important component of pay-for-performance metrics. As a result, according to the HIVBP program, the CMS makes value-based incentive payments to acute care hospitals based in part on the patient satisfaction survey. The Hospital Consumer Assessment of Healthcare Providers and Systems (HCAHPS) survey is a uniform, mandatory tool used to report publicly patients' satisfaction with inpatient management. The HCAHPS survey results are reported by the CMS. In addition, the CMS is coupling a certain amount of its funds with hospital HCAHPS performance. Medicare payments are initially reduced and then, based on the quality of healthcare provided, can be partially recovered as a bonus. Otherwise, the hospital can end up being penalized.[10] The HCAHPS survey consists of 27 questions in seven domains of inpatient management related to satisfaction with care, with some questions on patient demographics.

There are a number of questions in this survey that are directly or indirectly related to patients' perceptions of inpatient management of their pain. The questions directly concerning pain include following:

- Did you need medicine for pain?
- How often was your pain well controlled?
- How often did the hospital staff do everything they could to help you with your pain?

For each question, patients have the option of answering "never," "sometimes," "usually," or "always." Responses to the pain management domain of the HCAHPS survey are standardized and contribute to the overall patient satisfaction score, the individual physician's evaluation, and, eventually, the hospital's reimbursement. One earlier study summarized that an environment of good patient satisfaction is associated with better patient response to treatment, improved staff satisfaction and morale, reduced malpractice risk, and improved financial outcomes of the institution.[11] One study found, and we support this finding, that nurses' job satisfaction was reduced, though not uniformly, with an increased number of complaints and risk management episodes.[12,13] Several recent studies suggest that overall, while patient satisfaction is multifaceted and a puzzling outcome to define, patients' perceptions of pain management and healthcare providers' efforts to control their pain were associated with their satisfaction assessment. In one study involving 4349 patients, the odds of a patient being satisfied were almost five times greater if his or her pain was adequately controlled.[14]

Challenges and Controversies of Hospital Consumer Assessment of Healthcare Providers and Systems (HCAHPS) Survey

The strategy of evaluation of a healthcare provider and hospital, and of payment based on patient experience, is very important and, at first look, appears indisputable. A recent paper, "The Cost of Satisfaction: A National Study of Patient Satisfaction, Health Care Utilization, Expenditures, and Mortality," however, showed that this assumption is wrong. This national prospective cohort study of 51,946 patients showed that greater patient satisfaction was associated with greater mortality, along with other negative outcomes.[15] The limitations are especially obvious when looking at the management of opioid-tolerant patients, often referred to as the "most challenging patients treated in hospitals today."[9] A significant number of patients admitted to the hospital are opioid-dependent, and about 10% are opioid-tolerant (patients taking 60 mg PO of morphine equivalence for 7 days or longer, per FDA definition).[9,16] The HCAHPS does not separate out or recognize patients with low satisfactions scores who have chronic pain and/or substance use disorders prior to admission. These patients typically report moderate to severe baseline pain scores at home, which are typically much lower than their assessments of pain when presenting with an acute disease to the hospital. These patients consistently report lower satisfaction scores.[4]

When managing patients' pain, healthcare providers and hospitals are forced to choose between patient safety and the same patient's satisfaction as reflected in HCAHPS scores. A recent systematic review of 848 studies confirmed the notion that performance assessment based on the link between satisfaction and quality of healthcare has mixed and contradictory evidence.[17] It was postulated that satisfaction with healthcare quality should not be misrepresented as a measure of healthcare quality or patient safety.[18] With that, one may predict that pain management–related questions might be modified or possibly excluded from the forthcoming hospital surveys. The studies of better instruments to measure patient experience of healthcare quality in hospitals are forthcoming.[19] Still, questions regarding how to help chronic pain patients attain a better inpatient experience and how to manage their complaints will likely remain a priority.

Chronic Pain Patient Complaints: Communication Is Key

There are three common domains of patient complaints described in the literature: safety and quality of clinical care (33.7%), hospital healthcare delivery (35.1%), and problems in staff–patient relationships (29.1%).[20] While patient dissatisfaction often leads to a complaint (typically presented informally), it is less commonly presented as a grievance (formal written complaint).[21,22] Complaints are typically related to a minor problem that generally does not require any further investigation and can be quickly resolved by the same healthcare or housekeeping team, commonly within 24 hours, and a verbal rather than written response will suffice. A grievance typically represents a larger patient or family concern, filed in writing during admission or after discharge. The grievance requires additional investigation and a written response to the patient and/or family that includes detailed results of the investigation. Some studies have shown that in half the grievances against staff physicians there were breaches of practice standards.[23]

Chronic pain itself was noted to be a factor associated with increased complaints and litigation.[24] It corresponded to an increased frequency of angry responses from chronic pain patients, which is significant—about 5–10 times higher than in the general population.[25,26] Anger, mistrust, a focus on compensation, addiction, and some other patient variables were also strongly associated with thoughts of suing a physician.[27]

The exploration of anger development and of dissatisfaction among pain sufferers might offer ways to improve patient experience and provide evidence for more effective pain management.[28] Hospitals and healthcare teams should have explicit protocols and guidelines on management of chronic-pain and opioid-tolerant patients' complaints. The nature of these complaints and grievances from patients is not typically a failure of medical management but instead a failure to communicate with the patient. Regardless, such complaints should be reviewed thoroughly.

A qualified hospital representative should first evaluate whether the patient complaint or grievance can be resolved immediately, whether patient safety or quality of care has been compromised, and whether there was a possible breach of standard care. Second, it should be determined if there was hospital management or communication failure. The verbal (in the case of complaint) or written (in the case of grievance) response to a patient should typically begin with acknowledgement of the receipt of the complaint and apology for untoward patient experience (for a sample response, see Box 28.1). The details of any investigation, including both process and outcomes, should be described next, including reviewed documents and staff interviews. The conclusion of the response to the patient and/or family typically contains a brief summary of acknowledgement, apology, and appreciation. If the patient has a legitimate complaint, the hospital should take steps to avoid similar situations in the future and can comment on these steps in the response. It can be mentioned in the response that the hospital collects, tracks, and trends data on patient grievances and complaints as part of its quality improvement process. The reply must include detailed contact information, including the name and position of the person who conducted the investigation and prepared the response. In some cases, after consultation with hospital quality management service, staff may directly communicate back to the patient, apologize, indicate what steps they have taken to fix the situation, and state that the situation was challenging but presents a tremendous opportunity for quality improvement. In fact, proper communication has been shown to be key in improving chronic pain patient satisfaction during hospitalization.[9]

Balancing Adequate Pain Control with Patient Satisfaction: Special Techniques

Suggested approaches to balancing adequate pain control with patient satisfaction require attention to the three following domains: expectation management, clear algorithms of care, and early involvement of expert resources, such as pain services (Figure 28.2).[9]

Effective communication through courtesy and empathy, despite the apparent simplicity, are key in managing acute pain in patients with chronic pain ("acute on chronic" pain). Recent studies have demonstrated that patient satisfaction was more strongly associated with the perception that "caregivers did everything they could to control pain than with pain actually being well controlled."[9] The odds of a patient's being satisfied were almost 10 times greater if the staff enactment was appropriate. In other words, patient satisfaction has

Box 28.1 **Sample Reply Letter**

LETTERHEAD, Detailed info

Date

Mr./Ms. Patient Name
Patient Street Address
City, State (Province), Zip (Postal Code)

Dear Mr./Ms. Patient Name,

This letter is in response to the concerns you expressed (to our Patient Experience Specialist [fill in name of employee who spoke with patient]) or (in your letter) regarding your experience with [fill in name of physician/nursing staff/or department] (our surgery nursing team) following your hospitalization. [Start sentence with something specific to the complaint, for example: "In preparing this letter, I and other healthcare professionals have reviewed the medical documentation of your stay in the hospital from (date to date).] In your letter you noted that your pain was not adequately controlled during this admission. Specific to this hospital stay, you requested to have your pain medicine (hydromorphone 2-4 mg, every 2 hours as needed for pain) combined with your anti-anxiety medicine (lorazepam 0.5–1 mg every 4 hours as needed for anxiety) and your anti-nausea medicine (promethazine 25 mg every 6 hours as needed for nausea). We take the feedback from our patients very seriously and I want to assure you that your complaint has been filed formally. Your feedback has been brought to the attention of our [fill in department/leadership investigating complaint] (Surgical Services leadership) team. Our investigation demonstrated that the combination of these medications may decrease your level of consciousness and, in the case of the combination of opioid medicine (hydromorphone) with benzodiazepine (lorazepam), it may spontaneously suppress your ability to breathe. Simply put, this is not safe, and your safety is our, and your, number 1 goal.

Service excellence is very important to all of us at [name of the hospital] and we strive to provide excellent care every day for every patient. We value the comments and concerns expressed by our patients, and actively seek to identify and implement improvements in our practices as a result of your feedback. We apologize for the dissatisfaction you had with the care provided and for not meeting your expectations. We hope that you will continue to feel comfortable utilizing the services at our hospital.

Thank you for bringing this matter to our attention.

Sincerely,

Name
Title
Detailed contact info

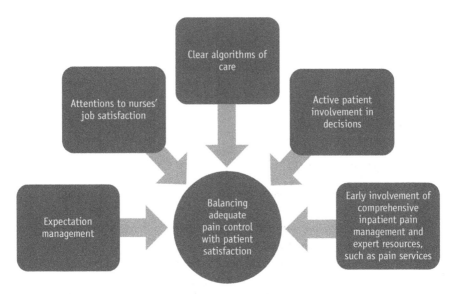

Figure 28.2 Suggested approaches to balancing adequate pain control with patient satisfaction.

been more intensely correlated with the *perception* that healthcare providers have done everything possible to control pain rather than with *actual pain scores*.

The pre-admission discussion is an important step in managing patients' expectations and creating a basis for their satisfaction with upcoming hospital admission. If possible, opioid doses should be decreased before hospital admission to ensure adequate responsiveness to inpatient opioid management. Chronic pain patients should be advised that application of routine acute pain management strategies may not be enough for them, and that they should ask about an inpatient chronic pain management consultation. Realistic expectations still need to be set, even in the face of a chronic pain consultation. These patients should be advised about the benefits of perioperative regional analgesia, use of adjunct medications, emotional support (psychology consult), spiritual counseling (chaplain consult), and even bedside complementary therapies. A combination of these strategies may be as important as, if not more important than, escalated doses of opioids. It has been suggested that "education of caregivers at every phase of hospital care on the need for early intervention with available expert resources, such as dedicated pain services, for this patient population may also help to reduce length of stay and readmission rates and improve overall patient satisfaction."[9] A recent multinational study showed that patients should be provided with information and be involved in pain treatment decisions to the level they wish (within conventional safety limits). Behaviors such as these will likely significantly improve patients' satisfaction with pain control.[29]

Summary

Pain control in patients with chronic pain remains challenging even in the in-hospital setting. These patients have more hospital admissions, longer hospital stays, and often avoidable trips to the emergency department. Good patient satisfaction is associated with better patient response to treatment, improved staff satisfaction and morale, reduced malpractice risk, and improved financial outcomes of the institution. Increased patient satisfaction, however, is associated with higher mortality rates, along with other negative outcomes. Higher doses of analgesics were associated with a worsened patient satisfaction. The pain scores themselves were not predictive of greater patient satisfaction. Suggested approaches to balancing adequate pain control with patient satisfaction requires attention to expectation management, clear algorithms of care, active patient involvement in decisions regarding their pain control, improved nurses' job satisfaction, and the early involvement of comprehensive inpatient pain management and expert resources, such as pain services.

References

1. Summary of HCAHPS Survey results. http://www.hcahpsonline.org/files/Report_December_2014_States.pdf Accessed December 28, 2014.
2. A call to revolutionize chronic pain care in America: an opportunity in health care reform. http://www.maydaypainreport.org/docs/A%20Call%20to%20Revolutionize%20Chronic%20Pain%20Care%20in%20America%2003.04.10.pdf Accessed December 30, 2013.
3. Gupta A, Lee LK, Mojica JJ, Nairizi A, George SJ. Patient perception of pain care in the United States: a 5-year comparative analysis of hospital consumer assessment of health care providers and systems. *Pain Physician*. 2014;17(5):369–377.
4. Danforth RM, Pitt HA, Flanagan ME, Brewster BD, Brand EW, Frankel RM Surgical inpatient satisfaction: what are the real drivers? *Surgery*. 2014;156(2):328–335.
5. Maher DP, Woo P, Padilla C. et al. Perioperative surgical management and HCAHPS outcomes: a retrospective review of 2758 patients. Abstract A3181. The American Society of Anesthesiologists' annual meeting, 2014. http://www.asaabstracts.com/strands/asaabstracts/abstract.htm;jsessionid=411E08C19AC156BDAFA1A48E2987B50F?year=2014&index=14&absnum=4773. Accessed October 15, 2014.
6. Bot AG, Bekkers S, Arnstein PM, Smith RM, Ring D. Opioid use after fracture surgery correlates with pain intensity and satisfaction with pain relief. *Clin Orthop Relat Res*. 2014;472(8):2542–2549.
7. Phillips S, Gift M, Gelot S, Duong M, Tapp H. Assessing the relationship between the level of pain control and patient satisfaction. *J Pain Res*. 2013;6:683–689.
8. Schwartz TM, Tai M, Babu KM, Merchant RC. Lack of association between press ganey emergency department patient satisfaction scores and emergency department administration of analgesic medications. *Ann Emerg Med*. 2014;64(5):469–481.
9. American Society of Anesthesiologits Committee News. Patients and their pain experience in the hospital: the HCAHPS imperative with payments at risk in value-based purchasing environment. https://www.asahq.org/For-Members/Publications-and-Research/Newsletter-Articles/2014/March-2014/committee-news-on-pain-medicine.aspx Accessed November 30, 2014.

10. Centers for Medicare & Medicaid Services. Medicare program; Hospital inpatient prospective payment systems for acute care hospitals and the long-term care hospital prospective payment system and fiscal year 2013 rates; Hospitals' resident caps for graduate medical education payment purposes; Quality reporting requirements for specific providers and for ambulatory surgical centers; Proposed rule. *Federal Register*. 2012;77(92):27870–28192.

11. Worthington K. Customer satisfaction in the emergency department. *Emerg Med Clin North Am*. 2004;22(1):87–102.

12. Cydulka RK, Tamayo-Sarver J, Gage A, Bagnoli D. Association of patient satisfaction with complaints and risk management among emergency physicians. *J Emerg Med*. 2011;41(4):405–411 [physicians].

13. Stelfox HT, Gandhi TK, Orav EJ, Gustafson ML. The relation of patient satisfaction with complaints against physicians and malpractice lawsuits. *Am J Med*. 2005;118(10):1126–1133.

14. Hanna MN, González-Fernández M, Barrett AD, Williams KA, Pronovost P. Does patient perception of pain control affect patient satisfaction across surgical units in a tertiary teaching hospital? *Am J Med Qual*. 2012;27(5):411–416.

15. Fenton JJ, Jerant AF, Bertakis KD, Franks P. The cost of satisfaction: a national study of patient satisfaction, health care utilization, expenditures, and mortality. *Arch Intern Med*. 2012;172(5):405–411.

16. FDA blueprint for prescriber education for extended-release and long-acting opioid analgesics. http://www.fda.gov/downloads/Drugs/DrugSafety/InformationbyDrugClass/UCM277916.pdf Accessed November 30, 2014.

17. Farley H, Enguidanos ER, Coletti CM, et al. Patient satisfaction surveys and quality of care: an information paper. *Ann Emerg Med*. 2014;64(4):351–357.

18. Wendling P. Patient satisfaction not always linked to hospital safety, effectiveness. ACS Surgery News Digital Network, May 5, 2014. http://www.acssurgerynews.com/index.php?id=15051&type=98&tx_ttnews[tt_news]=251961&cHash=da03e20e36. Accessed October 1, 2014.

19. Beattie M, Lauder W, Atherton I, Murphy DJ. Instruments to measure patient experience of health care quality in hospitals: a systematic review protocol. *Syst Rev*. 2014 Jan 4;3:4.

20. Reader TW, Gillespie A, Roberts J. Patient complaints in healthcare systems: a systematic review and coding taxonomy. *BMJ Qual Saf*. 2014;23:678–689.

21. Alexander AA. Complaints, grievances, and claims against physicians: does tort reform make a difference? *J Healthc Risk Manag*. 2010;30(1):32–42.

22. Jiang S, Wu Y. Chinese people's intended and actual use of the court to resolve grievance/dispute. *Soc Sci Res*. 2015;49:42–52.

23. Halperin EC. Grievances against physicians: 11 years' experience of a medical society grievance committee. *West J Med*. 2000;173(4):235–238.

24. Tsimtsiou Z, Kirana P, Hatzimouratidis K, Hatzichristou D. What is the profile of patients thinking of litigation? Results from the hospitalized and outpatients' profile and expectations study. *Hippokratia*. 2014;18(2):139–143.

25. Okifuji A, Turk DC, Curran SL. Anger in chronic pain: investigations of anger targets and intensity. *J Psychosom Res*. 1999;47(1):1–12.

26. Fishbain DA, Lewis JE, Bruns D. et al. Exploration anger constructs in acute and chronic pain patients versus community patients. 2011 AAPM Annual Meeting abstracts. http://www.painmed.org/library/posters/poster-179/. Accessed December 30, 2013.

27. Fishbain DA, Bruns D, Disorbio JM, Lewis JE. What patient attributes are associated with thoughts of suing a physician? *Arch Phys Med Rehabil*. 2007;88(5):589–596.

28. Trost Z, Vangronsveld K, Linton SJ, Quartana PJ, Sullivan MJ. Cognitive dimensions of anger in chronic pain. *Pain*. 2012;153(3):515–517.

29. Schwenkglenks M, Gerbershagen HJ, Taylor RS, et al. Correlates of satisfaction with pain treatment in the acute postoperative period: results from the international PAIN OUT registry. *Pain*. 2014;155(7):1401–1411.

29

Criteria for Discharge from the Hospital from the Chronic Pain Perspective

ANKIT MAHESHWARI AND RICHARD D. URMAN

KEY POINTS

- Chronic conditions, chronic opiate therapy, and polypharmacy—conditions commonly encountered in patients with chronic pain—are all predictors of readmission, medication errors, adverse reactions, and even death.
- Special attention must be paid while discharging a patient with chronic pain, keeping in mind that resolution of the chronic pain complaints may not be possible during hospitalization and should not be a criterion for discharge.
- Detailed discharge instructions, including relevant prescriptions and explanations on how to adjust the opioid regimen after discharge, and an appropriate follow-up appointment with the patients' chronic pain physician should be provided prior to discharge to reduce adverse events and decrease the chance of readmission.

Introduction

It is estimated that over 100 million adults in the United States have chronic pain conditions.[1] The number of patients with chronic pain admitted to hospitals is therefore high, and these patients often have multiple pain complaints apart from the primary reason for the hospitalization.[2] Patients with chronic pain may be hard to treat during hospitalization because clinicians are often faced with the challenge of differentiating acute from chronic pain. In addition, chronic pain is associated with tolerance, wind-up phenomenon,[3] and opioid-induced hyperalgesia,[4] which can make pain from acute events amplified (such as postsurgical pain). Addiction and dependence may be motivators for patients to continue reporting a high pain score in order to gain treatment with opiates. Standard discharge criteria for pain relief are not generalizable to the chronic pain patient. It may not be possible to alleviate chronic pain during hospitalization for an acute problem. Astute medication reconciliation and detailed discharge planning may reduce the risk of adverse reactions, uncontrolled pain, and readmission.

Assessment of Acute Pain in the Chronic Pain Patient

Simple measures of pain intensity such as the Visual Analogue Score (VAS), Numerical Rating Score (NRS), and Verbal Rating Score (VRS) are convenient and well-validated tools for use in hospitalized patients.[5-9] However, in patients with chronic pain conditions these unidimensional scores of pain intensity are frequently elevated chronically. Hospital discharge may often not be based on this score. Complex conditions such as addiction and dependence may have to be teased out or else may lead to overtreatment and extended hospitalizations. At the same time, assumptions must not be made about falsification of the self-report of pain because of the presence of addiction or dependence diagnoses; this may lead to gross undertreatment. Pain rating scales, which measure other dimensions of pain (affective and cognitive), and if the situation calls for it, assessment scales for addiction and dependence may be needed. Detailed discussion of these questionnaires is beyond the scope of this chapter. We recommend consultation with a specialist (pain, psychiatry, addiction) depending on the situation for both inpatient and outpatient treatment recommendations. For more information regarding pain assessment refer to Chapter 4.

Discharge Planning

Discharge planning is the development of a plan prior to a patient leaving the hospital to address the patient's post-discharge care. This includes evaluation of the patient, review of treatments and recommendations, medication reconciliation, and arrangement for post-discharge care.

Unplanned rehospitalizations are a significant cost to the healthcare delivery system; 20% of patients are readmitted within 30 days.[10]

A study has shown that a majority of elderly patients did not understand clearly after discharge why a new medication was added and why any changes were made to their pre-existing medications.[11] In patients with chronic pain who may also have other comorbidities, medication reconciliation is extremely important (Table 29.1).

Table 29.1 **Important Checkpoints for Medication Reconciliation**

Pre-admission medications	Check and reconfirm dose, route, and
Changes to pre-admission medications	frequency.
New medications	Affirm with the patient.
Check interactions	Inform the patient about these and
Check adverse reactions	when the patient should call the doctor.
Over-the-counter medications and herbal medications	Check for interactions.
Prescribe opiate medications based on previous prescription and next follow-up with prescriber	Use a prescription drug monitoring program (PDMP) in your state, such as OARRS (Ohio) or INSPECT (Indiana).

Opiates, antiepileptic drugs (membrane stabilizers), antidepressants, non-steroidal anti-inflammatory drugs, muscle relaxants, and topical preparations are now commonly used for treating chronic pain. Several interactions are possible and new medications during hospitalization need to be checked for these interactions. Controlled substances should be checked using prescription drug monitoring programs such as OAARS (in Ohio) and INSPECT (in Indiana), and enough prescription medication should be provided to the patient until he or she has follow-up with the pain practitioner (Table 29.2).

Chronic opioid therapy has been associated with hospital readmission and death.[12] Patients with chronic pain and patients treated with opiate pain medications are independent risk factors for readmission,[13] and so is polypharmacy.[14]

Thus it is imperative to check interactions at the time of discharge and educate patients (and caregivers) about adverse drug reactions. Chronic pain in the elderly is frequently accompanied by other comorbid conditions such as cancer, depression, diabetes mellitus, COPD, and congestive heart failure,[13,15] all of which increase the possibility of drug–drug interactions and risk of readmission. Demographic factors that may be used as predictors of risk of readmission and problems after discharge from a pain standpoint include prior hospitalization for the same (chronic pain) problem, black race, low health literacy, low socioeconomic status, and reduced social support. Discharge interventions that assess the need for social support and provide access and services have the potential to reduce chronic hospitalization.[16] Patients in this demographic may require special attention at the time of discharge.

Irritable bowel syndrome (IBS), Crohn's disease, ulcerative colitis, and sickle cell disease are examples of conditions in which pain control may be challenging and readmission can be expected. In a study of patients with IBS, it was found that the risk of readmission was 2.2-fold higher for patients who were not given opioid analgesia at the time of discharge. Whether patients were treated with opioids while in the hospital or not did not influence the rate of readmission.[17]

Table 29.2 **States and Provinces with Programs for Prescription Drug Monitoring**

Alabama	Maine	Oregon
Arizona	Maryland	South Carolina
Arkansas	Michigan	South Dakota
Colorado	Minnesota	Tennessee
Connecticut	Mississippi	Utah
Delaware	Montana	Washington
District of Columbia	Nebraska	West Virginia
Georgia	Nevada	Wyoming,
Idaho	New Jersey	Canada:
Illinois	New Mexico	British Columbia, Alberta,
Kansas	North Carolina	Saskatchewan, Manitoba, Ontario, Nova Scotia, Newfoundland and Labrador
Kentucky	North Dakota	New Brunswick*
Louisiana	Ohio	Prince Edward Island* Yukon**

Sources: www.PMPalliance.org and www.ccsa.ca.

* programs in development.

** linked in with the Alberta program.

In one study, patients with sickle cell disease had a mean pain score of 7 during their hospital (7 on an NRS scale of 0–10). The incidence of readmission within 1 month was 50%. This study suggests that improvement is needed in the management of pain during hospitalization and at discharge.[18] While there is no specific protocol or guideline to follow, the general principles of appropriate assessment and detailed discharge planning may improve outcome.

Patient Instructions and Discharge Checklist

Written instructions regarding medications and follow-up appointments should be provided to the patient upon discharge.

A discharge summary should include changes to medications and new medications in addition to the routine information regarding reason for hospitalization, diagnosis, and inpatient management.

The same principles of discharge apply when sending patients to a facility such as a nursing home for continuation of treatment. Chronic pain on its own is not an indication for discharge to a facility such as a nursing home or long-term acute care center, but the patient's overall level of function, if impaired by pain, may warrant such an admission at discharge.

Pediatric Patient Population

Pediatric patients with chronic pain have elevated readmission rates. Admissions for chronic pain are rising in this patient population and account for significant resource utilization. Pediatric patients with chronic pain are hospitalized with complex problems and several comorbid conditions. The most common admission diagnosis for chronic pain in this population is abdominal pain.[19] Assessment of the pediatric patient with chronic pain at discharge should include a detailed discussion with the parent and the child (if age appropriate) regarding medications. Discharge planning should include special attention to pain treatment and a detailed plan should be in place for outpatient follow-up.

An emerging concept of the perioperative surgical home holds the promise of reducing the risk of rehospitalization and may be of special value to patients of all age groups with complicated chronic conditions, including chronic pain.[20]

Summary

Chronic conditions, chronic opiate therapy, and polypharmacy are all predictors of readmission, medication errors, adverse reactions, and even death. These are all conditions commonly encountered in patients with chronic pain. Special attention must be paid while discharging a patient with chronic pain to reduce adverse events and rehospitalization. On the other hand, resolution of chronic pain complaints may not be possible during hospitalization and should not be a criterion for discharge. Detailed discharge instructions and an appropriate follow-up appointment with the patients' chronic pain physician should be provided prior to discharge.

References

1. Institute of Medicine of the National Academies Report. *Relieving Pain in America: A Blueprint for Transforming Prevention, Care, Education, and Research*. Washington DC: National Academies Press; 2011.
2. Souzdalnitski D, Halaszynski TM, Faclier G. Regional anesthesia and co-existing chronic pain. *Curr Opin Anaesthesiol.* 2010;23(5):662–670.
3. Angst MS, Clark JD. Opioid induced hyperalgesia: a qualitative systematic review. *Anesthesiology.* 2006;104(3):570–587.
4. Herrero JF, Laird JM, Lopez Garcia JA. Wind up of spinal cord neurones and pain sensation: much ado about something? *Prog Neurobiol.* 2000;61(2):169–203.

5. Joyce CRB, Zutshi DW, Hrubes V, et al. Comparison of fixed interval and visual analog scales for rating chronic pain. *Eur J Clin Pharmacol.* 1975;8:415–420.

6. Joshi GP, Viscusi ER, Gan TJ, et al. Effective treatment of laparoscopic cholecystectomy with intravenous followed by oral COX-2 specific inhibitor. *Ambul Anesthes.* 2004;98:336–342.

7. Chesney MA, Shelton JL. A comparison of muscle relaxation and electromyography biofeedback treatments for muscle contraction headache. *J Behavior Ther Exper Psychiatry.* 1976;7:221–225.

8. Kremer EF, Atkinson JH Jr, Ignelzi RJ. Measurement of pain: patient preference does not confound measurement. *Pain.* 1981;10:241–248.

9. Fox EJ, Melzack R. Transcutaneous electrical stimulation and acupuncture: comparison of treatment for low back pain. *Pain.* 1976;2:141–148.

10. Jencks SF, Williams MV, Coleman EA, et al. Re-hospitalizations among patients in the medicare fee-for-service program. *N Eng J Med.* 2009;360:1418.

11. Ziaeian B, Araujo KL, Van Ness PH, et al. Medication reconciliation accuracy and patient understanding of intended medication changes on hospital discharge. *J Gen Intern Med.* 2012;27(11):1513.

12. Mosher HJ, Jiang L, Sarrazin MSV, et al. Prevalence and characteristics of hospitalized adults on chronic opioid therapy. *J Hosp Med.* 2013;9(2):82–87.

13. Allaudeen N, Vidyarthi A, Maselli J, et al. Redefining readmission risk factors for general medicine patients. *J Hosp Med.* 2011;6(2):54.

14. Campbell SE, Seymour DG, Primrose WR, et al. A systematic literature review of factors affecting outcomes in older medical patients admitted to hospital. *Age Ageing.* 2004;33:110.

15. Kartha A, Anthony D, Manasseh CS, et al. Depression is a risk factor for rehospitalization in inpatients. *Prim Care Companion J Clin Psyciatry.* 2007;9:256.

16. Strunnin L, Stone M, Jack B, et al. Understanding rehospitalization risk: can hospital discharge be modified to reduce recurrent hospitalization? *J Hosp Med.* 2007;2:97.

17. Hazratjee N, Agito M, Lopez R, et al. Hospital readmission in patients with inflammatory bowel disease. *Am J Gastroenerol.* 2013;108:1024–1032.

18. Ballas SK, Lusardi M. Hospital readmission for adult acute sickle cell painful episodes: frequency, etiology and prognostic significance. *Am J Hematol.* 2005;79:17–25.

19. Coffelt TA, Bauer BD, Carroll AE. Inpatient characteristics of the child admitted with chronic pain. *Pediatrics.* 2013;132(2):422–429.

20. Vetter TR, Goeddel LA, Boudreaux AM, et al. The peri-operative surgical home: how can it make the case so everyone wins? *BMC Anesthesiol.* 2013;13:6.

Appendix

Opioid Conversion Table

PREPARED BY GLENN R. RECH

Opioid	IV Equivalent	Oral Equivalent	Elimination Half-life (hours)	Bioavailability (%) (oral)	Active Metabolite	Primary Metabolic Route	Primary Excretion Route
Morphine	10 mg	30 mg	2–4	17–33%	M6G, M3G	Hepatic: phase II conjugation	Renal
Hydrocodone	N/A	30 mg	3–4	N/A	Hydromorphone	Hepatic: phase I demethylation	Renal
Hydromorphone	2 mg	7.5 mg	2–4	35–80	H3G	Hepatic: phase II glucuronidation	Renal
Methadone	2–10 mg	2–10 mg	30–60	60–90	Unknown	Hepatic: phase I demethylation	Renal
Fentanyl • Lozenge • Buccal • SL tab	100–250 mcg	N/A	3–7	50 50–65 54	Unknown	Hepatic: phase I dealkylation	Renal
Fentanyl (transdermal)	12 mcg/h × 24 h	12 mcg/h × 24 h	20–27		Unknown	Hepatic: phase I dealkylation	Renal
Meperidine	75 mg	300 mg	3–4	30–60	Normeperidine	Hepatic: phase I demethylattion and phase II conjugation	Renal
Codeine	75 mg	300 mg	3–4	60–90	Morphine	Hepatic: phase I demethylation and phase II glucuronidation	Renal
Oxycodone	N/A	20 mg	2–6	40–100	Oxymorphone	Hepatic: phase II	Renal

Buprenorphine	0.3 mg	5 mcg/hr Transdermal patch	24–60	29 (SL)	B3G, NB3G	Hepatic: phase II dealkylation and glucuronidation	Feces
Naloxone	N/A	N/A	0.5–1.5	<1	N/A	Hepatic: phase II glucuronidation	Renal
Heroin	8 mg	12.5	2–3 min	38–53 (smoked)	Morphine, M6G	Hepatic	Renal
Oxymorphone	1 mg	10 mg	7–11	10	Unknown	Hepatic: phase II glucuronidation	Renal and feces

B3G, buprenorphine-3-glucuronide; H3G, hydromorphone-3-glucuronide; IV, intravenous; M3G, morphine-3-glucuronide; M6G, morphine-6-glucuronide; N/A, not applicable; NB3G, norbuprenorphine-3-glucoronide; SL, sublingual.

Sources: Lexi-Comp, accessed January 21, 2015; Rook et al. *Curr Clin Pharmacol.* 2006;1:109–118;

Duragesic package insert; University of Alberta, Multidisciplinary Pain Centre, Conversion Between Analgesics. http://www.uofapain.med.ualberta.ca/en/ForHealthProfessionals/OpioidConversionGuide.aspx, accessed January 27, 2015.

Index

Note: Page numbers followed by *f* and *t* indicate figures and tables, respectively. Numbers followed by *b* indicate text boxes.